The
Vegan
Cook's Bible

Pat Crocker

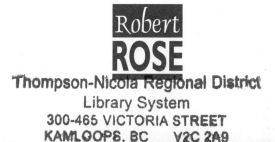

Robert
ROSE

Thompson-Nicola Regional District
Library System
300-465 VICTORIA STREET
KAMLOOPS, BC   V2C 2A9

For complete cataloguing information, see page 371.

Disclaimers

The Vegan Cook's Bible is intended to provide information about the preparation and use of
whole foods and whole food ingredients. It is not intended as a substitute for professional medical
care. The publisher and authors do not represent or warrant that the use of recipes or other information
contained in this book will necessarily aid in the prevention or treatment of any disease or condition,
and specifically disclaim any liability, loss of risk, personal or otherwise, incurred as a consequence,
directly or indirectly, of the use and application of any of the contents of this book. Readers must assume
sole responsibility for any diet, lifestyle and/or treatment program that they choose to follow. If you have
questions regarding the impact of diet on health, you should speak to a health-care professional.

The recipes in this book have been carefully tested by our kitchen and our tasters. To the best of our
knowledge, they are safe and nutritious for ordinary use and users. For those people with food or other
allergies, or who have special food requirements or health issues, please read the suggested contents of
each recipe carefully and determine whether or not they may create a problem for you. All recipes are
used at the risk of the consumer.

We cannot be responsible for any hazards, loss or damage that may occur as a result of any recipe use.

For those with special needs, allergies, requirements or health problems, in the event of any doubt,
please contact your medical adviser prior to the use of any recipe.

Design and Production: PageWave Graphics Inc.
Editor: Carol Sherman
Recipe Editor: Jennifer MacKenzie
Contributor: Paulina Zettel
Proofreader: Karen Campbell-Sheviak
Indexer: Gillian Watts
Photography: Colin Ericson
Food Styling: Kathryn Robertson
Prop Styling: Charlene Ericson
Illustrations: Kveta

Cover image: Udon Noodles with Tofu and Gingered Peanut Sauce (page 304)

We acknowledge the financial support of the Government of Canada through the Book Publishing
Industry Development Program (BPIDP) for our publishing activities.

Published by Robert Rose Inc.
120 Eglinton Avenue East, Suite 800, Toronto, Ontario, Canada M4P 1E2
Tel: (416) 322-6552 Fax: (416) 322-6936

Printed in Canada
1 2 3 4 5 6 7 8 9 CP 17 16 15 14 13 12 11 10 09

Contents

To our beautiful green planet,
mother earth, provider of all.

Acknowledgments

More than any other, this book has been a collaborative effort involving my family and friends. My dear husband was excitedly anticipating becoming a full-time vegan along with me for the intense eight months of recipe development and testing. I think he was pleasantly surprised by the tremendous range and quality of recipes that are available to vegans and I am happy to see that he will continue to enjoy the benefits of a vegan diet.

My daughter, now 20 years old and starting her own life's journey, sipped, supped and helped select the dishes that were sophisticated enough to make it onto the final pages.

I am blessed to know and work with Nettie Cronish. Nettie embraces a vegetarian way of living and is vibrant proof of the benefits it bestows.

Thanks to my book club, each member of which blithely ignored lights, tripods, extension cords, camera and kitchen clutter to become part of the ongoing quest to find the right taste combination. Their comments, enthusiasm and suggestions are much appreciated.

Carol Sherman and I have developed a fine working relationship and I am always in awe of her brilliant talent and ability to move a manuscript along towards a professional end product. Thanks also to Jennifer MacKenzie, who tested the recipes, and Gillian Watts for her copy editing and indexing skills.

Bob Dees and Marian Jarkovich at Robert Rose have a strong commitment to producing high-quality health books. Thanks to the dedication and vision they bring to every book in their outstanding collection.

It has been almost four decades since Frances Moore Lappe penned *Diet for a Small Planet* (New York: Ballantine Books, 1971) and awakened in me an understanding and deep appreciation for our miraculous life-sustaining earth. Her book has been an important flash point for change all the way along the food chain.

Introduction

My goal in accepting the challenge of developing a strictly vegan recipe and resource book was to design recipes so good that everyone who enjoys food — non-vegan and non-vegetarian cooks included — would scramble to make and taste them.

As a creative food writer, culinary herbalist and cookbook author, I work with food and develop new recipes on a regular basis and I am always striving for tempting dishes that are bold, innovative, fresh and easy and above all deliriously delicious. It is a tall order for all cooks. For vegans, it can be overwhelming.

I am not a vegan. I am not even a strict vegetarian. I would characterize my eating style as flexitarian. That is, I enjoy organic fruits, vegetables, herbs and dairy products on a regular basis but include a small amount of organic lamb, chicken, beef and fish once or twice a week.

It doesn't necessarily take a strict vegan to develop fine vegan recipes. In my view, one needs to love food and have an intuitive understanding of how to create really good-tasting food before one can begin to work within the limits of a vegan regime. My recipes are based on honest ingredients with no "imitations." For example, I do not attempt a vegan angel food cake, because that beautifully light confection relies on a dozen egg whites for its very existence. Instead, I am pleased to present Spiced Apple Cake — a dessert classic that happily satisfies vegan guidelines while finishing off a meal in style.

This book takes away the worry of trying to make non-vegan recipes work. That is because the dishes herein are not simply non-vegan recipes reworked. They are original recipes that hold the divineness of plant foods at their core. They are spanking new with a new perspective and a healthy respect for today's sophisticated palates. And they celebrate the very best of organic fruits, herbs and vegetables.

Eat well — Be well, Pat Crocker
www.riversongherbals.com

Being Vegan

"...veganism gives us all the opportunity to say what we 'stand for' in life. The ideal of healthy, humane living is now easy with modern transport bringing us vegan foods from all over the world.

    Join us and add decades of health to your life, with a clear conscience as a bonus."

    — FROM AN INTERVIEW WITH DONALD WATSON, FOUNDER OF THE VEGAN SOCIETY AND ORIGINATOR OF THE WORD "VEGAN," AUGUST 11, 2004.

Veganism: A philosophy and way of living that seeks to exclude the exploitation of animals for entertainment, food, consumer products, or any other use by humans.

The term "vegan" first came into use in 1944 when the British Vegan Society coined it from the first three and last two letters of word "vegetarian." It originally meant "non-dairy vegetarians" but has since come to represent a philosophy and a lifestyle as well as a diet, all of which have well-defined parameters.

While animal rights issues are central to the vegan ethic, mainstream consumers are beginning to support the Green Movement and moving towards veganism as they learn more about how many resources are consumed and how much pollution is generated by factory farming. Clearly, with every *E. coli* and mad cow item in the news, people are thinking more about and making conscious changes to the food on their plates. And they are gravitating to foods that sustain healthy, fit bodies — plant foods low in the cholesterol-forming saturated fats, drugs and synthetic hormones found in industrial meat.

To me, veganism means a humane, responsible and connected way of living that shows reverence and respect for all life and the planet that sustains it. Vegan cooking is the act of preparing strictly plant food with care and conscience.

Nutrients and the Vegan Diet

It is clear to both Canadian and American dietitians that both vegetarians and vegans can satisfy their nutrient requirements (including protein) through a varied diet.

"Appropriately planned vegetarian diets are healthful, nutritionally adequate and provide health benefits in the prevention and treatment of certain diseases," according to a joint statement by the Dietitians of Canada and the American Dietetic Association.[1]

It is generally agreed that a wide variety of plant foods eaten over the course of a day can provide all the essential amino acids (protein) required by individuals and that even athletes can meet their protein requirements

---

[1] Position of the American Dietetic Association and Dietitians of Canada: Vegetarian Diets. *Canadian Journal of Dietetic Practice and Research* 64, no. 2 (Summer 2003).

with a vegan diet. Taking vitamin C–rich foods together with sprouting beans, grains and seeds and eating fermented soy foods (miso and tempeh) may improve iron and zinc absorption. Dried fruits are recommended because they contain almost six times more iron than do other fruits. Vegans need to avail themselves of high-calcium foods such as leafy greens and sea vegetables in order to meet daily needs; some soy and rice milks are fortified with calcium. Vitamin D requirements for light-skinned vegans can usually be met in the summertime by 15 minutes of exposure to sunlight, but northern and dark-skinned vegans should seek vitamin D-fortified foods, especially in the winter. Good sources of linolenic acid (flaxseed and flaxseed oil) are important to a vegan diet. Vitamin B_{12}, which is not found naturally in plant foods, should be insured by eating foods fortified with B_{12} or by taking a B_{12} supplement. If they are not consuming $\frac{1}{2}$ teaspoon (2 mL) of iodized salt per day, vegans should also eat iodine-rich sea vegetables or take supplements.

Vegan diets offer the advantage of less saturated fat; lower cholesterol intake; and more vitamins, minerals and phytonutrients from the abundance of fruits and vegetables in daily meals. As always, it is best to check with a nutritionist or health care professional when making significant changes to your diet.

Daily Vegan Guidelines
In general terms, here are some suggestions for the variety and amount of foods that represent a well-planned daily vegan diet.
- 2 to 4 servings of green, red, orange, yellow or white vegetables
- 2 to 3 servings of leafy greens and sea vegetables
- 4 to 8 servings of whole grain bread, pasta, rice and fortified cereals
- 2 to 3 servings of dried beans peas, lentils, tofu, tempeh, nuts and seeds
- 2 to 4 servings of fresh or frozen fruit
- 1 to 2 servings of dried fruit
- 2 to 3 servings of fortified non-dairy milk
- 8 glasses of water

Possible Supplementation
Vitamin B_{12}
Vitamin D
Calcium

Healthy Body Systems

Healthy Living

Today, the big killers in Western societies are the cancers, cardiovascular disease, diabetes and hypertension, most of which are preventable by diet. Immunity and obesity play a role in either reducing or elevating disease, and they in turn are both affected by the foods we eat.

Doctors, scientists, naturopaths, nutritionists and medical herbalists all agree: to be healthy and prevent disease, a healthy lifestyle is essential. Following these guidelines will maintain and help restore good health:

Guidelines to Good Health

- Limit alcohol consumption — post-menopausal women who drink less than one drink per day can decrease the risk of dying of breast cancer by up to 30%
- Exercise — moderate daily physical activity can lower cancer risk, boost the immune system, help prevent obesity, decrease estrogen and insulin growth factor (IGF), improve overall health and emotional well-being
- Do not smoke — smoking is related to one-third of all cancers and 80% of all lung cancer
- Eat well — a healthy diet is the best defense against disease.

Guidelines to Eating Well

- Eat a minimum of five servings of fruit and vegetables every day
- Focus on the most colorful fruit and vegetables, such as red peppers, dark greens, oranges, carrots, apricots, blueberries
- Choose whole grains over processed grains and white flours
- Limit refined carbohydrates, such as pastries, sweetened cereals, soft drinks, candy, salty snacks
- Cook with olive or organic canola oil
- Avoid trans-fats found in many margarines, baked and convenience products
- Limit intake of saturated fats and cholesterol found in meats and dairy products
- Add avocados, natural nuts, seeds, cold water fish (cod, sardines, salmon) to the diet
- Control portion sizes

The body may be characterized by seven major systems: Cardiovascular (the heart and its components); Digestive (stomach, pancreas, bowels); Endocrine (glands and hormones); Immune (protective cells); Musculoskeletal (muscles, bones, joints, connective tissue); Nervous (the brain, spinal cord and nerves); and Respiratory (nose, trachea, bronchial tubes, lungs). Each system has a role to play in keeping the body disease-free. And each system responds positively to specific whole foods.

In the following pages, you will find information on each system, including its importance to our health, what kinds of problems we develop when the systems break down, and the diet and lifestyle changes we need to make to keep each system working at top capacity. As you read about each system, check the corresponding table listing "Best foods" and how they affect the system. Use the "Top 10 Best Bets" to focus action that will bring the problems you may be experiencing back into a healthy balance. As you do so, you will see in some cases, fish is included as a Best Bet. This is because some body systems (for example, cardiovascular) require omega-3 fatty acids for disease prevention and cold water fish are the best sources.

As always, check with a health-care specialist if you are experiencing health problems.

Cardiovascular System

Healthy Cardiovascular System

The cardiovascular system consists of the heart, the blood, the arteries and veins. The heart is a muscular organ responsible for pumping oxygenated blood that has just come from the lungs, and for delivering it via the arteries to all body tissues and organs. The body's tissues and organs depend on this oxygen and other nutrients to function. The heart is also responsible for bringing de-oxygenated blood back from the body via the veins to the heart so this blood can be sent to the lungs to get more oxygen.

Cardiovascular Disease

Atherosclerosis, high cholesterol, high blood pressure

Cardiovascular disease — or heart disease, as it is most commonly called — is an illness that pertains to the heart and the blood vessels. Atherosclerosis is the most common precursor to heart disease.

Atherosclerosis occurs when fatty deposits build up on the inside of the arteries, restricting blood flow to the organs supplied by the arteries. If this narrowing and decreased blood flow happens in the coronary arteries, the arteries that supply the heart muscle itself, coronary heart disease occurs. Coronary heart disease has few signs or symptoms, until the arteries become severely occluded, resulting in tissue death and a heart attack.

With repeated heart attacks, the heart becomes weakened and the few areas that are still functioning are left to do most of the work. This inefficiency creates a backup of blood in the heart, lungs and other tissues. This is called congestive heart failure, and can result in difficult breathing even at rest and eventually heart failure and death.

Atherosclerosis also affects other organs and tissues, such as the brain and the legs and feet. If the occlusion happens in the brain, an area of the brain tissue dies and a stroke results. If the legs and feet are restricted of blood and oxygen, we get diminished peripheral circulation, pain with walking and even swelling and ulcerations of the legs.

For years, high cholesterol has been named as the culprit for the presence of fatty deposits inside of the arteries. But in fact, it is the presence of oxidized cholesterol in the bloodstream that can turn the fatty deposits in the arteries into harder plaques and eventually occlusion. This is why antioxidants in our foods are so important. It is also important to note that there are different types of cholesterol. LDL or low-density lipoprotein, is the "bad" cholesterol, the one that gets oxidized and causes the damage. On the other hand, HDL or high-density lipoprotein, is the "good" cholesterol and protects against heart disease.

Another important risk factor for heart disease is a high level of homocysteine. Homocysteine seems to reduce the integrity of the artery walls, as well as cause direct damage to the arteries. Vitamins B_6 (pyridoxine), B_{12} and folic acid help break down homocysteine in the body and keep levels low.

High blood pressure can damage the inside of the artery walls, starting the plaque build-up process and leading to heart disease. It is also much harder work for the heart to pump blood through a system with higher pressure, leading to heart disease and stroke.

Many risk factors contribute to high blood pressure, high levels of oxidized LDL cholesterol and atherosclerosis. The good news is that most of these risk factors can be controlled with diet, exercise and lifestyle modifications.

Optimizing Cardiovascular Function

To protect the cardiovascular system from disease, we need to maintain a healthy body weight, eat an antioxidant-plentiful diet, educate ourselves on the types of fats we should and should not consume, exercise regularly and learn how to cope with stress.

Increase antioxidant-rich foods

Antioxidants are responsible for preventing oxidation of LDL cholesterol inside the arterial walls. This makes it essential for preventing heart disease as it stalls the blockage of the arteries and allows oxygenated blood to be delivered to the organs. Vitamin C is especially important because it prevents the formation of free radicals, which damage the arterial walls, but it also helps heal the damaged areas before the plaque formation process begins. Numerous studies have shown antioxidants such as vitamin E, selenium and coenzyme Q10 to be efficient in both the prevention and treatment of heart disease.

Best foods

- Polyphenols: extra virgin olive oil
- Bioflavonoids (quercetin): strawberries, onions, apples, green and black tea
- Vitamin C: oranges, strawberries, kiwifruit, red bell peppers, sweet potatoes, broccoli, kale
- Vitamin E: wheat germ, almonds, sunflower seeds, cooked organic soybeans
- Selenium: Brazil nuts, garlic, cooked barley, brown rice, oatmeal, tofu
- Coenzyme Q10: soy oil, mackerel, sardines, peanuts

Increase intake of whole foods that are high in soluble and insoluble fibers

Fruits and legumes are high in soluble fiber, vegetables and whole grains are high in insoluble fiber, and most foods have a combination of both. Soluble fiber, which forms a gel-like compound when dissolved in water, helps eliminate excess cholesterol by binding the cholesterol in the bowels and getting it ready for elimination. Oats in particular contain beta-glucans, which bind cholesterol, and have a significant impact on preventing heart disease. Insoluble fiber, which does not dissolve in water, aids in lowering cholesterol by forming bulk in the stool, and helping to move the bowels.

Best foods

- Legumes (beans, such as black, kidney, lima, pinto, navy, white) and lentils, chickpeas, split peas
- Rolled oats (large flake whole oats/not quick-cooking or instant varieties) and oat bran
- Fruits (apples, oranges, pears), fruit pectin
- Ground flaxseeds

Increase unsaturated fats in your diet

Foods high in unsaturated fatty acids are an important part of a heart healthy diet. Research studies have shown that gamma-linolenic acid (GLA), an omega-6 fatty acid found in evening primrose oil, can decrease LDL levels and increase HDL levels, reducing the risk for atherosclerosis. GLA has also proven to decrease blood pressure levels.

Please note that along with increasing unsaturated fats in your diet, you should also avoid saturated fats (found in animal products such as meats and dairy products) and trans fats (which occur from the hydrogenation process of oils for some margarines and fast foods to make them more stable and increase shelf life). Research shows that trans fats elevate LDL cholesterol and reduce HDL cholesterol

Best foods
- Extra virgin olive oil, evening primrose oil, nuts and seeds, flaxseed oil, fresh fish

Learn stress management techniques and keep stress levels low

When people are under stress, they form more free radicals, which cause more LDL cholesterol oxidation. Stress also stimulates the release of adrenaline, which can create more clots and increase the thickness of the blood. Clots are the start of plaque formation and increase the risk of atherosclerosis. They can also get lodged and lead to a heart attack or stroke. Daily relaxation techniques and learning some stress coping mechanisms can protect against heart disease.

It has also been found that with deep breathing, the body eliminates more sodium than with shallow breathing. This means that deep-breathing techniques can help reduce blood pressure levels by having an effect on water retention.

Best techniques
- Daily relaxation techniques, deep-breathing, rest, hobbies

Exercise regularly and maintain a healthy weight

Exercising regularly helps maintain a healthy body weight, lowers stress and anxiety, and lowers blood pressure levels — all essential components of a heart disease prevention program. Exercise also helps decrease LDL levels and elevate HDL cholesterol levels in the blood, protecting against heart disease. Aim for at least 20 minutes, three times a week. Before starting on a new exercise routine, consult your physician.

Best exercises
- Yoga, brisk walking, swimming, bicycling, dancing

Top 10 Best Bets for Heart Health

❶ Broiled or baked fish: Fish oils contain omega-3 fatty acids that help prevent heart disease and stroke. Studies have shown that there is a difference in health benefits between different types of cooking methods for fish. For example, broiled or oven-baked fish lower the risk of stroke, while fried fish or fish burgers increase the risk of stroke.

❷ Garlic: Garlic contains thioallyls, including allicin, which help platelet aggregation and blood pressure, decreasing the risk for heart disease and stroke.

❸ Soy foods and other beans: Soy isoflavones, the active constituents in soy foods, help protect the cardiovascular system. Soy foods can significantly lower LDL cholesterol levels by decreasing cholesterol and absorption of bile acid from the gastrointestinal tract, but they also decrease the oxidative damage to LDL with their strong free-radical scavenging potential. Look for organic, non-genetically modified soy.

❹ Pomegranate: This delicious and fun-to-eat fruit is important due to its benefits on the cardiovascular system. Pomegranate juice has been shown to reduce the oxidation of LDL cholesterol, protect the arteries from becoming thicker and reduce the development of atherosclerosis. Even though the mechanism of the pomegranate's action is not completely understood, the strong antioxidant potential from its polyphenol compounds may be partly responsible for the benefits.

❺ Extra virgin olive oil: Olive oil is an essential part of the Mediterranean diet, which has been shown to reduce blood pressure and improve lipid profiles, even compared to a lower-fat diet. Olive oil is also a source of antioxidant and anti-inflammatory polyphenols and is high in monounsaturated fats.

❻ Whole oats and oat bran: Whole oats and oat bran are an easy and inexpensive way to achieve a healthy heart. Oats contain beta-glucan, a soluble fiber that binds cholesterol in the bowels and prevents it from being reabsorbed into the bloodstream.

❼ Celery: Celery contains a compound called 3-n-butyl phthalide, which benefits the cardiovascular system. Four ribs of celery per day can help to reduce blood pressure levels.

❽ Apples: Apples are rich in pectin, a soluble fiber that is effective in lowering cholesterol levels, as well as an antioxidant against the oxidation of LDL.

Apples are also rich in the bioflavonoid quercetin, a multipurpose nutrient that contributes to heart health. Quercetin acts as an antioxidant by scavenging free radicals to inhibit LDL damage inside the arteries, and also by regenerating the levels of vitamin E. Quercetin has anti-inflammatory and antihistaminic properties that help control inflammation and allergic reactions anywhere in the body.

❾ Asparagus and leafy greens: Asparagus and leafy green vegetables are high in folate, essential for the lowering of homocysteine levels. High homocysteine levels are an independent risk factor for cardiovascular disease and stroke. Keep in mind that vitamins B_6 and B_{12} are also important factors for controlling the levels of homocysteine in the blood, and that vitamin B_{12}, which is found mostly in animal products, is hard to find in a vegetarian diet.

❿ Tea and cocoa: Tea and cocoa are good providers of bioflavonoids. Studies show that drinking an average of 3 cups (750 mL) of brewed black tea per day can have a long-term positive effect on the cardiovascular system. Similarly, when consumed in moderation, flavonoid-rich chocolate or cocoa can be a component of a heart-healthy diet.

Foods that Protect the Heart

Best Foods that Protect the Heart	Cardiovascular System Benefits	Comments
FRUITS		
Citus: • Kiwifruit • Oranges • Strawberries • Mandarins • Pomegranate • Lemons • Grapefruit	Rich in vitamin C and bioflavonoids, which are antioxidants. Contain pectins. Kiwifruit also contains vitamin E, a powerful antioxidant. Strawberries contain quercetin, a bioflavonoid.	Kiwifruit has proven to be one of the most nutrient-dense fruits. Caution: Grapefruit juice can interfere with some medications.
• Apples	Pectin in apples clean up and bind cholesterol in the intestines, preventing it from being absorbed into the bloodstream. Also high in quercetin.	Studies show that pectin, the soluble fiber found in apple peel, is comparable in results to cholesterol-lowering drugs.
Orange/Yellow: • Apricots • Mangoes	Contain carotenoids and vitamin C, which are antioxidants. Apricots and mangoes are rich in potassium, which helps control blood pressure.	Choose firm and bright orange-colored apricots.
• Bananas	High in potassium, which helps keep blood pressure in check.	
Blue/Purple: • Blueberries and other berries • Purple grapes • Plums	Contain anthocyanins, which destroy free radicals. Also high in pectin and vitamin C.	Frozen berries carry all the heart-health benefits that fresh berries do.
VEGETABLES		
Red Nightshades: • Tomatoes • Red bell peppers	Rich in lycopene, a potent antioxidant. High in vitamin C and beta-carotene.	Lycopene is fat-soluble and must be eaten with a fat in order to be absorbed. Lycopene is also found in processed tomato products, such as tomato juice, ketchup and pizza sauce.
Orange/Yellow: • Carrots • Yams • Sweet potatoes • Pumpkin and other winter squashes	Contain carotenoids, which make LDL cholesterol less susceptible to oxidation.	
Green: • Spinach • Swiss chard • Asparagus • Dandelion greens • Other dark leafy greens	Contain folic acid, essential for lowering homocysteine levels. Contain magnesium, calcium and potassium, which help control blood pressure. Asparagus is high in folate, which helps reduce homocysteine levels.	1 cup (250 mL) of leafy vegetables is equal to one serving.

Best Foods that Protect the Heart	Cardiovascular System Benefits	Comments
VEGETABLES (cont.)		
Cruciferous Family: • Broccoli • Cabbage • Cauliflower	Broccoli contains large amounts of vitamin C and beta-carotene, both powerful antioxidants. All contain folic acid and potassium.	
• Celery	Contains 3-n-butyl phthalide and high amounts of potassium to help with lowering blood pressure.	4 ribs of celery per day can help reduce blood pressure levels.
Allium Family: • Garlic • Onions • Chives	Allicin in garlic lowers blood pressure and reduces blood clotting. Yellow or red onions are high in quercetin.	Released during crushing, allicin gives garlic its characteristic smell. Eat garlic raw and cooked.
LEGUMES		
• Beans • Organic soybeans • Lentils • Peas • Chickpeas	Legumes are a source of soluble fiber that can help eliminate excess cholesterol through the bowels. Rich in flavonoids, which prevent LDL oxidation and damage to the artery lining.	For soy foods, see page 102. 1 cup (250 mL) of cooked soybeans contains 25% of recommended daily fiber and 1 oz (30 g) of protein. Soy products contain phytoestrogens, which may act like weak estrogens in the body. Consult with your naturopathic doctor or nutritionist before consuming large amounts of soy.
WHOLE GRAINS		
• Whole oats and oat bran • Brown rice • Pot barley • Whole ancient grains: spelt, kamut, amaranth	Beta-glucans in oats bind cholesterol molecules in the bowel for elimination. They can lower LDL levels without lowering HDL levels.	Whole grains, such as whole oats and brown rice, contain more fiber than processed flours, pasta, crackers and breads.
NUTS AND SEEDS		
Nuts: • Almonds • Brazil nuts • Walnuts	Nuts contain monounsaturated fats, vitamin E and fiber. They help decrease LDL while leaving HDL unchanged. Brazil nuts, high in selenium, are antioxidant.	Buy raw or dry-roasted nuts and seeds. Choose an unsalted variety; salt can increase blood pressure.
Seeds: • Flaxseeds • Sesame seeds • Sunflower seeds • Pumpkin seeds	Flaxseeds are high in omega-3 oils, fiber and calcium, and help decrease LDL cholesterol, platelet stickiness and blood pressure. Sesame seeds are an excellent source of vitamin E.	Flaxseeds must be ground to maximize absorption and digestion. Once ground, they go rancid quickly, especially if not refrigerated. Best to purchase small quantities of whole flaxseeds, store in the refrigerator and grind fresh just before using.

Best Foods that Protect the Heart	Cardiovascular System Benefits	Comments
FATS AND OILS		
Cold-pressed oils: • Extra virgin olive oil • Grapeseed oil • Flaxseed oil • Avocados	Olive oil, grapeseed oil and avocados contain heart-healthy monounsaturated fats. Grapeseed oil contains significant amounts of vitamin E and, unlike many fats, increases HDL levels.	Look for cold-pressed, less refined oils that are packaged in dark glass containers. Keep oils in the refrigerator to keep them from going rancid.
HERBS AND SPICES		
• Cayenne • Ginger • Garlic	Cayenne stimulates blood flow and strengthens the heart beat and metabolic rate. Ginger can lower cholesterol and decrease stickiness of platelets.	
OTHER		
• Beer • Chocolate • Coffee • Black tea • Wine	Black tea and red wine contain quercetin. Beer is rich in bioflavonoids from the fermented grains. Phenols in dark chocolate and red wine are antioxidant.	Caution: Caffeine and alcohol consumption can increase blood pressure levels. Consume in moderation. Not recommended during pregnancy and lactation.

Digestive System

Healthy Digestive System

The digestive system is responsible for mixing the food we eat and breaking it down into smaller molecules that our body can absorb and use. Digestion starts at the mouth with chewing and breaking carbohydrate molecules down with the aid of enzymes found in saliva. Food then travels down the esophagus into the stomach, where hydrochloric acid, also known as HCl, and digestive enzymes break down proteins and allow for the absorption of some substances. Most digestion and absorption of nutrients take place in the small intestine, with the help of the liver and gall bladder, which provide bile, and the pancreas, which provides digestive enzymes. Food molecules, such as monosaccharides (carbohydrate units), amino acids (protein units) and fatty acids, as well as vitamins, minerals and water are absorbed into the bloodstream and lymphatic system, while indigestible foods (mostly fiber) continue down to the large intestine and eventually get eliminated.

The entire digestive system is lined with mucous membranes. Mucous membranes act as a barrier and are responsible for mucous secretions that aid in the digestive process. A smooth muscle layer also exists in the entire digestive tract and is responsible for mixing and breaking food down, as well as propelling food downwards through the digestive tract.

Digestive Problems

Heartburn, constipation, inflammatory bowel disease, colon cancer

Heartburn is one of the most common digestive complaints. It can be a symptom of gastric reflux, a hiatal hernia or a gastric or duodenal ulcer. Determining the cause of heartburn is important, as these conditions can be easily treated but can become serious if not attended to.

Another common indicator of suboptimal digestive function is constipation. Constipation occurs when bowel movements are infrequent or difficult, causing bloating, headaches or hemorrhoids, to name a few symptoms. Constipation can be caused by a lack of fiber or water in the diet, stress, or perhaps disease.

Constipation can be an indicator of other digestive system diseases. For example, constipation alternating with diarrhea can be one of the symptoms of irritable bowel syndrome (IBS). Other symptoms of IBS include abdominal pain and cramps, excess gas and bloating. IBS can be caused by sensitivity to foods and is often associated with emotional stress — and it can be extremely disabling.

Inflammatory bowel disease (IBD) includes two conditions with chronic inflammation of the bowels: Crohn's disease and ulcerative colitis. In these conditions, inflammation of the bowel can result in such symptoms as diarrhea, bleeding, cramping and a feeling of urgency. The cause of these conditions is not known. Consult a physician if you are suffering from any of the above symptoms.

The digestive system is also susceptible to cancer. Colon cancer is the second most common form of cancer, and one that can be easily prevented with a healthy lifestyle and regular bowel movements. Colon cancer is treatable, but early detection and treatment are crucial. If you experience a change in bowel habits, blood in the stool, unexplained weight loss or fatigue, consult your physician.

Optimizing Digestive Function

To protect the digestive system from disease and allow for optimal digestive function, we need to maintain healthy mucous membranes, and to heal them when necessary; create and maintain a healthy intestinal flora; eat a diet rich in fiber and antioxidants; drink plenty of water; eat fresh foods, which are rich in digestive enzymes, instead of frozen or prepared foods; and eliminate foods that irritate the bowel or cause inflammation. As the digestive system is closely linked with the nervous system, daily routines and stress-management techniques are also beneficial for digestive function.

Eat foods that create and maintain a healthy lining of the digestive tract

The lining of the digestive tract is responsible for choosing what is absorbed into the body and what gets eliminated, so it must be intact. The digestive process breaks food down into smaller molecules that are checked by the immune system as they are absorbed. If digestion is poor and food is not broken down properly, or the mucous membranes become increasingly permeable ("leaky gut"), molecules pass through the barrier in a larger form, and the immune system recognizes them as foreign invaders. This hypersensitivity of the immune system can create a number of symptoms that can manifest in any part of the body.

You can maintain the health of the digestive tract's lining by promoting repair of intestinal cells, reestablishing a healthy bacterial flora and decreasing inflammation. Foods such as cabbage are high in glutamine, an amino acid that helps regenerate and repair the cells of the digestive tract. Probiotics — the healthy bacteria that populate the intestines — and fiber help maintain a healthy intestinal environment and crowd out toxic bacteria. Fish oils and quercetin from apples and onions help decrease the inflammatory response, minimize damage to the digestive lining and dampen food sensitivity reactions.

Best foods
- Fish oils, whole grains (brown rice, rye, spelt, quinoa, millet)
- Fruits (apples, blueberries, blackberries, grapes)
- Vegetables (cabbage, onions, red bell peppers)
- Legumes (beans, peas, lentils)

Eat foods that create and maintain a healthy bacterial environment in the intestines

Friendly bacteria in our intestines are an important part of a healthy digestive system. They are responsible for crowding out pathogens and maintaining a beneficial acid-base balance (a balanced pH in the digestive tract is created by many factors, one being the production of lactic acid by "friendly bacteria,") that helps prevent infection from bacteria, viruses, yeast and parasites. Friendly bacteria optimize digestion by producing digestive enzymes. They also make B vitamins and vitamin K and protect against food allergies by maintaining a healthy immune system in the digestive tract.

When we eat a diet that is rich in processed foods and chemicals or take antibiotics to treat infection, the population of healthy bacteria is reduced. We can increase this by supplementing with probiotics and by eating foods that contain prebiotics. Prebiotics are vegetable fibers or complex sugars, which the healthy bacteria depend on for survival. These carbohydrate compounds, including fructooligosaccharides (FOS) are found in foods such as fruits, vegetables, whole grains and legumes.

Best foods
- Garlic, onions, asparagus, leeks, artichokes, natural yogurt

Eat a diet rich in fiber and increase water intake

Fiber is the part of plant food that goes through the digestive tract undigested. It is necessary to clean the digestive tract by collecting dead cells and debris, and also helps prevent cholesterol and excess hormones from being reabsorbed back into the bloodstream. In general, both soluble and insoluble fibers help with these functions. Insoluble fiber is necessary to form bulk and stimulate the muscles of the digestive tract to move the bowels. Soluble fiber acts as a food source for friendly bacteria in the intestinal tract. Together with proper intake of water, all these factors help maintain a healthy digestive tract and protect against digestive system diseases, such as constipation, hemorrhoids and colon cancer. In fact, insufficient fiber contributes to a large percentage of digestive disorders. Fiber can come from many foods, such as whole grains, fruits and vegetables, nuts and seeds, and beans and other legumes. Most processed foods and animal products are devoid of fiber.

Best foods

- Whole grains (brown rice, rye, oats, millet, buckwheat, quinoa, spelt, whole wheat)
- Fruits (apples, pears, oranges, berries, peaches, dates, fresh or dried figs, prunes)
- Vegetables (carrots, celery, leafy greens and cruciferous vegetables, such as cabbage, broccoli, cauliflower)
- Seeds (sesame seeds, sunflower seeds, pumpkin seeds, flaxseeds)
- Nuts (almonds, hazelnuts, walnuts)
- Legumes (beans, lentils, peas, chickpeas, organic soybeans)

Eat foods that promote digestion

Digestion depends on different substances to break foods down, prepare them for absorption and help the body to utilize them. For example, starting at the mouth, salivary glands produce saliva, which can initiate the digestion of carbohydrates. Then hydrochloric acid (HCl) in the stomach helps dissolve food particles and activates other enzymes. Similarly, in the small intestine, digestive enzymes produced by the pancreas and bile from the liver and gall bladder help emulsify fats, break down carbohydrates, proteins and fats, and get them ready for absorption. See Top 10 Best Bets for foods that stimulate the release of saliva and enhance the production of HCl and the release of digestive enzymes and bile into the digestive tract. Foods high in enzymes (bananas, papaya, mangoes, pineapple) along with a nutritionally dense diet, can ensure healthy body functions.

Best foods

- Cider vinegar, bitter foods (dandelion greens and other bitter greens), lemon juice, "live" (sprouted) foods, bananas, pineapple, papaya, unpasteurized honey, sauerkraut, natural yogurt

Practice stress-management techniques and regular bowel habits

Conditions such as heartburn and irritable bowel syndrome (IBS) are closely linked with the nervous system. It is also helpful to establish a daily routine that includes a regular time for bowel elimination. This encourages daily bowel movements and decreases the incidence of constipation. Managing stress and following a daily routine can help maintain a healthy digestive system, increase the frequency of bowel movements and reduce the risk for colon cancer.

Best techniques

- Yoga, breathing exercises, daily bowel routine (in this case, an overall daily routine is helpful for stress management), regular bowel habits, counseling for emotional stress

Top 10 Best Bets for Digestive Health

❶ **Cabbage:** Cabbage is rich in glutamine, an amino acid used by the intestinal cells as their principal fuel source. Glutamine helps the cells repair and regenerate themselves and prevents undigested foods from passing through the intestinal lining. Cabbage is also used to make sauerkraut through the process of fermentation. Sauerkraut helps populate the intestinal micro flora and contains digestive enzymes.

❷ **Onions:** Onions are essential for digestive health. Onions are a source of quercetin, which helps decrease hypersensitivity in the intestines. This helps to protect the lining of the digestive system from irritation and protect the body from food sensitivities. Onions are also a source of fructooligosaccharides (FOS), a complex sugar that acts as a prebiotic and feeds the healthy bacteria in our digestive system.

❸ Apples and apple cider vinegar: Apples are high in pectin, a soluble fiber that absorbs 100 times its weight in water. Pectin from apples helps calm the intestinal tract during diarrhea and prevents constipation. Quercetin, a flavonoid found in apples, helps stabilize immune reactions and decrease inflammation and irritation of the digestive system.

Apple cider vinegar helps increase production of hydrochloric acid (HCl) in the stomach. HCl helps break food particles down and activates other enzymes to digest proteins. As part of the immune system, HCl helps kill food pathogens before they reach the rest of the digestive system.

❹ Garlic: Garlic is a source of FOS, which helps nourish the healthy bacteria in our digestive system and maintain an optimal environment in our intestines. Garlic is also a powerful antimicrobial that protects against parasites, yeast, viruses and bacteria that could be harmful to our health when they populate our digestive tract.

❺ Fennel and caraway seeds: Fennel and caraway seeds help stimulate digestion and appetite. In Asian countries, they are also commonly chewed after a meal to relieve bloating, flatulence and colic, and even to freshen the breath.

❻ Peppermint: Peppermint is one of the most effective digestive herbs. It helps relax the stomach and intestines when they suffer from cramping and spasms, and it helps relieve nausea. This also means that peppermint can relax the esophageal sphincter. When relaxed, the sphincter can open and food and stomach acids from the stomach can travel upward to the esophagus and cause symptoms of heartburn. If you suffer from gastric reflux, avoid peppermint.

❼ Dandelion greens and other bitter greens: Dandelion greens and other bitter greens are indispensable to optimize digestion. These bitter foods help stimulate the release of bile from the gall bladder and digestive enzymes from the pancreas, enhancing digestive function. The greens can be eaten in a salad to increase appetite before the main course of a meal.

❽ Pineapple and papaya: Pineapple and papaya contain bromelain and papain, digestive enzymes that can complement the enzymes already produced by the body. These enzymes help break foods down in the digestive tract and can decrease symptoms of food sensitivities, as well as reduce bloating and flatulence after a meal.

❾ Brown rice: Brown rice and other whole grains are a source of insoluble fiber. Insoluble fiber increases bulk in the stool and helps prevent constipation and protect against colon cancer. Brown rice is an ideal food for people who suffer from IBS, IBD or constipation, in part because, unlike wheat, rye and spelt, brown rice is a gluten-free grain that does not seem to cause intestinal irritation or allergic reactions in patients with gluten sensitivity. In addition, brown rice contains phytic acid, which seems to protect against colon cancer.

❿ Beans and other legumes: Beans and other legumes are an excellent source of soluble fiber. Soluble fiber is a food source for friendly bacteria in the intestines, which then produce short chain fatty acids. These fatty acids create an optimal pH balance in the digestive tract and protect the lining of the digestive tract against colon cancer.

Foods that Protect the Digestive System

Best Foods for Protecting the Digestive System	Digestive System Benefits	Comments
FRUITS		
Citrus: • Oranges • Mandarins • Lemons • Grapefruit • Kiwifruit • Strawberries	Contain pectin and other soluble fiber, which provide food for healthy intestinal bacteria and protect against constipation and other digestive diseases.	Lemon juice can increase the release of HCl, helping with protection against pathogens, break down of proteins and absorption of nutrients.
• Apricots • Peaches • Pears • Apples	Contain pectin and other soluble fiber that prevent constipation and colon cancer. Apples contain quercetin, which helps decrease irritability in the digestive tract.	Most fruits and vegetables contain a mixture of soluble and insoluble fibers.
• Fresh or dried figs • Prunes	Help increase bowel frequency and prevent bowel toxicity and colon cancer.	Prunes are high in fiber; prune juice is not. (Prune juice is a natural laxative, but it does not contain fiber and does not have all the other benefits of a high-fiber food like prunes.)
Tropical fruits: • Bananas • Pineapple • Papaya	These tropical fruits are loaded with natural digestive enzymes that enhance the break down of foods in the digestive tract.	Take digestive tropical fruit drinks one hour before a meal.
Berries: • Blueberries • Blackberries • Grapes	Berries contain flavonoids, which help maintain the health of the lining in the digestive tract.	
VEGETABLES		
Green: • Spinach • Swiss chard • Asparagus • Dandelion greens • Endive • Other dark leafy greens	Dandelion greens and other bitter greens help improve digestion by stimulating the release of bile and digestive enzymes.	Raw foods are more difficult to digest. Steaming, covered, or sautéing briskly can make foods easier to digest without much loss of nutritive value.
Cruciferous Family: • Broccoli • Cabbage • Sauerkraut • Cauliflower	Sauerkraut contains healthy intestinal bacteria and digestive enzymes. Cabbage contains glutamine — an energy source for intestinal cells — and helps prevent a "leaky gut."	Sauerkraut is made of finely sliced cabbage that is fermented by various lactic acid bacteria, including *Lactobacillus*.

Best Foods for Protecting the Digestive System	Digestive System Benefits	Comments
VEGETABLES (cont.)		
Allium Family: • Garlic • Onions	Garlic, onions and asparagus contain fructooligosaccharides (FOS) or prebiotics. Onions contain quercetin, which helps decrease intestinal irritability and immune system hypersensitivity.	Garlic is an important antimicrobial for all the systems and fights against bacteria, viruses, yeast and parasites.
LEGUMES		
• Beans • Organic soybeans • Lentils • Peas • Chickpeas	Legumes are a source of soluble fiber, which feeds healthy intestinal bacteria.	Soaking beans for 8 hours before cooking makes them easier to digest.
WHOLE GRAINS		
• Oats (soluble fiber) • Brown rice • Pot Barley • Buckwheat • Quinoa • Whole wheat • Spelt • Rye	Whole grains are a source of insoluble fiber; they increase bulk and help prevent constipation. Contain phytic acid, which protects against colon cancer.	Whole grains containing gluten can be irritating to people with IBS, and cannot be tolerated by people with Crohn's disease.
NUTS AND SEEDS		
Nuts: • Almonds • Brazil nuts • Walnuts • Hazelnuts • Pine nuts	Nuts contain fiber. Brazil nuts are high in selenium, an antioxidant that helps protect against colon cancer.	
Seeds: • Flaxseeds • Sesame seeds • Sunflower seeds • Pumpkin seeds	Flaxseeds are high in omega-3 fatty acids, which help decrease inflammation, and lignins, an insoluble fiber that creates bulk for the stool and prevents constipation.	Lignins in flaxseeds also help maintain optimal levels of estrogen in the body. Flaxseeds must be freshly ground to avoid rancidity and maximize absorption and digestion.
FATS AND OILS		
Cold-pressed oils: • Extra virgin olive oil • Grapeseed oil • Flaxseed oil • Avocados	Oils are necessary for the absorption of fat-soluble vitamins A, E, D and K.	Adding a capsule of vitamin E into your oil container helps prevent oxidation and rancidity.

Best Foods for Protecting the Digestive System	Digestive System Benefits	Comments
HERBS AND SPICES		
• Cayenne • Ginger • Turmeric • Cumin • Coriander (dried or fresh Cilantro) • Fennel • Peppermint • Caraway seeds	These herbs and spices enhance digestion, help flush toxins out of the body and help improve absorption and assimilation of nutrients. Ginger can stimulate digestion.	Eat or make tea with ginger. Take a slice of fresh ginger 30 to 60 minutes before a meal for optimal digestion. Peppermint can relax the esophageal sphincter and stimulate symptoms of acid reflux.

A Note about Food Combining

One short-term method of relieving indigestion, flatulence, fatigue, food allergies and, in some cases, inflammatory bowel and peptic ulcer, is to follow a discipline of eating certain foods in a set order. This order is as follows:

Fruits Alone
Fruits require the least time and energy for the body to digest and because of this it is recommended that fruit be eaten before a meal or at least two hours after a meal. Fruits are best taken alone at breakfast or as small, between-meal snacks.

Proteins with Non-starchy Vegetables
Protein foods (fish, eggs, nuts, seeds, dairy products, soy products) take the longest and use up the most of the body's effort to digest. When fruit or starchy vegetables are eaten before or with proteins, they break down and ferment long before the proteins are digested. This causes the digestive problems listed earlier. It is best to eat protein foods with non-starchy vegetables (leafy greens, asparagus, broccoli, cabbage, celery, cucumber, onion, sweet bell peppers, sea vegetables, tomatoes, zucchini).

Whole Grains with Non-starchy Vegetables
Whole grains and non-starchy vegetables are complex carbohydrates that break down at about the same rate, providing the body with a slow and steady supply of starches and sugars for fuel. If eaten together, they are best without fruit or protein.

Starchy Vegetables, Legumes and Refined Grains in Small Amounts, Alone
Squash, legumes, pasta, refined grains, beets, parsnips, carrots, sweet potatoes and pumpkin are starchy carbohydrate foods that break down faster than protein foods and other carbohydrates but not as quickly as fruits. It is recommended that starchy carbohydrates be eaten in small amounts, away from other foods.

Endocrine System

Healthy Endocrine System

The endocrine system consists of endocrine glands and the hormones produced by these glands, which work together to serve as one of the body's main control systems. Hormones are chemicals that carry messages through the blood. To do this, hormones travel from the endocrine glands in which they are produced to the target cells where they will perform their function. For example, the thyroid gland produces and secretes thyroid hormones (thyroxine or T4, and triiodothyronine or T3), which control the body's metabolic rate. The adrenal glands, located on top of the kidneys, secrete a number of hormones, including cortisol, which is released in response to stress and can help balance the immune system. Epinephrine, also known as adrenaline, and norepinephrine are also released in response to stress and can have an effect similar to that of sympathetic nerves (the "fight or flight" response).

Some organs have a function in more than one body system. For example, the pancreas, which secretes digestive enzymes as part of the digestive system, also performs an endocrine function by releasing the insulin and glucagon responsible for balancing blood sugar.

The reproductive organs are also part of the endocrine system. In females, the ovaries manage the functioning, growth and development of the female reproductive system, including the breasts, via hormones such as estrogen and progesterone. In males, the testes produce testosterone, which is responsible for the functioning, growth and development of the male reproductive system.

The hypothalamus in the brain and the pituitary gland just below it control many of these glands through hormones they secrete. Hormonal feedback can signal to these glands to produce more or less hormones that help keep the body's functions in balance.

Many other glands and organs are part of the endocrine system and no doubt many others remain to be discovered.

Endocrine Disorders

Hormone imbalance, hyperthyroidism, hypothyroidism, diabetes

Most endocrine disorders occur when too much or too little of a hormone is produced by an endocrine gland, when the target cell exerts a reduced response, or in some cases, when our body cannot properly eliminate excess hormones.

Hyperthyroidism is a condition where the thyroid gland secretes too much of the thyroid hormone, creating symptoms of an increased metabolic rate. On the other hand, in hypothyroidism, there is too little of the active thyroid hormone, giving rise to such symptoms as fatigue, weight gain, cold intolerance and other signs of low metabolic function. Hypothyroidism can be caused by mineral deficiencies, as minerals are essential to produce and activate the thyroid hormone, or by a destruction of thyroid cells due to inflammatory disease.

Adrenal glands produce cortisol, which has potent anti-inflammatory and immunosuppressive properties important for normal immune responses. However, under constant stress, cortisol is overproduced and the body's immune system can be suppressed, leading to an increased risk of infections. Also, as part of the blood glucose-regulating system, increased cortisol and epinephrine production due to chronic stress can lead to higher blood glucose and insulin levels and subsequent weight gain.

In Type 1 diabetes, the pancreas does not produce enough insulin, whereas in Type 2 diabetes, the target cells resist insulin. In both cases, glucose cannot enter the cells and there is an elevation of blood sugar levels that can lead to serious complications. For people with diabetes, diet is critically important to help restore insulin sensitivity, control blood sugar levels and prevent complications.

In the reproductive system, an excess of estrogen that is unbalanced by progesterone can be linked with many female disorders, such as menstrual difficulties, endometriosis, fibrocystic breasts, infertility and breast cancer. Estrogen and progesterone balance is affected by many factors, including the use of oral contraceptives and hormone replacement therapy, diet and chemicals in food and the environment. In males, testosterone is released from the testes and converted into the hormone dihydrotestosterone (DHT), which stimulates the synthesis and growth of prostate cells. High levels of DHT can cause benign prostatic hyperplasia or prostate cancer.

What makes the endocrine system so complex is that most times hormones act in concert with one another to produce their physiologic effects, and the improper function of one can deeply affect the function of others.

Optimizing Endocrine Function

Eat a diet rich in complex carbohydrates

The glycemic index (GI) is a dietary guide that ranks foods based on how they affect blood sugar levels. It is often used by people with diabetes to help them choose foods that do not increase blood sugar levels rapidly. Foods with a high GI rating increase blood sugar levels at a fast rate, which an individual with too little insulin (Type 1 diabetes) or insulin-resistant cells (Type 2 diabetes) may not be able to tolerate. In general, simple carbohydrates, found in foods such as pasta, breads and crackers made with refined flours, as well as in soft drinks and candy, have a high GI. Foods that contain complex carbohydrates, fat and proteins have a low GI and will slow the absorption of sugar into the bloodstream. The GI should be utilized with other tools, as it does not take into consideration the fat content or the type of fat a food contains.

In particular, the fiber contained in complex carbohydrates is capable of slowing down the digestion and absorption of blood sugar and increasing insulin sensitivity, therefore giving it a low score on the GI scale. Water-soluble fiber is the most beneficial type for blood sugar control. Fruits and legumes are the best sources of water-soluble fiber. Soluble and insoluble fibers also encourage regular bowel movements, which helps eliminate excess estrogen from the body and prevent an estrogen/progesterone imbalance and breast cancer.

Best foods
- Whole grains (oats, brown rice, barley, quinoa, spelt, kamut, whole wheat)
- Legumes (beans, soybeans, chickpeas, lentils)
- Fruits (pears, apples, oranges, plums)
- All vegetables except white potatoes and parsnips
- Nuts and seeds (almonds, cashews, walnuts, sesame seeds, sunflower seeds, pumpkin seeds, ground flaxseeds)

Eat a diet rich in essential fatty acids

Essential fatty acids are precursors to all hormones and therefore constitute an indispensable part of a diet that promotes a healthy endocrine system.

Omega-3 fatty acids are part of cell membranes, where insulin receptors are located. Insulin receptors become more responsive to insulin when there are more omega-3 fatty acids in the cell membrane. Therefore, omega-3 fatty acids can help prevent insulin resistance and diabetes.

Best foods
- Fish oils (wild salmon, mackerel, albacore tuna, sardines, herring), flaxseed oil, soy oil, hempseed oil, canola oil, walnuts

Eat foods rich in minerals

Minerals are important in every aspect of endocrine function. For example, iodine is a component of thyroid hormones T4 and T3, and it must be obtained from the diet. T4 and some T3 are produced and released by the thyroid gland and travel to tissues where these hormones act in the body. Within the cell, T4 is converted to T3, the most active form. This conversion depends on the minerals zinc, copper and selenium.

Chromium, vanadium, manganese and zinc are essential for regulating blood sugar, either by increasing the production of insulin, by increasing the target cell's sensitivity to insulin or by acting on enzyme systems of glucose metabolism. That is why these minerals are important in the prevention of diabetes.

Minerals such as selenium and manganese are antioxidants, prevent damage to the cell's DNA and decrease the risk of cancer.

Best foods

- Zinc: black-eyed peas, pumpkin seeds, tofu, wheat germ
- Copper: nuts, legumes, potatoes, vegetables, cereal grains (oats and wheat)
- Selenium: Brazil nuts, yeast, whole grains
- Chromium: brewer's yeast, grains, some beers
- Vanadium: cereal grains, parsley, mushrooms, corn, soy foods
- Manganese: nuts, wheat germ, wheat bran, leafy green vegetables, beet tops, pineapple, seeds
- Iodine: iodized salt, sea vegetables (kelp), vegetables grown in iodine-rich soil

Learn ways of coping with stress

When a person suffers from stress, cortisol and adrenaline are released from the adrenal glands. These adrenal hormones can then trigger the pancreas to release glucagon, which is responsible for increasing blood sugar levels when the body demands more sugar to be available as an energy source. This usually happens when a person has not eaten in a while or in stress situations ("fight or flight" response) by a process called glycolysis, where stored glycogen is broken down into glucose molecules and released into the blood stream. This response is ideal during a state of crisis, but can be detrimental to the endocrine system over a long period. It is important to keep in mind that sugar and caffeine tend to stimulate the adrenal glands and it is best to consume these products in moderation, especially at times of high stress.

Techniques that induce a relaxation response and prevent the release of excess stress hormones from the adrenal glands can be beneficial.

Best methods

- Daily routine, meditation, prayer, breathing exercises, physical exercise, counseling

Exercise

The benefits of exercise for the endocrine system cannot be overstated. Exercise can decrease insulin resistance, and it increases the concentration of chromium in the tissues, helping the body maintain normal blood sugar levels. Exercise can help increase metabolic rate, energy and endurance, and for many people it helps achieve a proper body weight. Maintaining an ideal body weight is an important factor for prevention of diabetes. Exercise can help stimulate blood and lymphatic circulation, essential for the transport of hormones and elimination of excess hormones. Exercise also reduces secretions of stress hormones from the adrenal glands in response to psychological stress.

Best exercises

- Weight lifting, brisk walking, jogging, bicycling, swimming, dancing, yoga, racquet sports (such as tennis), team sports

Top 10 Best Bets for Endocrine Health

❶ Cruciferous vegetables: Cruciferous vegetables, such as broccoli, cauliflower, kale, Brussels sprouts and bok choy contain a phytochemical called indole-3-carbinol, which induces the break down of estrogen into its harmless metabolites, decreasing the risk for breast cancer.

❷ Sea vegetables: Sea vegetables, such as nori, arame, kelp, dulse and kombu, contain iodine, an essential mineral that is needed for the production of thyroid hormones. As part of thyroid hormones, iodine helps increase metabolism and reduce the risk of symptoms of hypothyroidism.

❸ Pumpkin seeds: Pumpkin seeds are high in zinc, a mineral essential for the normal function of the male reproductive system. Zinc is associated with proper testosterone levels, sperm production and sperm motility. Maintaining adequate levels of zinc may help prevent male infertility. Eat a handful of raw pumpkin seeds daily.

❹ Stevia: Stevia is an extract from the plant *Stevia rebaudiana*. The extract has 200 times the sweetness of sugar and contains no calories. It is a safe alternative for people with diabetes as it does not raise blood sugar levels and has glucose-lowering properties. Stevia extract can be used to sweeten foods and drinks. (See also Herbs, page 122)

❺ Soy foods: Soybeans contain phytoestrogens, chemicals that are plant-based and similar in structure to estrogen. Although the research is conflicting and inconclusive, the phytoestrogens found in soy (genistein and daidzein), act like weak estrogens and may help block estrogen's cancer promoting effect. Soybeans and soy foods should only be consumed if they are organic and non-genetically modified.

❻ Onions and garlic: Onions and garlic have blood sugar-regulating properties. They contain sulfur, which aids in liver detoxification and elimination of excess hormones. Garlic is also high in selenium, a potent antioxidant that can help prevent cancer.

❼ Ground flaxseeds: Ground flaxseeds are a source of omega-3 fatty acids and phytoestrogens. Lignins, the phytoestrogens found in flaxseeds, stand out in their ability to regulate the menstrual cycle in women. They have been shown to be mildly estrogenic or anti-estrogenic, depending on the body's need to balance hormones.

❽ Brewer's yeast: Brewer's yeast is the dried, powdered form of the *Saccharomyces cerevisiae* fungus used in the brewing process. It is the highest source of chromium, a mineral that works in conjunction with insulin to promote the uptake of glucose by the target cells. For this reason, chromium is essential for blood sugar regulation and diabetes prevention.

❾ Citrus fruits: Citrus fruits are a rich source of vitamin C. Vitamin C is stored in high concentration in the adrenal glands and helps in the production of adrenal hormones. In addition, vitamin C increases insulin's response to sugar, thus helping lower blood sugar levels. Vitamin C is also an antioxidant that can help prevent breast and prostate cancer.

❿ Spinach: Spinach is one of the best sources of alpha-lipoic acid, a vitamin-like nutrient that is very important for glucose metabolism and prevention of diabetes. Alpha-lipoic acid is also an antioxidant that helps prevent free-radical damage and decreases the risk of cancer. Spinach is also a source of many minerals that can be beneficial for endocrine function.

Foods that Protect the Endocrine System

Best Foods for Protecting the Endocrine System	Endocrine System Benefits	Comments
FRUITS		
Citrus: • Oranges • Mandarins • Lemons • Grapefruit • Kiwifruit • Strawberries	Contain soluble fiber, which helps control blood sugar levels. Contain vitamin C and bioflavonoids, antioxidants that can help reduce the risk of cancer. Vitamin C in particular is essential for the production of stress hormones by the adrenal glands.	Fructose, the natural sugar found in fruits, is first absorbed in the digestive tract and then has to be converted into glucose, so it does not increase blood sugar levels as rapidly as other simple sugars obtained from the diet.
• Apricots • Peaches • Pears • Apples	Contain pectin and other soluble fiber, the most beneficial type of fiber for the control of blood sugar levels.	Most fruits and vegetables contain a mixture of soluble and insoluble fibers and can slow down the absorption of sugar.
Berries and grapes: • Blueberries • Blackberries • Raspberries • Grapes	Berries and grapes are a rich source of bioflavonoids. These are antioxidants and help prevent breast and prostate cancer.	Bioflavonoids help the body use vitamin C. They are found in highest concentration in the skin or peel of fruits and vegetables.
VEGETABLES		
Green: • Spinach • Swiss chard • Dandelion greens	Rich in many minerals needed for optimal endocrine function, including iodine, selenium and manganese. Spinach is a source of alpha-lipoic acid, an important nutrient for glucose metabolism.	
Red Nightshades: • Bell peppers • Tomatoes	Tomatoes are the best source of lycopene, a strong antioxidant that helps protect cells against damage and plays an important role in cancer prevention.	Lycopene is a carotene that gives tomatoes their deep red color.
Cruciferous Family: • Broccoli • Cabbage • Sauerkraut • Cauliflower • Kale • Bok choy	Cruciferous vegetables contain indole-3-carbinol, a chemical that helps break down estrogen into its harmless metabolites.	Cooking destroys indoles, so eat these foods raw or lightly steamed.
Sea Vegetables: • Nori • Arame • Kelp • Dulse • Kombu	Contain minerals, including iodine, calcium and iron. Iodine is needed for the production of thyroid hormones.	Caution: Do not consume sea vegetables if you have a hyperthyroid condition. Also, hijiki may contain high levels of inorganic arsenic, a carcinogen, and food safety agencies in many countries, including Canada and Britain, have cautioned against its consumption.

Best Foods for Protecting the Endocrine System	Endocrine System Benefits	Comments
VEGETABLES (cont.)		
Allium Family: • Garlic • Onions	Garlic and onions can help regulate blood sugar levels.	
LEGUMES		
• Beans (kidney, adzuki, mung) • Lentils • Peas (black-eyed) • Chickpeas	Legumes are a source of soluble fiber, which helps eliminate excess estrogen through the bowels. Black-eyed peas and tofu are rich sources of zinc, essential for endocrine system function.	Consult with your naturopathic doctor or nutritionist before consuming large amounts of soy.
WHOLE GRAINS		
• Whole oats • Brown rice • Pot Barley • Buckwheat • Quinoa • Whole wheat • Spelt • Rye	Barley is the grain with the lowest glycemic index (GI) rating, which means it is highly efficient at slowing the rate at which sugar is absorbed into the blood stream.	Whole grains score lower in the GI scale in comparison to refined carbohydrates.
NUTS AND SEEDS		
Nuts: • Almonds • Brazil nuts • Walnuts • Hazelnuts • Pine nuts	Nuts contain fiber, which helps control blood sugar levels. Nuts are high in minerals, such as zinc and manganese, essential for the functioning of the endocrine system.	Try natural nut butters without added hydrogenated oils, sugar or salt.
Seeds: • Flaxseeds • Sesame seeds • Sunflower seeds • Pumpkin seeds	Seeds are high in fiber and unsaturated fats, which help control blood sugar levels. Sesame seeds are a source of iodine, a component of thyroid hormones. Pumpkin seeds are high in zinc, needed for all aspects of insulin metabolism and male reproductive system.	Try natural seed butters without added hydrogenated oils, sugar or salt.

Best Foods for Protecting the Endocrine System	Endocrine System Benefits	Comments
FATS AND OILS		
Cold-pressed oils: • Flaxseed oil • Soybean oil • Hempseed oil • Canola oil • Avocados	Flaxseed and hempseed oils are rich sources of omega-3 fatty acids, necessary for the production of all hormones.	Do not cook with flaxseed oil (or any of the oils listed at the left), but use them unheated, in small amounts with foods such as cooked vegetables, salads, beans, grains or smoothies.
HERBS AND SPICES		
• Turmeric • Sage	Turmeric has antioxidant and antitumor activity, helping prevent against cancer. Sage balances endocrine glands.	Add turmeric to stir-fries, soups or curry dishes. Caution: Sage should not be consumed during pregnancy. Sage contains steroid-like factors and can encourage miscarriage.
• Brewer's yeast	Best source of chromium, a mineral that works closely with insulin and helps increase insulin sensitivity, reducing the risk of diabetes.	Do not confuse brewer's yeast with baking yeast or nutritional yeast.

Immune System

Healthy Immune System

The immune system consists of a complex collection of cells found throughout the body. These cells are responsible for protecting the body against infection, as well as for constant surveillance and destruction of the cancer cells.

The skin and mucous membranes, along with chemical substances like mucous, tears and stomach acid, are also an important part of the immune system, acting as front-line barriers that prevent foreign materials and pathogenic organisms from entering and harming the body.

When the immune system does not work optimally, we see an increased risk for infections and cancers, as well as the development of allergies and inflammatory disease.

Support and enhancement of the immune system through consumption of whole foods, proper intake of water, regular moderate exercise and mental relaxation can increase the body's resistance to colds, flus and cancers, and keep allergies and inflammation in check.

Immune System Disorders

Frequent and chronic infections, cancer, inflammation, allergies

Frequent and chronic infections may include anything from a common cold, flu, ear infections and urinary tract infections to more serious illnesses, such as herpes virus infections, bronchitis and pneumonia. Viruses, bacteria, fungi and parasites can all cause infections, especially when they do not meet adequate resistance from a weakened immune system.

Similarly, cancer risk increases when there is damage to a cell's DNA and the immune system's DNA repair or cancer surveillance systems are not functioning at an optimal level. DNA can be damaged by free radicals produced inside the body or by elements from the external environment, such as chemicals, radiation or viruses.

Another way the body defends itself is through inflammation. Inflammation is a normal immune system response responsible for destroying invaders or setting the stage for tissue repair. When the immune system is out of control, inflammation can become chronic and cause pain and damage body tissues.

Allergies are the body's exaggerated response to foreign invaders. This reaction is usually a manifestation of a leaky gut (an increase in permeability of the lining of the digestive tract, which allows undigested food particles to enter the bloodstream and be recognized as foreign invaders or antigens — see Digestive System, page 20), and/or excessive allergens overtaxing the immune system. Maintaining a whole foods diet can have a profound effect on the management of allergies.

Optimizing the Immune System

To optimize the functioning of the immune system, we need to choose foods that increase antioxidant levels, boost cellular immunity and enhance mucous membrane integrity, maintain proper levels of stomach acid and other body secretions, and stabilize immune reactions.

Eat five to nine servings of fruit and vegetables daily

Antioxidants in fruit and vegetables, nuts, seeds and whole grains act as a defense mechanism against free radicals by collecting the free electron that floats outside some oxygen-containing molecules. This action makes the molecule more stable and prevents it from damaging the cell's DNA. Beta-carotene, lycopene and other carotenoids, vitamin E, vitamin C, selenium and glutathione are some of the best antioxidants we can find in our foods. Many of these substances have antihistamine properties (vitamin C) and tumor destruction abilities (selenium). Studies also show that carotenoids can boost immune cells. Green tea is also an excellent antioxidant with antimicrobial properties.

Best foods

- Beta-carotene, lycopene and other carotenoids: carrots, tomatoes, red and orange bell peppers, sweet potatoes, pumpkin and other winter squashes, kale, spinach, apricots, mango
- Vitamin E: wheat germ, almonds, sunflower seeds, cooked organic soybeans
- Vitamin C: oranges, strawberries, kiwifruit, red bell peppers, sweet potatoes, broccoli, kale
- Selenium: Brazil nuts, garlic, barley, brown rice, oatmeal, tofu
- Glutathione: watermelon, avocados, cruciferous vegetables

Increase foods that are high in lean protein

The body uses amino acids, the building blocks of protein, to assemble immune cells and immunoglobulins responsible for fighting infections. These building blocks are also essential for skin and mucous membrane integrity and as biological enzymes. Enzymes are needed for chemical reactions in the body, including antioxidant and detoxification systems.

Best foods

- Legumes (beans, peas, lentils, organic soybeans)
- Nuts and seeds (ground flaxseed, sesame seeds, sunflower seeds, almonds, cashews)
- Fresh fish

In particular, soy foods, which are rich in protein, are also high in phytoestrogens, plant derived estrogens that may protect against some cancers by blocking estrogen's cancer-promoting effect. (See Caution, page 102.)

Best foods

- Organically, non-genetically modified soybeans, tofu, soy milk

Increase unsaturated fats in your diet

Reducing trans-fats and saturated fats can boost immune function because these fats appear to impair the immune system. Omega-3 and omega-6 polyunsaturated fatty acids are anti-inflammatory (omega-3) and help protect against cancer. They also help with the absorption of fat-soluble vitamins, such as vitamins A and E. Phytosterols, or plant-based oils, also help reduce inflammation. Of particular benefit are sterols and sterolins, which can be found in abundance in nuts and seeds.

Best foods

- Avocados, olives and extra virgin olive oil, nuts and seeds (especially flaxseeds and flaxseed oil), fresh fatty fish (salmon, halibut, sardines)

Learn stress-management techniques and keep stress levels low

When our body is exposed to constant high levels of stress, our adrenal glands produce higher levels of the hormone cortisol. Cortisol is the body's natural corticosteroid, which in normal amounts helps keep allergies and inflammation under control. At high levels, however, cortisol is an immune suppressant, causing the body to have a reduced ability to fight infections.

Best techniques

- Regular moderate exercise, daily relaxation techniques, deep breathing, daily routine, rest

Top 10 Best Bets for Immune Health

❶ Soy foods: High in protein, complex carbohydrates and phytonutrients, organic, non-genetically modified soy products are a favorite food for disease prevention. Although the research is conflicting and inconclusive, the soy phytoestrogens, genistein and daidzein may protect women against some forms of cancer by blocking estrogen receptors. Some studies show that a diet rich in phytoestrogens may also reduce the risk of prostate cancer in men. Look for organic, non-genetically modified soybeans and soy foods. (See Caution, page 102)

❷ Cruciferous vegetables: Broccoli, cauliflower, cabbage, Brussels sprouts, kale and collard greens are part of the cruciferous, or Brassica, family. These are a favorite because they provide a wide range of nutrients, including indoles. Indole-3-carbinol has the ability to convert a harmful estrogen molecule into its non-harmful metabolites, thereby protecting against some forms of cancer.

❸ Flaxseed oil: Flaxseed oil is an excellent choice because it is one of the few sources rich in omega-3 polyunsaturated fatty acids. Polyunsaturated fatty acids from flaxseed oil are converted to EPA (eicosapentaenoic acid), the active molecule also found in fish oils, which acts to inhibit the inflammatory cascade. Studies show that using flaxseed oil in foods reduces the substances that contribute to inflammation. So, add flaxseed oil to salads and soups or blend a small amount in smoothies in the morning. Remember not to heat flaxseed oil, and keep it refrigerated in a dark bottle to prevent rancidity.

❹ Shiitake mushrooms: Time and time again, shiitake mushrooms have been reported to have cancer-preventing properties. Mycochemicals, the active constituents in shiitake mushrooms, may stop the growth of tumors by suggesting a programmed death to the individual cancer cells.

❺ Tomatoes: Lycopene, found abundantly in tomatoes, plays a crucial role as an antioxidant in our bodies, providing protection against some forms of cancer (including lung and prostate) and boosting the immune system. Lycopene is also found in tomato juice and pizza sauce. In fact, processed and cooked tomato products contain a more bioavailable form of lycopene than do raw tomatoes.

❻ Avocados: This simply delicious fruit — among the most studied and documented foods — proves to be one of the best in providing symptom relief for patients with osteoarthritis. Avocados are high in the antioxidant glutathione and rich in monounsaturated fats.

❼ Brown rice: Rice is a staple of the diet in Asia, where the incidence of breast and colon cancer is below that of the Western world. Rice can offer protection against cancer, including breast and colon cancers, when eaten unprocessed instead of in its white form. Brown rice is also extraordinary in that it has low allergenic potential when compared to other grains. This makes it less of a burden for our immune system, which is overtaxed by many other allergens and pollutants.

❽ Blueberries: Blueberries are a rich source of anthocyanins, which destroy free radicals in the body. In fact, studies put blueberries at the top of the list of best antioxidant foods, especially on the basis of typical serving sizes.

❾ Green tea: Polyphenols in green tea have significant antioxidant, anti-inflammatory and antimicrobial properties. Even with moderate consumption (2 cups/500 mL per day), green tea has the ability to protect against oxidative damage of the DNA in the cells, lowering the risk of cancer.

⑩ **Pumpkin seeds:** Pumpkin seeds are high in zinc, a mineral that boosts immunity, protects against free radicals and is needed for wound repair. Zinc helps prevent recurrent infections, and reduce the duration of cold symptoms. Pumpkin seed oil can also be used to destroy parasites in the intestinal tract.

Foods that Enhance the Immune System

Best Foods for Enhancing Immune System	Immune System Benefits	Comments
FRUITS		
Citrus: • Oranges • Mandarin • Lemons • Grapefruit	Rich in vitamin C and bioflavonoids, which are antioxidants and protect against cancer.	Whole fruit is best; otherwise, use freshly squeezed juices. Caution: Grapefruit juice can interfere with some medications.
Orange/Yellow: • Mangoes • Apricots • Peaches	Contain carotenoids and vitamin C, which are antioxidants. Enhance immune system function.	Choose locally grown fruits when possible.
Blue/Purple: • Blueberries and other berries • Purple grapes • Plums	Contain anthocyanins, which destroy free radicals.	Blueberry season runs from May though September; otherwise, choose frozen ones to use in your cooking.
VEGETABLES		
Red Nightshades: • Tomatoes • Red bell peppers	Rich in the antioxidant lycopene. High in beta-carotene, which has immune cell-boosting properties.	Lycopene is fat-soluble and must be eaten with a fat in order to be absorbed.
Orange/Yellow: • Carrots • Yams • Sweet potatoes • Pumpkin and other winter squashes	Contain carotenoids rich in antioxidants and support the immune system.	Eat carrots lightly steamed for better nutrient absorption.
Green: • Spinach • Swiss chard • Asparagus • Dandelion greens • Other dark leafy greens	Contain folic acid, essential for healthy cell reproduction and genetic material (DNA) replication.	1 cup (250 mL) of leafy vegetables is 1 serving.
Cruciferous Family: • Broccoli • Cauliflower • Brussels sprouts • Cabbage • Kale • Collard greens	Contain glutathione, a powerful antioxidant. Contain indoles, which eliminate excess estrogens and carcinogens, helping in cancer prevention.	Eat raw or lightly steamed.

Best Foods for Enhancing Immune System	Immune System Benefits	Comments
VEGETABLES (cont.)		
Allium Family: • Garlic • Onions and chives	Contain allyl sulfides, which destroy cancer cells and support immune function. Contain antimicrobial properties.	Use garlic and onions daily in your cooking, raw or cooked.
Mushrooms: • Shiitake • Maitake • Enoki	Powerful immune-boosting and antiviral properties.	Enjoy them in soups and salads. Can be found dried. Rehydrate them in boiling water and keep the soaking liquid for a rich and nutritious soup.
LEGUMES		
• Beans • Organic soybeans • Lentils • Peas • Chickpeas	Beans are high in protein, soluble fiber and complex carbohydrates. Soybeans contain phytoestrogens, plant-derived estrogens that may protect against some cancers.	Soy products include tofu, tempeh, organic soybeans and soymilk. Use dried peas and beans in soups, salads and dips. Must be soaked before cooking.
WHOLE GRAINS		
• Brown rice • Whole oats • Barley	Whole grains are important for their B vitamin content. Many contain high amounts of the antioxidant selenium. Brown rice seems to be less allergenic than other grains.	Choose whole grains rather than refined products and flours. The hull, removed during processing, contains most of the nutrients.
NUTS AND SEEDS		
Nuts and nut butters: • Brazil nuts • Almonds • Walnuts	High in protein, fiber and unsaturated fats needed for healthy immune function.	Nut and nut butters add protein to salads, snacks and soups. Nuts are an incomplete source of protein; complete the protein by eating with a grain.
Seeds and seed butters: • Sunflower seeds • Pumpkin seeds • Sesame seeds • Flaxseeds	Contain essential fatty acids (EFAs), needed for healthy immune function. Flaxseeds contain omega-3 fats, which have anti-inflammatory properties. Pumpkin seeds are high in zinc, essential for boosting cellular immunity and thymus gland development.	Eat the seeds whole or freshly ground daily. Try seed butters. Flaxseeds must be ground.

Best Foods for Enhancing Immune System	Immune System Benefits	Comments
FATS AND OILS		
Cold-pressed oils: • Extra virgin olive oil • Flaxseed oil	Flaxseed oil contains omega-3 essential fatty acids (EFAs), which have anti-inflammatory properties.	Look for cold-pressed, less refined oils that are packaged in dark glass containers. Keep oils in the refrigerator to keep them from going rancid.
HERBS AND SPICES		
• Fennel • Ginger • Turmeric • Rosemary • Thyme • Sage	Most herbs are antioxidant. Turmeric has anti-inflammatory properties. Thyme has 75 identified antioxidants.	Use fresh or dried in cooking on a regular basis
OTHER		
• Beer • Coffee • Tea • Wine	Rich in bioflavonoids. Green tea is a rich source of the catechin epigallocatechin gallate (EGCG) that seems to offer antigen-fighting abilities.	Consume in moderation. Not recommended during pregnancy and lactation. Limit coffee to one cup per day and substitute green tea for the other times when coffee might be consumed.

Musculoskeletal System

Healthy Musculoskeletal System

Muscles, bones, joints and connective tissue make up the musculoskeletal system, responsible for the movement of the human body and its individual parts. The musculoskeletal system also gives structure to the body and physically protects the internal organs.

Nutrition is very important in the management of this system. For example, muscle contraction and relaxation depend on minerals like calcium and magnesium to perform movements and maintain an upright posture and balance. Bones also need minerals to maintain their density and withstand the pulling forces created by the muscles and the impact of accidents and falls.

Another important part of the musculoskeletal system is the joints, such as the hip, knees and elbows. Within the joints, the ends of the bones are covered with cartilage and are surrounded by synovial fluid, a lubricating fluid, which allows smooth and frictionless motion where two bones meet.

Musculoskeletal Disorders

Arthritis, osteoporosis, low back pain, muscle spasms and cramps, sprains and strains

Muscle cramping and spasms can occur with dehydration and if minerals such as calcium, sodium, potassium and magnesium are not in the proper balance. This can cause simple cramping of the calf muscle or can aggravate existing conditions, such as low back pain. Low back pain can also be due to misalignment of the spine or other parts of the skeleton, nerve impingement, injury and chronic inflammation.

Inflammation also occurs during arthritis. There are many types of arthritis, some with more inflammation than others. For example, osteoarthritis, the most common type, is characterized by wear and tear at the joints, wearing down of the joint cartilage, and causing changes in the bone. Although minimal, osteoarthritis consists of some inflammation at the joint and in surrounding tissues. Symptoms can be stiffness and pain at the joint and eventually restricted joint function. On the other hand, rheumatoid arthritis is an autoimmune condition characterized by chronic inflammation that can affect the joints as well as other areas of the body. Rheumatoid arthritis can give symptoms of inflammation at the joint, such as pain, redness, swelling and eventually deformity, but also generalized symptoms of fatigue, weakness and low-grade fever. Regardless of the cause and the differing symptoms and location, nutrition is essential to repair and build cartilage and decrease inflammation.

Unlike arthritis, osteoporosis is mostly symptom-free, which is why people at increased risk must get regular bone-density checks. In osteoporosis, the bone density is diminished and the bones become brittle and susceptible to fractures. The density of the bone depends on many nutrients, such as calcium, magnesium and zinc, for the strength to withstand trauma, perform movement and provide support.

Optimizing Musculoskeletal Function

To maintain the musculoskeletal system in top shape, we need to eat foods that are high in vitamins and minerals, foods that help us maintain a balanced acid-base environment, and foods that deal with inflammation. Of course, regular exercise is just as important as eating well.

Eat foods that are high in minerals

Foods such as leafy green vegetables, nuts and seeds, legumes and grains are loaded with minerals that are essential for the functioning of the muscles, the building of bones and the maintenance of healthy joints. For example, calcium and magnesium are essential for muscle contraction and relaxation. Calcium, magnesium, zinc and many trace minerals, such as boron, manganese and copper, are needed to build strong bones and prevent the risk of fractures with osteoporosis.

Best foods
- Calcium: leafy green vegetables, broccoli, almonds, canned fish bones (sardines, salmon), tofu, soymilk, corn tortillas
- Magnesium: nuts and seeds, grains, beans, dark green vegetables
- Zinc: pumpkin seeds, black-eyed peas, tofu, wheat germ
- Boron: raisins, prunes, almonds
- Manganese: nuts and seeds, wheat, leafy green vegetables, beet tops, pineapple
- Copper: nuts, legumes, cereals, potatoes

Eat foods that are high in vitamins

Many vitamins essential for lowering the risk of osteoporosis can be found in foods such as leafy green vegetables, cruciferous vegetables and fish. For example, vitamin D, which is converted to its active form by the ultraviolet rays of the sun, helps increase the absorption of the calcium that is important for keeping bones strong.

Vitamin K helps mineralize bone during bone formation. Increasing the levels of vitamin K can decrease the risk of osteoporosis. This is easily achieved by increasing the consumption of leafy green vegetables.

B vitamins, especially vitamins B_6 (pyridoxine), B_{12} and folate, are needed to decrease homocysteine levels in the blood. High levels of homocysteine are detrimental in cardiovascular disease, as well as increasing the risk of osteoporosis by interfering with bone formation.

Best foods
- Vitamin D: sunlight, cod liver oil
- Vitamin K: leafy green vegetables (kale, collard greens, beet greens, parsley, broccoli, spinach)
- B vitamins: B_6: chickpeas, halibut
- B_{12}: fish, leafy green vegetables, grains

Eat foods that alkalinize the diet

When we eat a diet rich in fruits and vegetables, especially leafy greens, the body's acid-base (or pH) balance is at normal levels and calcium remains in the bones. On the other hand, when we eat a diet high in protein, refined sugars and soft drinks, as is common in our society, the pH of the body decreases and becomes too acidic. To buffer this high acidity, calcium from the bones is leached into the bloodstream, decreasing the density of the bone and increasing risk of osteoporosis and bone fractures.

Refined sugars, a high-protein diet and soft drinks (high in phosphates) can also increase the excretion of calcium in the urine.

Best foods
- String green beans, bananas, dandelion greens, grapes, fresh or dried figs, prunes, raisins, Swiss chard
- Also almonds, asparagus, avocados, beets, carrots, cranberries, kale, pomegranate, raspberries, spinach

Eat foods that decrease inflammation

Whole foods are especially important for the musculoskeletal system, which deals with trauma such as sprains and strains; and cases of chronic inflammation, such as arthritis. Fish oils are high in omega-3 fatty acids, which redirect the inflammation cascade and ease such symptoms as pain, swelling and stiffness.

Best foods
- Fish (salmon, mackerel, albacore tuna, sardines, herring), ground flaxseed and flaxseed oil, hemp seeds and hemp seed oil

Participate in a regular exercise routine

When a bone is exposed to repetitive physical stresses, its mass will increase over time. An increase in bone mass makes the bone stronger and less susceptible to fracture. Weight-bearing exercises, such as when the bones make contact with the ground while supporting body weight or when the muscles pull on the bone to make a movement, are an excellent way to place physical stress on bones. For example, walking is considered a weight-bearing exercise as compared to swimming. Swimming is still a good form of cardiovascular exercise, but it does not entail supporting the body's weight against the forces of gravity and contact with the ground. Lifting light weights is another safe way to increase bone density and decrease the risk of osteoporosis.

Exercise is also excellent for maintaining a healthy body weight. And it helps reduce pain and stiffness, increase circulation, and keep muscles toned to support the joints and prevent injuries.

Best exercises
• Brisk walking, weight training, yoga, jogging, swimming

Top 10 Best Bets for Musculoskeletal Health

❶ **Almonds:** Almonds are high in calcium and, like other nuts, high in magnesium. These minerals are important for contraction and relaxation of muscle and mineralization of bone. Almonds are a great all-round nutritious snack that is high in protein and monounsaturated fats.

❷ **Tofu:** Tofu has been the staple food of Asian cultures. It is made from curdled soy milk, the milky liquid extracted from cooked and ground soybeans. Tofu is an excellent source of high-quality protein, calcium (check the label first to see if calcium was added as a coagulant), iron and zinc. With its high mineral content, tofu is a great food to prevent against loss of bone mass and risk of fractures with osteoporosis.

Tofu, like all other soybean products, contains phytoestrogens (isoflavones), plant-based estrogens that may help to prevent osteoporosis, especially in post-menopausal women. Whenever possible, choose calcium sulfate (over magnesium sulfate) as the coagulating additive in tofu.

❸ **Cruciferous vegetables:** Broccoli, cabbage, cauliflower, Brussels sprouts and especially kale are very high in an easily absorbed form of calcium. Calcium, along with other minerals, is essential for maintaining high-bone density, helping decrease the risk of osteoporosis. Calcium is also essential for muscle contraction and nerve conduction.

Cruciferous vegetables are also high in vitamin C, which protects the joints against free-radical damage created during inflammation and helps stop the progression of arthritis by repairing and building new cartilage in the joints.

❹ **Leafy greens:** Vitamin K, found in leafy green vegetables, such as collard greens, Swiss chard, dandelion greens and beet greens, helps bind calcium to the bone matrix and reduce the excretion of calcium in the urine. Leafy green vegetables are also high in calcium and folic acid. Leafy greens are also beneficial because they create an alkaline environment in the body and prevent calcium extraction from the bones, thus protecting the body from osteoporosis.

❺ **Fish oils:** There is growing evidence that omega-3 fats are beneficial in the prevention and treatment of arthritis. Omega-3 fatty acids, found in fish and flaxseed oil, have anti-inflammatory properties. Fish oils in particular contain the fatty acids in their final form and help control inflammation, while fatty acids from flaxseed oil must be converted in the body before they can perform their anti-inflammatory function.

6 Turmeric: Turmeric can halt the enzyme that produces inflammation and inhibits the break down of cortisone in the body, which makes turmeric a great anti-inflammatory. Cortisone, the body's own anti-inflammatory steroid, helps reduce inflammation. Through these means, turmeric can help decrease the symptoms of arthritis and prevent further damage to the cartilage in the joints.

7 Ginger: Ginger is anti-inflammatory in two ways. One way it decreases inflammation is by inhibiting the enzymes that promote inflammation. This helps terminate the inflammation cascade and prevent swelling and pain. Ginger also helps make white blood cells more stable so they release fewer inflammation mediators. This means that ginger can help diminish the destruction of cartilage and reduce symptoms of arthritis.

8 Citrus fruit: Citrus fruits, such as oranges, grapefruit, lemons, limes and mandarins, are alkalinizing to the body. Foods that alkalinize are beneficial in preventing osteoporosis because the body no longer needs to take calcium from the bones to buffer acidity. Vitamin C from citrus fruits is also essential for building cartilage in the joints and other connective tissue. This can help with the progression of osteoarthritis and the repair of muscles, tendons and ligaments after surgery or injury. Vitamin C has anti-inflammatory, antihistaminic and antioxidant properties.

9 Sunlight: Ultraviolet light from the sun converts 7-dehydrocholesterol in the skin into vitamin D_3. Vitamin D_3, which is converted to its more active forms in the liver and kidneys, stimulates the absorption of calcium through the digestive tract and the kidneys. This process is essential in the prevention of osteoporosis. People who live farther away from the equator, have darker skin or use a sunscreen with SPF 8 or higher may need longer exposure to the sun to get the same benefits.

10 Nuts and seeds: Nuts and seeds are an excellent source of magnesium, a mineral that is just as important for bone formation as is calcium, making it an essential nutrient for the prevention and treatment of osteoporosis. Magnesium from nuts and seeds is also essential for muscle relaxation, and can prevent muscle spasms and pain in such conditions as chronic low back pain.

Foods that Enhance the Musculoskeletal System

Best Foods for Enhancing Musculoskeletal System	Musculoskeletal System Benefits	Comments
FRUITS		
Citrus: • Oranges • Lemons • Limes • Grapefruit • Kiwifruit • Strawberries	Rich in antioxidants essential to prevent damage to inflamed joints. Citrus fruits alkalinize the body and inhibit the calcium loss from bones. Rich in vitamin C, which helps build and repair cartilage and connective tissue.	Choose oranges that do not look perfect and are not spongy in texture. Perfect-looking oranges likely have been treated with preservatives, pesticides and colorings. Spongy texture may indicate that the fruit is soft inside and either damaged or not fresh.
• Pineapple • Papaya • Mangoes • Apricots • Melons (cantaloupe, honeydew, watermelon)	Contain vitamin C, which helps build and repair cartilage in joints.	
Blue/Purple: • Blueberries and other berries • Purple grapes • Plums	Contain anthocyanins, which destroy free radicals and prevent further damage to the joints.	Choose blueberries that are dark blue, plump, firm, dry and free from stems and leaves.
VEGETABLES		
Nightshades: • Tomatoes • Potatoes • Peppers (bell peppers, hot peppers) • Eggplant	Contain vitamin C and carotenoids.	Avoiding nightshade vegetables, which contain solanine, may bring relief to some arthritis patients.
Leafy green vegetables: • Spinach • Swiss chard • Dandelion greens • Beet greens	Contain folate, which helps decrease homocysteine levels, a risk factor for osteoporosis. Leafy green vegetables help alkalinize the diet and keep calcium in the bones. Source of vitamin K for mineralization of bone.	Vitamin K is not available as a supplement. High doses can interfere with the effect of some pharmaceutical drugs.
Cruciferous Family: • Broccoli • Cauliflower • Brussels sprouts • Cabbage • Kale • Collard greens	High in calcium needed for muscle contraction and bone formation.	Collard greens have leaves that are relatively tough in texture. Cook for 8 to 10 minutes on medium heat. Use as a substitute for cabbage. Great for juicing.

Best Foods for Enhancing Musculoskeletal System	Musculoskeletal System Benefits	Comments
LEGUMES		
• Beans • Organic soybeans • Lentils • Peas • Chickpeas	Beans are high in magnesium for muscle relaxation and bone building. Soybeans contain phytoestrogens, which may help protect women against osteoporosis. Tofu is a great source of calcium, as this mineral is often added to help set the tofu.	Generally, soy milk is fortified with calcium and other minerals. Soft tofu is ideal for blending into smoothies, creamy soups and dressings. Consult with your naturopathic doctor or nutritionist before consuming large amounts of soy.
WHOLE GRAINS		
• Brown rice • Whole oats • Barley	Whole grains are important for their B vitamin content, which helps keep homocysteine levels low and decrease the risk of osteoporosis.	Choose whole grains rather than refined products and flours. The hull, removed during processing, contains most of the nutrients.
NUTS AND SEEDS		
Nuts and nut butters: • Brazil nuts • Almonds • Walnuts	Contain magnesium, essential for muscle relaxation; and preventing some forms of low back pain. Magnesium is also needed for making energy in the body.	Eat 10 raw almonds per day. Try almond butter.
Seeds and seed butters: • Sunflower seeds • Pumpkin seeds • Sesame seeds • Flaxseeds	Seeds are high in magnesium and zinc (pumpkin seeds), which are necessary for bone mineralization.	Eat the seeds whole or freshly ground daily. Try seed butters.
FATS AND OILS		
Cold-pressed oils: • Extra virgin olive oil • Flaxseed oil • Hemp seed oil • Canola oil	Flaxseed oil and hemp seed oil contain omega-3 essential fatty acids (EFAs), which have anti-inflammatory properties. Canola oil is a source of vitamin K, needed for bone formation.	Vitamin K is a fat-soluble vitamin that must be eaten with a source of fat in order to be absorbed. Vitamin K is also produced by the healthy bacteria in the intestines.
HERBS AND SPICES		
• Ginger • Turmeric	Ginger is highly effective at decreasing pain and inflammation. Turmeric has anti-inflammatory properties.	One teaspoon (5 mL) of ground turmeric blended in a smoothie will help prevent post-exercise cramping.

Nervous System

Healthy Nervous System

The nervous system is a highly complex system made up of two main parts, the central and the peripheral nervous systems, which together allow us to respond to our internal and external environments. The central nervous system consists of the brain and the spinal cord, while the peripheral nervous system is made up of nerves (sensory and motor) and connects the central nervous system with other parts of the body.

The peripheral nervous system is responsible for receiving information, such as taste, sound or hormone levels, from the internal and external environments and for relaying that information to the central nervous system via peripheral sensory nerves. The spinal cord and brain integrate this information in the central nervous system and generate a response, which is then sent to other parts of the body via the peripheral motor nerves. For example, the peripheral sensory nerves might relay information about a song on the radio to the spinal cord and the brain. A response would then be sent through the peripheral motor nerves to make a movement to turn up the radio.

Of course, not all responses are conscious. The peripheral nervous system also consists of the autonomic nervous system, which controls internal organs and glands, such as the heart, or the thyroid gland, which is responsible for the body's metabolism. Through this system, consisting of sympathetic and parasympathetic responses, the body can maintain an internal balance and react to different stimuli based on the needed responses. For example, a sympathetic or "fight or flight" response is created when you are frightened or stressed. This response causes your heart rate to increase. In contrast, a parasympathetic response allows you to perform such functions as relaxing and digesting your food after a meal. These two parts of the autonomic nervous system act on the same organs and glands, but have opposing effects, helping maintain balance in the body.

Individual nerve cells (neurons) use neurotransmitters, chemicals that allow them to communicate with each other and with other cells in the body. For example, the neurotransmitter seratonin is involved in memory, emotions, wakefulness, sleep and temperature regulation. Acetylcholine allows for communication between the nervous system and the muscles to create a movement. An imbalance of neurotrasmitters can result in dysfunction in the nervous system, which is why neurotransmitters are often the target of pharmaceutical and recreational drugs.

Nervous System Disorders

Depression and seasonal affective disorder (SAD), memory loss and decreased cognitive function

Depression is a condition that occurs when there is an imbalance of neurotransmitters in the brain. It can be characterized by a loss of interest or pleasure in usual activities and a lack of energy. It can also affect appetite, with either a decrease or increase, and subsequent changes in body weight. Depression can be quite debilitating and can trigger feelings of worthlessness or even thoughts of death or suicide.

Seasonal affective disorder (SAD) is a form of depression that occurs with diminished exposure to sunlight in the winter months. This disorder may result in the general symptoms of depression, and also an increase in sleep, appetite and perhaps body weight.

Anxiety is a devastating psychiatric disorder that can consist of feelings of agitation, nervousness, fearfulness, irritability or shyness. Other symptoms may include heart palpitations, flushing of the face, sweating, shallow breathing or even fainting. Both anxiety and depression can be caused by psychological factors; a physical cause, such as trauma or illness; nutrient deficiencies; or the side effects of medications.

As a result of normal living and aging, the nervous system suffers from oxidation of its cells, improper nutrient status and a decrease in blood circulation. These and other factors can lead to a decline in neurotransmitter levels, a decrease in the number of connections between neurons and an actual decrease in brain size, leading to a decrease in cognitive function and memory loss.

Optimizing the Nervous System

To help maintain optimal nervous system functioning, you must eat whole foods that are rich in vitamins and minerals and that help maintain constant blood sugar levels. It's also important to engage in regular physical exercise, go outside to catch some sunlight and practice relaxation techniques.

Eat a diet rich in complex carbohydrates

The brain relies on a constant supply of glucose as its primary source of energy. Glucose is one of the building blocks of carbohydrates. However, there are a few other things to take into consideration. Carbohydrates can come in two forms — simple and complex. Simple carbohydrates, when broken down in the digestive tract, are absorbed rapidly into the bloodstream and can cause a quick rise in blood sugar. This rapid increase in blood sugar can lead to symptoms of hyperactivity or anxiety and is followed by a rapid decline or sugar "crash," which can give symptoms of fatigue, irritability or depression. Pasta, breads, crackers and cereals made of refined products, candy and soft drinks are examples of simple carbohydrates. These foods are also devoid of nutrients, such as vitamins and minerals.

On the other hand, complex carbohydrates contain fiber, which slows down the rate at which sugar is absorbed into the body, allowing for a more constant level of blood sugar that can help stabilize mood patterns. Complex carbohydrates are found in whole grains, beans and other legumes, fruits and vegetables, and nuts and seeds. Proteins and fats can also help slow down the absorption of sugar into the bloodstream.

It is also important to note that caffeine can affect blood sugar levels in a negative manner and can cause symptoms of hyperactivity, depression, fatigue, irritability, insomnia or anxiety.

Best foods
- Whole grains, legumes (beans, soybeans, chickpeas, lentils)
- All fruits and vegetables
- Nuts and seeds (almonds, cashews, walnuts, sesame seeds, sunflower seeds, pumpkin seeds)

Eat a diet rich in omega-3 fatty acids

The nervous system, including the brain, contains a high concentration of omega-3 fatty acids, which cannot be made in the body and must be obtained from the diet. Omega-3 fatty acids, such as those obtained from flaxseed oil and fish oils, are not only components of all cell membranes, including nerve cells (neurons), but they also help regulate nerve cell function and signal transmission. The brain and neurons are highly dependent on the quality of the fats from the diet, and this factor can impact behavior, mood and mental function.

Omega-3 fatty acids have also been proven to have some effect through their anti-inflammatory function, preventing the production of inflammatory mediators that might be linked with mood disorders.

Best foods
- Fish oils (salmon, mackerel, albacore tuna, sardines, herring), flaxseed oil, organic soy oil, hempseed oil, canola oil, walnuts

Eat a diet rich in B vitamins

B vitamins are essential for the functioning of the nervous system. For example, the brain needs vitamin B_1 (thiamin) to be able to use glucose as fuel. Without vitamin B_1, the brain cannot function properly and can lead to symptoms of anxiety, irritability, fatigue and depression. B_1 also inhibits an enzyme that breaks down neurotransmitters, thereby boosting their levels in the brain. Vitamins B_6 (pyridoxine), B_{12} and folic acid are absolutely essential for the manufacturing of mood-regulating neurotransmitters, such as melatonin, seratonin and dopamine, which may be why these vitamins seem to have antidepressant effects. Vitamin B_{12} is also involved in the production of the myelin sheath, the fatty covering of the neurons that helps protect them and speed up the conduction of nerve impulses.

Foods such as whole grains, legumes and fish are good sources of B vitamins. It is also interesting that refined carbohydrates and some prescription medications, including oral contraceptives and antidepressants, can deplete the body's levels of B vitamins. If you are taking prescription medications, check with your health professional to see what foods you should be eating to prevent deficiencies.

Best foods

- Vitamin B_1: whole wheat, sweet potatoes, peas, beans, fish, peanuts
- Vitamin B_6: potatoes, bananas, legumes (lentils, chickpeas) fish (halibut), whole grains (rice)
- Vitamin B_{12}: fish (and other animal products), spirulina (blue-green algae), seaweed
- Folate: lentils, pinto beans, rice, leafy green vegetables

Learn ways of coping with stress

The stress of everyday life or stress caused by a major life event can produce a sympathetic response known as a "fight or flight" response. The nervous system here works in conjunction with the endocrine system by signaling to the adrenal glands to release adrenalin and other stress-related hormones. These hormones can alter blood sugar levels and change moods accordingly. In fact, excess or ongoing stress, can create feelings of irritability, fatigue, insomnia, depression or anxiety.

Techniques that induce a relaxation response and switch the nervous system from sympathetic to parasympathetic mode help optimize your nervous system.

Best techniques

- Meditation, prayer, breathing exercise, physical exercises, counseling

Get plenty of exercise

Exercise is one the most powerful antidepressants available and has repeatedly proven to decrease feelings of anxiety, depression and fatigue. Exercise increases endorphins, neurotransmitters that give a sense of well-being and elevate mood. It can also help increase self-image, self-confidence, mental performance and happiness.

Physical activity can benefit the nervous system in many different ways. For example, group exercises or sports can help elevate mood by creating a feeling of belonging. Other exercises give you a chance to "play" and can also be an excellent channel to let out frustrations and anger. Exercise can make you feel productive if lawn mowing, vacuuming or other types of yard or housework make up part of your work-out routine. Similarly, activities such as hiking or cross-country skiing can take you outdoors, breathing fresh air and enjoying different scenes. Any of these forms of physical activity are a step toward achieving a balanced nervous system.

Best exercises

- Weight lifting, brisk walking, jogging, bicycling, swimming, dancing, yoga, lawn mowing, vacuuming, racquet sports (such as tennis), team sports

Top 10 Best Bets for Nervous System Health

1 Fish: The human brain is more than 60% fat, the majority being omega 3-fatty acids, which cannot be made in the body and must be obtained from the diet. Fish oils are the best source of omega-3 fatty acids. These fatty acids are essential for regulating mood and emotions and preventing depression. Fish oils are also beneficial for attention and memory.

Fish oils are also an excellent source of B vitamins, including vitamin B_{12}, which can be hard to find in a vegetarian diet. B vitamins are necessary for neurotransmitter and myelin sheath production, nerve conduction and utilization of fuel by the brain.

2 Whole grains: Among the most important nutrients for the proper functioning of the nervous system is the group of B vitamins. B vitamins can be found in whole grains, such as whole wheat, whole oats, barley and brown rice. B vitamins are responsible for the manufacture of neurotransmitters and the proper use of fuel by the brain.

Whole grains also help maintain stable moods and energy levels throughout the day by helping to control blood sugar levels.

3 Spirulina or blue-green algae: Spirulina, or blue-green algae, is a microscopic plant that is found in some lakes. Spirulina is a rich source of protein, as it contains amino acids essential for neurotransmitter production. It also contains vitamins, minerals and essential fatty acids. Spirulina can provide small amounts of vitamin B_{12}, which helps produce red blood cells and myelin, helping to increase oxygen to the brain and the speed of nerve impulses.

4 Oats: Oats are one of the best foods for nourishing the nervous system. They can be used specifically to prevent debility and exhaustion caused by anxiety and depression. Oats can help relax the nervous system in conditions, such as insomnia, anxiety and stress. Oats can also help with the symptoms of drug withdrawal, especially nicotine withdrawal in smoking cessation. Oats are a rich source of B vitamins and contain fiber, which can help control blood sugar levels.

5 Brewer's yeast: Brewer's yeast is the dried, powdered *Saccharomyces cerevisiae* fungus used in the brewing process. Brewer's yeast is an extraordinary source of B vitamins, which help maintain a healthy nervous system. It is also the best source of chromium, a mineral that is essential for blood sugar regulation.

6 Blackstrap molasses: Molasses is a by-product of the manufacture of sugar. Blackstrap molasses is mostly sugar, but unlike refined sugars, it contains significant amounts of vitamins and minerals. In particular, blackstrap molasses is a source of B vitamins, calcium, magnesium and iron. These nutrients help with the production of brain neurotransmitters and general nervous system functioning.

7 Chocolate: Chocolate consumption has been linked with the release of seratonin in the brain, a neurotransmitter that is thought to produce feelings of pleasure. Caution: Chocolate contains small amounts of caffeine and most likely contains sugar, substances that can lead to blood sugar fluctuations and mood changes. Consume dark chocolate in moderation.

8 Exercise: Exercise is a very important component of a healthy nervous system. Exercise helps increase the circulation of blood, oxygen and glucose to the brain, which can help sharpen your cognitive skills such as memory. It also helps increase self-confidence and self-image, and by stimulating the release of endorphins, it can elevate mood.

9 Barley: The glycemic index (GI) is an index that ranks foods on how they affect blood sugar levels. Barley is exceptional because it has the lowest GI rating of any grain. This means that when eating barley, blood sugar levels remain relatively constant and so does the supply of glucose to the brain. The low GI of this food means it can help prevent mood fluctuations that may occur with anxiety, depression, hyperactivity or premenstrual syndrome in women.

10 Nuts and seeds: Nuts and seeds are a source of protein that when broken down provide amino acids, the building blocks for neurotransmitters. B vitamins, also found in these foods, help with the production of these neurotransmitters and make glucose available to the brain for fuel. Nuts and seeds also contain fiber, which helps keep blood sugar levels constant. Magnesium, calcium, zinc and selenium, found in a variety of nuts and seeds, may help prevent neurological disorders.

Foods that Protect the Nervous System

Best Foods for Protecting the Nervous System	Nervous System Benefits	Comments
FRUITS		
Citrus: • Oranges • Mandarins • Lemons • Grapefruit • Kiwifruit • Strawberries	Contain fiber, which helps control blood sugar levels. Contain vitamin C and bioflavonoids, required to synthesize neurotransmitters and as antioxidants for the nervous system.	Fruit juice contains large amounts of fructose, a natural sugar, and it does not contain fiber. Fruit juice can raise blood sugar levels rapidly.
• Apricots • Peaches • Pears • Apples	Contain pectin and other soluble fiber that can help control blood sugar levels. Pears contain B vitamins, and can help optimize nervous system function.	Most fruits and vegetables contain a mixture of soluble and insoluble fibers and have the ability to slow down the absorption of sugar.
Berries and grapes: • Blueberries • Blackberries • Raspberries • Red grapes	Red grapes are a great source of B vitamins, and like berries are rich sources of bioflavonoids. These protect brain cells against oxidation, and some nervous system disorders.	
VEGETABLES		
Green: • Spinach • Swiss chard • Dandelion greens • Endive • Other dark leafy greens	Leafy green vegetables contain folate, essential for the manufacture of neurotransmitters and optimal function of the nervous system.	Lightly steam these vegetables to reduce nutrient loss and increase nutrient absorption.

Best Foods for Protecting the Nervous System	Nervous System Benefits	Comments
VEGETABLES (cont.)		
Cruciferous Family: • Broccoli • Cabbage • Sauerkraut • Cauliflower • Kale • Bok choy	Cruciferous vegetables contain large amounts of vitamin C, a powerful antioxidant that helps protect the nervous system and restore normal levels of neurotransmitters.	Note that oral contraceptives, antibiotics, stress, pregnancy, infection and surgery can increase the need for vitamin C.
LEGUMES		
• Beans (lima, navy, organic soybeans) • Lentils • Peas • Chickpeas	Legumes are a source of soluble fiber. Soybeans are a good source of vitamins B_1, B_3, B_5 and B_6, which help prevent anxiety and depression. Lima and navy beans contain folate.	Soaking beans for 8 hours and rinsing well before and after cooking makes them easier to digest.
WHOLE GRAINS		
• Whole oats • Brown rice • Pot Barley • Buckwheat • Quinoa • Whole wheat • Spelt • Rye	Barley is one of the best whole grains for controlling the rate at which glucose is absorbed into the bloodstream. All whole grains are a good source of B vitamins.	
NUTS AND SEEDS		
Nuts: • Almonds • Brazil nuts • Walnuts • Hazelnuts • Pine nuts	Nuts contain fiber, which helps control blood sugar levels and contain B vitamins. They also contain amino acids, the building blocks for mood-regulating neurotransmitters. Brazil nuts are high in selenium, which can elevate mood and decrease anxiety.	Magnesium, which is found in abundance in nuts, may help prevent depression and other neurological disorders.
Seeds: • Sesame seeds • Sunflower seeds • Pumpkin seeds	Seeds are high in fiber, and fats, which help control blood sugar levels. Contain amino acids, the building blocks for mood-regulating neurotransmitters.	Zinc found in pumpkin seeds may help prevent depression.

Best Foods for Protecting the Nervous System	Nervous System Benefits	Comments
FATS AND OILS		
Cold-pressed oils: • Flaxseed oil • Soy oil • Hempseed oil • Canola oil • Avocados	These oils are a source of omega-3 fatty acids, which are an essential component of the nervous system and necessary for its function. Avocados are a good source of B vitamins.	Other vegetable oils, such as sunflower and safflower oils, are higher in omega-6 fatty acids, another type of essential fatty acid that must be obtained from the diet. These vegetable oils contain little omega-3 fatty acids.
OTHER		
• Blackstrap molasses	Contains B vitamins, essential for nervous system function. Also a source of magnesium, required for neurotransmitter production.	1 cup (250 ml) molasses can be used as a substitute for 1 cup (250 mL) liquid honey, $\frac{1}{2}$ cup (125 mL) brown sugar or 1 cup (250 mL) dark corn syrup or 1 cup (250 mL) pure maple syrup.
• Brewer's yeast	A good source of B vitamins, including B_1, B_3, B_5, B_6 and folate.	Do not confuse brewer's yeast with baking yeast or nutritional yeast.
• Spirulina (blue-green algae) Seaweed	A source of vitamin B_{12}, otherwise hard to find in a vegetarian diet. Essential for the manufacture of neurotransmitters and myelin sheath and for nerve conduction.	Hydrochloric acid (stomach acid) and intrinsic factor (a protein that binds vitamin B_{12}) are both produced by the stomach cells and aid its absorption in the large intestine.

Respiratory System

Healthy Respiratory System

The respiratory system is responsible for the exchange of oxygen and carbon dioxide between the external environment and the blood. The air that we breathe travels in through the nose, past the pharynx and larynx, down the trachea, into the bronchi and bronchioles and eventually reaches its destination, the lungs. In the lungs, the exchange of gases occurs in tiny air sacs called alveoli, where oxygen from the air enters the bloodstream and carbon dioxide from the bloodstream enters the air to be expelled. Through the actions of inspiration and expiration, the air flows in and out of the lungs providing all body cells with the fresh supply of oxygen essential to them for survival.

The respiratory system is also responsible for protecting the body against microbes, toxic chemicals and foreign matter. This is achieved with the help of cilia, tiny hair-like structures that sweep mucous and foreign materials out of the system. The cilia also work with the immune system to produce mucous and perform phagocytosis (engulfing pathogens and debris).

Respiratory System Disorders

Asthma and allergies, respiratory tract infections, lung cancer

Asthma is the most common illness associated with the respiratory system. It is an inflammatory condition of the lungs and airways in which swelling, smooth muscle contraction and excess mucous production create acute breathing difficulties. Someone who suffers from asthma might experience a feeling of tightness and constriction of the chest, with shortness of breath, wheezing and coughing. It is believed that asthma, like allergies, is a hypersensitivity disorder and therefore greatly linked to the immune system.

The respiratory system is the most susceptible to infection because it is directly exposed to the external environment. Therefore, respiratory infections, such as colds, sinusitis, bronchitis and pneumonia, also greatly depend on the immune system. Here, the immune system is responsible for protecting the respiratory system by producing mucous, attacking foreign invaders and developing a proper response to fight pathogens once they enter the body.

The respiratory system is also susceptible to cancer. Lung cancer is the most prevalent form of cancer today and can affect one or both lungs. Smoking is the biggest risk factor for lung cancer, so quitting smoking is a valuable method in its prevention. Other methods include eating a vitamin-rich diet, which can help reduce the risk of cancer, but there is also the chance that cancer will come back once treated.

Optimizing the Respiratory System

To protect the respiratory system from disease, we need to heal and moisten the mucous membranes, keep the cilia healthy and functioning well, strengthen and restore the balance of the immune system (see Immune System, page 34), and eliminate possible environmental triggers and foods that produce mucous and irritate the respiratory tract.

Eat foods that moisten the respiratory tract and thin excess mucous

Proper water intake helps keep the mucous membranes in the respiratory tract moist and capable of resisting infection. Water also helps thin mucous that builds up in your respiratory passageways and causes congestion. Vegetable broths and hot herbal teas can also be beneficial for maintaining hydration and clearing congestion. Warm drinks also help the cilia move to clear pathogens and foreign materials from the system.

Spices and flavoring agents, such as garlic, cayenne and horseradish, can also help get things moving by thinning mucous and stimulating the respiratory tract.

Humidifiers that moisten the air can help the respiratory system by preventing the mucous membranes from becoming dry and prone to infection, especially in the winter months.

On the same note, avoid foods and beverages that stimulate production of excess mucous (dairy products, sugar), dehydrate the body or irritate the respiratory passageways (alcohol, coffee).

Best foods

- Plenty of filtered water, hot herbal teas (peppermint, fennel, thyme), homemade vegetable broths

Eat a diet rich in antioxidants

In general antioxidants help prevent damage of the respiratory system by protecting against free radicals and boosting immune function. Antioxidants are also important in the prevention of cancer.

Vitamin A helps maintain healthy mucous membranes in the mouth, nose, sinuses and lungs, as well as the cilia in the respiratory passageways. This helps protect the passageways from virus and bacteria. Vitamin A also helps boost the immune system.

Vitamin C has an antihistaminic effect that can benefit asthma and allergy sufferers. It also protects against infection, helps heal wounds and strengthens the adrenal glands, essential glands for fighting allergic reactions and inflammation.

Vitamin E helps maintain healthy mucous membranes and is a powerful antioxidant.

Quercetin, a bioflavonoid, has anti-inflammatory and antihistaminic properties.

Histamine is the substance that is released during an allergic reaction causing symptoms of itching and swelling. Quercetin can help with allergies, asthma and respiratory infections.

Best foods

- Beta-carotene (converted in the body into vitamin A): apricots, carrots, cantaloupe, pumpkin and other winter squashes
- Vitamin C: bell peppers, broccoli, cantaloupe, cauliflower, kale, kiwi, oranges, strawberries, sweet potatoes, tomatoes
- Vitamin E: almonds, hazelnuts, walnuts, sunflower seeds, vegetable oils
- Quercetin: apples, red and yellow onions, black tea, tomatoes

Eat foods that contain essential fatty acids

Asthma, allergies and respiratory infections are associated with inflammation of the respiratory tract. Foods that are high in omega-3 fatty acids, such as fish oils and flaxseed oil, have anti-inflammatory properties that can keep allergies and asthma in check. Essential fatty acids along with other unsaturated fats help keep mucous membranes healthy and resistant to infection.

Best foods

- Fresh fish (salmon, mackerel, albacore tuna, sardines, herring)
- Flaxseeds and flaxseed oil, borage oil, evening primrose oil

Breathe good-quality air and do breathing exercises

The quality of the air we breathe is directly related to the condition of the lining of the respiratory tract. If the air we breathe is polluted with pollens, dust, dander, mold, smoke, bacteria and viruses, it can cause chronic irritation and inflammation of our airways and lungs. If you live or work in a polluted environment, use air filters to purify the air.

Breathing exercises increase the amount of oxygen that enters our system and the amount of carbon dioxide that is eliminated via the lungs.

Best techniques
- Use air filters, vacuum and clean carpets frequently, check homes and basements for mold, dust frequently, practice abdominal breathing

Top 10 Best Bets for Respiratory Health

❶ Sprouted seeds and grains: According to traditional Chinese medicine, sprouted seeds and grains are alive and full of chi (life energy). These foods help strengthen the body's chi along with the lungs and respiratory system.

❷ Fish oils: Fish oils, high in omega-3 fatty acids, have anti-inflammatory properties that could help relieve asthmatic patients. Studies have shown that when asthma patients consume more fish oils, they are able to breathe more easily and use less medication.

❸ Garlic: The antibacterial properties of garlic have been tested and proven to be effective against the bacteria that cause pneumonia. Garlic can also be used to fight viruses and fungal infections that target the respiratory system.

❹ Pumpkin seeds: Studies have found that people who suffer from allergic asthma and other allergies have a deficiency of zinc. Pumpkin seeds are an excellent source of zinc, which may help reduce the incidence of allergies and asthma as well as boosting the immune system to protect against infection. Have a handful per day as a snack.

❺ Yellow and red onions: Yellow and red onions contain quercetin, a bioflavonoid that has antioxidant, anti-inflammatory and antihistaminic properties. Quercetin also seems to protect the lungs against viral infections, such as those caused by the flu virus, due to its antioxidant properties.

❻ Ginger: Ginger extracts have been shown to have antimicrobial activity against bacteria and viruses that cause respiratory infection. Ginger is also an antioxidant and has anti-inflammatory properties. Make a ginger tea by slicing and slightly bruising fresh gingerroot and adding the slices to boiling water. Continue to boil the water until it looks darker in color. Let it steep and enjoy with a bit of lemon.

❼ Almonds: Almonds are high in calcium, and like all other nuts, are a great source of magnesium. Calcium and magnesium are essential for muscle contraction and relaxation, even for the smooth muscle in the respiratory airways. Almonds also contain monounsaturated fats and are a good source of protein. Delicious and satisfying as a mid-afternoon snack.

❽ Berries: Berries contain anthocyanins, which destroy free radicals, and are high in vitamin C. Vitamin C is a natural antioxidant and anti-inflammatory. Vitamin C is also antihistaminic, as it makes mast cells (the cells that contain histamine) more stable during allergic reactions. Vitamin C in berries is essential in the prevention of allergies, asthma and inflammation and helps boost the immune system.

❾ Cruciferous vegetables: Broccoli, cauliflower, cabbage, Brussels sprouts and bok choy are part of the cruciferous family. They contain cancer-fighting chemicals and other minerals important for health. Cabbage, with its high glutamine content, is beneficial for the building and repair of mucous membranes, including the mucous membranes in the respiratory tract. This helps keep allergens, and pathogens from attacking the body.

⑩ Thyme and Oregano: Thyme has a high content of volatile oils that are powerful agents for fighting infections. Thyme can be used to soothe sore throats and calm irritating coughs by helping reduce spasm reactions. It is also used for bronchitis, whooping cough and asthma. It can be taken as a delicious and refreshing tea.

Oregano is a powerful antioxidant with potent antibacterial, antifungal and antiparasitic properties, which make it useful for treating swollen glands, asthma, cough, earache and viral infections. The essential oil is effective both internally and externally. Take oregano oil diluted in herbal tea or water.

Foods that Protect the Respiratory System

Best Foods for Protecting the Respiratory System	Respiratory System Benefits	Comments
FRUITS		
Citrus: • Oranges • Mandarins • Lemons • Grapefruit • Kiwifruit • Strawberries	Rich in vitamin C and bioflavonoids, which are antioxidants. Vitamin C containing foods are anti-inflammatory and antihistaminic, helping reduce allergic-type reactions including asthma and allergies.	Caution: Grapefruit juice can interfere with some medications. Strawberries are heavily sprayed; choose organic when possible.
Orange/Yellow: • Apricots • Mangoes • Cantaloupe	Contain carotenoids and vitamin C, which are antioxidants. Beta-carotene helps maintain healthy mucous membranes of the respiratory tract.	When buying cantaloupe, choose fruit that is thick, with a coarse surface and veins standing out. Avoid fruit with mold.
Blue/Purple: • Blueberries and other berries • Purple grapes • Plums	Contain anthocyanins, which destroy free radicals. Also high in pectin and vitamin C.	Choose well-colored, plump grapes that are firmly attached to their stems.
VEGETABLES		
Red Nightshades: • Tomatoes • Red bell peppers	Rich in the antioxidant lycopene. High in vitamin C and beta-carotene, which help keep mucous membranes intact and control allergic reactions.	Lycopene is fat-soluble and must be eaten with a fat in order to be absorbed.
Orange/Yellow: • Carrots • Yams • Sweet potatoes • Pumpkin and other winter squashes	Contain carotenoids, which maintain resistance in mucous membranes and cilia to protect against infections and foreign materials.	
Green: • Spinach • Swiss chard • Asparagus • Dandelion greens • Other dark leafy greens	Contain magnesium, which helps decrease bronchial reactivity and constriction in asthma sufferers.	1 cup (250 mL) of these leafy vegetables is equal to one serving.

Best Foods for Protecting the Respiratory System	Respiratory System Benefits	Comments
VEGETABLES (cont.)		
Cruciferous Family: • Bok choy • Broccoli • Brussels sprouts • Cabbage • Cauliflower • Kale	Broccoli contains large amounts of vitamin C, beta-carotene and calcium. Calcium is a mineral needed for smooth muscle relaxation of the respiratory tract.	Broccoli sprouts have high amounts of cancer fighting nutrients.
Allium Family: • Chives • Garlic • Onions	Yellow or red onions are high in quercetin, an antihistaminic compound that helps reduce allergy symptoms. Garlic has antimicrobial properties that help the body fight infections.	Allicin, which is released during crushing, gives garlic its characteristic smell. Research indicates that for optimum benefit, garlic should be crushed and allowed to sit for a few minutes before using. Eat garlic raw or cooked.
LEGUMES		
• Beans (lima, pinto, organic soy) • Lentils • Peas (black-eyed peas) • Chickpeas	A source of protein essential for building and repairing tissues and immune cells to fight infection. A source of zinc, essential for resisting infection and tissue repair.	
WHOLE GRAINS		
• Whole oats • Brown rice • Barley • Whole wheat • Quinoa • Millet	Grains are a source of selenium, a strong antioxidant that works along with vitamin E. High in B vitamins, including B_6, which nourishes the adrenal glands.	Brown rice, quinoa and millet are less allergenic, so choose these grains, especially when the body is fighting an infection to prevent excess mucous formation.
NUTS AND SEEDS		
Nuts: • Almonds • Walnuts • Brazil nuts • Hazelnuts • Pecans	Nuts contain monounsaturated fats, vitamin E and magnesium. Almonds are a good source of calcium. Magnesium and calcium help relax the smooth muscle of the respiratory airways.	Buy raw or dry-roasted nuts and seeds. Choose an unsalted variety.
Seeds: • Flaxseeds • Sesame seeds • Pumpkin seeds • Sunflower seeds	Flaxseeds are high in omega-3 oils, which are anti-inflammatory. Sesame and sunflower seeds are an excellent source of vitamin E, a fat-soluble antioxidant. Pumpkin seeds are high in zinc, essential for immune function.	Sunflower seeds, pumpkin seeds and sesame seeds are excellent mixed together and eaten as a snack. Make your own trail mix.

Best Foods for Protecting the Respiratory System	Respiratory System Benefits	Comments
FATS AND OILS		
Cold-pressed oils: • Extra virgin olive oil • Flaxseed oil • Borage oil • Evening primrose oil • Avocados	Flaxseed, borage and evening primrose oil have been known to offset inflammation.	Do not use flaxseed oil for cooking. Use in salads, smoothies or over vegetables.
HERBS AND SPICES		
• Thyme • Peppermint • Ginger • Parsley • Oregano • Cumin • Mustard • Basil • Sage	Ginger is antiviral, antioxidant and anti-inflammatory. Peppermint stops coughs and releases congestion. Thyme helps clear the respiratory passageways and fight infection. Caution: Peppermint can relax the stomach sphincter and stimulate acid reflux.	
OTHER		
• Beer • Chocolate • Coffee • Tea • Wine	Tea and red wine contain quercetin. Beer is rich in bioflavonoids from the fermented grains. Phenols in dark chocolate and red wine are antioxidant.	Caution: Caffeine and alcohol can dehydrate and irritate the respiratory tract. Not recommended during pregnancy and lactation.

Whole Foods

Whole Foods for Health

There is no doubt about it. What you eat affects not only who you are and what you can accomplish, but also how you look and feel, including your overall health and vitality. Eating a variety of whole, fresh foods including fruit and vegetables is essential. As developed countries produce more and more refined and processed foods — foods like sugar-coated breakfast cereals, fat and chemical-laden, frozen and convenience foods and empty-calorie snack foods — there is also an increase in "modern" diseases. According to the 1988 U.S. Surgeon General's Report on Nutrition and Health, dietary choices are a factor in two-thirds of all deaths from coronary heart disease, stroke, atherosclerosis, diabetes and some cancers.

Whole foods are our first line of defense against those diseases. Whole foods are those foods that are as close to their natural state as possible. They are full of the essential vitamins, minerals, proteins, enzymes, complex carbohydrates and phytonutrients that combine to keep us active, alert and free from disease. What follows is a comprehensive outline of whole foods — foods that contain the optimum healing compounds so vital for human health.

For many reasons, locally grown, organic whole foods are the best possible foods we can choose for our family. Most notably, children are most vulnerable to pesticides, fertilizers, ionizing radiation and growth hormones, but everyone deserves to enjoy food that is produced without these human and environmental hazards. Farmers who use renewable resources, along with soil and water conservation practices, produce organic food in order to preserve a healthy environment for future generations. Most organic farms sell food locally. Their consumers are their friends and neighbors. Organic living provides a practical and painless first step that everyone can take towards a healthier lifestyle and planet.

MESSAGE FROM THE SURGEON GENERAL

I am pleased to transmit to the Secretary of the Department of Health and Human Services this first Surgeon General's Report on Nutrition and Health. It was prepared under the auspices of the Department's Nutrition Policy Board, and its main conclusion is that over consumption of certain dietary components is now a major concern for Americans. While many food factors are involved, chief among them is the disproportionate consumption of foods high in fats, often at the expense of foods high in complex carbohydrates and fiber — such as vegetables, fruits, and whole grain products — that may be more conducive to health.

— C.Everett Koop, M.D., Sc.D., Surgeon General, U.S. Public Health Service

Fruits

Apples

Malus pumila

Actions: Tonic, digestive, diuretic, detoxifying, laxative, antiseptic, lower blood cholesterol, antirheumatic, liver stimulant.

Uses: Fresh apples help cleanse the system, lower blood cholesterol levels, keep blood sugar levels up, and aid digestion. The French use the peels in preparations for rheumatism and gout as well as in urinary tract remedies. Apples are useful components in cleansing fasts because their fiber helps eliminate toxins. Apples are good sources of vitamin A and also contain vitamins C, B_2 (riboflavin) and K. Apples are high in the phytonutrients pectin and boron and are a good source of proanthocyanidins, which may contribute to maintenance of urinary tract and heart health.

Buying and Storing: Look for blemish-free apples with firm, crisp flesh and smooth, tight skin. Because of the widespread use of pesticides on apples, choose organic whenever possible or peel before using. Apple orchards produce seasonal gluts and since apples have excellent keeping qualities, local varieties may be available out of season. Keep in a cool dry and dark place (or the produce drawer of your refrigerator) for 1 month or more.

Culinary Use: Apples can be blended with most fruits and many vegetables. They add natural sweetness and lots of fiber and texture to both sweet and savory dishes. Not all sweet, crisp and delicious eating apple varieties are as good when cooked. Cox's Orange Pippin, Jonathan, Gravenstein or Baldwin apples are varieties that can be eaten raw and used as an ingredient in cooked dishes.

One apple, peeled and cored yields approximately 1 cup (250 mL) roughly chopped fruit. Homemade or commercially canned, unsweetened applesauce may be used in recipes as a natural sweetener.

Recipes:
- Chickpea Stuffing (page 158)
- Creamy White Sauce (page 149)
- Fruit Purée (Butter Replacement) (page 139)
- Moroccan Pumpkin Soup (page 193)
- Orange-Spiked Power Cereal (page 340)
- Spiced Apple Cake with Coconut Pecan Glaze (page 358)
- Vegetable Stock (page 137)

Apricots

Prunus armeniaca

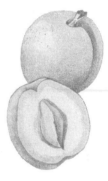

Actions: Antioxidant, anticancer.

Uses: Apricots are very high in beta-carotene, a precursor of vitamin A. Vitamin A may prevent the formation of plaque deposits in the arteries, thus preventing heart disease. Three small fresh apricots deliver 2,770 IU and $\frac{1}{2}$ cup (125 mL) dried contains 8,175 IU of vitamin A. Also high in B_2 (riboflavin), potassium, boron, iron, magnesium and fiber, apricots have virtually no sodium or fat. Fresh or dried apricots are especially recommended for women because they are a good source of calcium and an excellent source of vitamin A. Apricots help normalize blood pressure, heart function and maintain normal body fluids.

Buying and Storing: Choose firm, fresh apricots that range from dark yellow to orange. Keep in a dry cool place for up to 1 week. Dried apricots have the highest protein content of all dried fruit. Buy naturally sun-dried, sulphur-free dried fruit whenever possible, and without exception, if given regularly to children. The sulphur dioxide gas used to fumigate dried fruit (to keep the bright colors) is poisonous and if taken in excess can cause severe alimentary problems and possibly genetic mutations.

Culinary Use: Leave the peel on fresh apricots if organic but do not use the seeds. Peel in the same way as peaches, by pouring boiling water over and allowing them to cool enough to slip the skins off. Lemon juice will prevent browning.

Dried apricots are an excellent source of natural sugar and are generally sweeter than fresh fruit so use them to reduce refined sugar in sauces and cooked fruit recipes. Substitute 2 dried apricot halves for each fresh apricot. Canned apricots in unsweetened juice may also be used in dessert recipes and smoothies.

Recipes:
- Apricot Coulis (page 363)
- Apricot Milk (page 143)
- Apricot Tamarind Marmalade (page 183)
- Braised Greens with Cherries and Pine Nuts (v) (page 223)
- Christmas Sugarplums (page 361)
- Citrus Wheat Berries and Greens (page 323)
- Garlic Greens with Chickpeas and Cumin (page 219)
- Mini Mushroom Burgers with Apricot Tamarind Marmalade (page 168)
- Moroccan Chickpea Tagine (page 230)
- Orange-Spiked Power Cereal (page 340)
- Roasting Vegetables and Fruit (page 132)
- Yellow Coconut Curry Sauce (page 155)

Bananas

Musa cavendishii, syn. *M. chinensis*

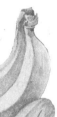

Actions: Boost immunity, lower cholesterol, prevent ulcers, antibacterial.

Uses: Due to their ability to strengthen the surface cells of the stomach lining and protect against acids, bananas are recommended when ulcers (or the risk of ulcers) are present. High in potassium and vitamin B_6 (pyridoxine) bananas help prevent heart attack, stroke and other cardiovascular problems.

Buying and Storing: Look for ripe bananas that are soft to the touch, yellow from neck to bottom and that are only very slightly speckled. Store in a cool dry and dark place.

Culinary Use: Bananas are peeled and added to salads and desserts just before serving whenever possible. Brushing bananas with lemon juice will prevent browning. Over-ripe bananas (very darkly speckled, almost solid brown) may be used in quick breads, puddings and sauces. Plantains are larger and green, usually used for cooking baked goods or in Caribbean and African dishes.

To Freeze Bananas: For freezing, choose fully yellow bananas with no bruises or brown spots. Peel and cut each into four chunks and arrange on a baking sheet. Freeze in coldest part of the freezer for 30 minutes. Transfer to one large or several individual resealable freezer bags. Seal and store in freezer for up to 6 months. Four frozen chunks are equal to one whole fresh banana. Use frozen bananas in baked goods and smoothies.

Recipes:
- Baked Bananas with Garlic Citrus Caramel Sauce (page 357)
- Baked Plantain and Peanut Stew (page 249)
- Baked Rice Pudding with Roasted Peaches (page 348)
- Egg Replacement (page 145)
- Orange Creamsicle (page 336)
- Pomegranate Smoothie (page 337)
- Red Lentil and Buckwheat Waffles (page 322)
- Sweet Potato, Bean and Wild Rice Quesadillas (page 292)
- Tropical Banana Tahini Smoothie (page 337)
- Tropical Fruit with Orange Liqueur (page 355)
- Tropical Nog (page 334)

Blackberries

Rubus species

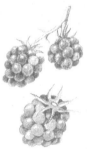

Actions: Antioxidant.

Uses: Blackberries are an excellent source of vitamin C and fiber. They have high levels of potassium, iron, calcium and manganese.

Buying and Storing: Choose plump berries with dark, glossy color and firm flesh. Fresh blackberries are best used immediately (if necessary, store for 1 day only in the refrigerator). Wash just before using.

Culinary Use: Use blackberries in all recipes that call for blueberries, raspberries or strawberries. Blackberries combine well with other berries, apples and peaches in pies, jams, puddings and soufflés.

Recipes:
- Açai Mocktail (page 336)
- Strawberry Pecan Crisp (page 352)

Black Currants

Ribes nigrum

Actions: Antioxidant, antibacterial, boost immunity, promote healing, antidiarrheal, anticancer.

Uses: Black currant flesh is extremely high in vitamin C. Three ounces (90 grams) contain 200 mg of vitamin C. Black currant skins and the outer layers of their flesh contain anthocyanins, a flavonoid, proven to prevent the development of bacteria such as E. coli. Black currants (especially the seeds) are high in gamma linolenic acid (GLA), important for heart health and a number of body functions. Although red currants are not as common as black, they have similar properties.

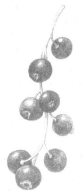

Buying and Storing: Black (or red) currants are not widely available but are sometimes found in midsummer at farmers' markets. While not as fragile as blackberries or raspberries, fresh currants must be stored in the refrigerator and will keep up to 1 week. Wash just before using.

Culinary Use: Remove the tiny stems before cooking fresh black currants. Fresh currants are usually simmered in water until tender before being used in recipes. Dried currants are not generally the dried version of fresh currants, but tiny raisins from the small seedless grapes of Corinth. Soak dried currants in water before using in baked goods or compotes.

Blueberries

Vaccinium species

Actions: Antidiarrheal, antioxidant, antibacterial, antiviral.

Uses: High concentrations of tannins are found in blueberries. Tannins kill bacteria and viruses and help prevent (or relieve) bladder infections. Anthocyanosides in blueberries protect blood vessels against cholesterol buildup. Anthocyanidins bolster cellular antioxidant defenses and may contribute to maintenance of brain function. Blueberries are high in pectin, vitamin C, potassium and natural aspirin and add extra fiber to the diet.

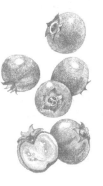

To Prevent Bladder Infections: Add at least $^1/_2$ cup (125 mL) fresh or frozen blueberries to smoothies, cereals or salads and take daily for a minimum of 3 weeks.

Buying and Storing: A silvery bloom on blueberries indicates freshness. Choose plump, firm, dark blue berries with smooth skin. Pick over and discard split or soft berries. Blueberries are best used immediately but can be stored in the refrigerator for up to 3 days. Wash just before using.

Culinary Use: The flavor of blueberries can be tart, especially in wild varieties, so combine with sweeter fruits (apples, apricots, bananas, pineapple) in order to avoid adding sugar to recipes. Frozen, canned or dried blueberries can be used when fresh are not available without sacrificing their medicinal qualities.

Recipes:
- Açai Mocktail (page 336)
- Pomegranate Smoothie (page 337)
- Strawberry Pecan Crisp (page 352)

Cantaloupe

See Melons

Cherries

Prunus species

Actions: Antibacterial, antioxidant, anticancer.

Uses: Cherries are high in ellagic acid, a potent anticancer agent. They are also high in vitamins C and A, biotin and potassium. Black cherry juice (from the Morello variety) protects against tooth decay unless sweetened. Cherries are a good source of anthocyanidins.

Buying and Storing: Choose sweet varieties and look for dark red, firm, plump, tight-skinned, glossy fruit with the stems attached. Whole ripe cherries are best used immediately but will keep in the refrigerator for up to 2 days.

Culinary Use: Wash, cut in half and remove stones. Sweet cherries such as the Bing variety range from pale yellow to deep purple-red and are juicy-sweet. The bitter, dark-skinned cherries are used mainly for jam that will be sweetened. When fresh cherries are not available, use pitted frozen, dried, or canned in recipes.

Recipes:
- Christmas Sugarplums (page 361)
- Citrus Wheat Berries and Greens (page 323)
- Roasting Vegetables and Fruit (page 132)
- Whole-Grain Power Bars (page 341)

Citrus Fruits

Citrus species
oranges, lemons, limes,
grapefruit, tangerines

Actions:
Antioxidant,
anticancer.

Uses: All citrus fruits
are high in vitamin C
and limonene, which is
thought to inhibit breast
cancer. Red grapefruit is
high in cancer-fighting
lycopene. Oranges are a
good source of choline, which
improves mental functioning.
The combination of carotenoids, flavonoids,
terpenes, limonoids and coumarins make citrus
fruits a total cancer-fighting package.

Buying and Storing: Plump, juicy citrus fruits
that are heavy for their size and yield slightly to
pressure are best. Although citrus fruits will keep
for at least a couple of weeks if kept moist in the
refrigerator, they are best if used within a week.
Look for organic citrus fruits because they are not
injected with gas for transportation.

Culinary Use: Make fresh citrus juice with a
citrus press or juicing machine. Lemon or lime juice
adds a fresh, sharp-tasting edge that complements
many vegetable dishes and tones down the cloying
sweet taste of other fruits. One half of a lemon or
lime yields about 3 tbsp (45 mL) of juice. Sauces
and dressings use various citrus juices. Whole or
sliced citrus fruit is used in salads, desserts and
some main dish recipes.

 Buy organic citrus fruit and wash the peel with
food-safe soap if using the rind. Candied citrus peel
is used in cakes, cookies and fruit compotes.
Canned oranges or grapefruit and their juice may be
used in most dishes, such as sauces and compotes,
that call for those fruits.

Caution: Grapefruit juice can interfere with some
medications.

Recipes:
- Baked Bananas with Garlic Citrus Caramel Sauce
  (page 357)
- Broccoli Lemon Rice (page 317)
- Chocolate Cake with Lemon Cream (page 354)
- Christmas Sugarplums (page 361)
- Citrus Beets (page 221)
- Citrus Greens with Fig Dressing (page 209)
- Citrus Wheat Berries and Greens (page 323)
- Fruited Rice Spring Rolls (page 351)
- Garlic Citrus Caramel Sauce (page 357)
- Lemon Cream (page 362)
- Lemon Cream Rice Pudding (page 355)
- Lemon Sauce (page 362)
- Maple and Orange–Glazed Eggplant (page 214)
- Orange Creamsicle (page 336)
- Orange-Spiked Power Cereal (page 340)
- Spiced Lemon Rice (page 315)
- Sweet Lemon Rice (page 349)
- Tropical Fruit with Orange Liqueur (page 355)

Cranberries

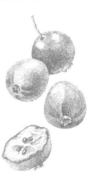

Vaccinium macrocarpum

Actions: Antibacterial,
antiviral, antioxidant,
anticancer.

Uses: The proanthocyanidins
in cranberries make them
extremely useful in urinary
and bladder infections. Whole
cranberries or juice work in
the same way as elderberries to
prevent the barbs on the bacteria from
attaching to the cells of the bladder or urinary tract,
rendering them ineffective in causing infection. Best
used as a first step in preventing urinary tract and
bladder infection, cranberry juice does not take the
place of antibiotic drugs, which are more effective in
eliminating bacteria once an infection has taken
hold. High in vitamins C and A, iodine and calcium,
cranberries also prevent kidney stones and deodorize
the urine.

 To Prevent Bladder Infections: Add at least
$1/2$ cup (125 mL) cranberries to smoothie recipes
or fruit salads and take every day for a minimum
of 3 weeks.

Buying and Storing: Choose bright red, plump
cranberries that bounce. Keep fresh cranberries in a
cold, dark place or produce drawer of the refrigerator
for 2 to 3 weeks. Cranberries may be frozen whole in
a freezer bag. Wash just before using.

Culinary Use: Unless used in small quantities or combined with very sweet fruits, their tartness makes it appropriate to use fresh cranberries with honey, stevia or other sweeteners. Cook fresh cranberries in a small amount of water or juice before combining with other ingredients in recipes. Canned whole cranberries or cranberry sauce are high in sugar so dried, fresh or frozen cranberries are preferred.

Recipes:
- Baked Cranberry Tofu with Creamed Asparagus and Leeks (page 270)
- Braised Greens with Cherries and Pine Nuts (v) (page 223)
- Cranberry Baked Beans (page 235)
- Whole-Grain Power Bars (page 341)

Crenshaw Melon

See Melons

Dates

Phoenix dactylifera

Actions: Boost estrogen levels, laxative.

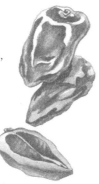

Uses: Dates are good sources of boron, which prevents calcium loss, so important in the fight against osteoporosis and weakening of bones. Dates contain vitamins A, B_1 (thiamin), B_2 (riboflavin), C and D and valuable mineral salts as well as fiber.

Buying and Storing: Dried dates are widely available and keep in a cool dark place for a couple of months. Fresh dates may be found in Middle Eastern markets when in season. Buy firm, plump, fresh dates with dark shiny skins. Fresh dates will keep for several days in the refrigerator.

Culinary Use: High in sugar (60% in fresh and 70% in dry), dates sweeten and add fiber to stews, tagines, salads, baked goods, puddings, grain dishes and desserts. Golden or dark brown in color, fresh dates are very different from dried and are becoming more and more common in upscale supermarkets. Use fresh dates in appetizer and salad recipes to show off their superior flavor and texture.

Recipes:
- Almond Milk (page 140)
- Apricot Tamarind Marmalade (page 183)
- Berry Chia Smoothie (page 337)
- Chilled Chia Chai (page 335)
- Christmas Sugarplums (page 361)
- Citrus Greens with Fig Dressing (page 209)
- Date Milk (page 143)
- Date Molasses (page 147)
- Fruit Purée (Butter Replacement) (page 139)
- Maple Baked Beans (page 269)
- Orange-Spiked Power Cereal (page 340)
- Spiced Apple Cake with Coconut Pecan Glaze (page 358)
- Spinach Cream Gazpacho (page 200)
- Sweet Potato Curried Cauliflower Soup (page 192)
- Tomato Grilling Sauce (page 152)
- Walnut Milk (page 142)

Elderberries

Sambucus species

Actions: Increase perspiration, diuretic, laxative.

Uses: Elderberries support detoxification by promoting bowel movements, urination, sweating and mucus secretion. They are effective in combating viruses, such as those that cause colds and flu. Elderberries work in the same way as cranberries, by providing protection from the barbs that puncture the body's cell walls. Viruses slide off and are eliminated before they can enter the cells and cause damage.

Buying and Storing: Elderberries are still mainly harvested from the wild (although some are now grown commercially in the United States and Canada). They are usually available at farmers' markets from mid- to late summer. Look for plump, deep, purple-black berries with tight, shiny skin and firm flesh. Use immediately or if necessary, store for 1 day in the refrigerator. Wash just before using.

Culinary Use: Elderberries add a dark blue color to foods. Their taste can be sweet or slightly tart. Use fresh or frozen elderberries, or small amounts of elderberry syrup, or elderberry jam in puddings, sauces, dressings, salads, beverages and vegetable dishes. Elderberries may be used in place of blueberries or raspberries in recipes.

Figs

Ficus carica

Actions: Antibacterial, anticancer, antiulcer, digestive, demulcent, laxative.

Uses: Figs contain benzaldehyde, a cancer-fighting agent. They are also high in potassium, B vitamins, calcium and magnesium, and are naturally sweet.

Buying and Storing: Dried figs are readily available in supermarkets throughout the year. In summer and early fall, some supermarkets and most Middle Eastern food markets carry fresh figs. There are over 700 varieties of figs and they range in color from green to purple or dark brown. Choose soft, plump fresh figs with thin skins that yield to a gentle touch. Fresh figs are delicate but keep in a cool dark place for several days.

Culinary Use: Fresh figs contain 12% sugar and are best eaten whole, with cheese or fruit. Cook with dried figs, which contain about 50% sugar. Dried figs are used to sweeten and thicken dressings, puddings and sauces. Figs can be substituted for apricots and dates in most recipes.

Recipes:
• Christmas Sugarplums (page 361)
• Citrus Greens with Fig Dressing (page 209)
• Fig Milk (page 143)
• Fig Spread (page 181)

Gooseberries

Ribes grossularia

Actions: Protect skin and gums, laxative.

Uses: High in vitamin C, potassium and pectin, gooseberries are often added to jams to make them set.

Buying and Storing:
Once found in many home gardens, gooseberries are now sometimes found at farmers' markets in early summer. Be sure to use dessert varieties (early ripening amber and yellow varieties) and look for plump, bright, almost transparent berries with tight, shiny skin and firm flesh. Use immediately or if necessary, store for 1 day in the refrigerator. Wash just before using.

Culinary Use: Refreshingly tart-sweet, gooseberries add depth to the sweet taste of seasonal berries and bananas. Red-skinned and green gooseberries are too tart to use raw and require sweetening when cooked.

Grapefruit

See Citrus Fruits

Grapes

Vitis vinifera

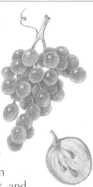

Actions: Antioxidant, antiviral, anticancer.

Uses: Grapes contain large amounts of ellagic and caffeic acids, which deactivate carcinogens. Grapes are a good source of potassium. The flavonoids in grape juice protect the heart, and the resveratrol found in red wine and red grape juice has a protective effect on the cardiovascular system. Grapes are also high in boron, a substance that helps maintain estrogen levels and may be instrumental in preventing osteoporosis.

Buying and Storing: Organic grapes are preferred due to the high amounts of pesticides used on commercial crops. Look for bright color, firm flesh and unwrinkled skin. Wash grapes in food grade hydrogen peroxide or vinegar because they are heavily sprayed. Store in the produce drawer of refrigerator for 3 or 4 days.

Culinary Use: Grapes are sweet and their mild taste blends with most fruit in salads and desserts. Grapes are generally used raw but may be added to tagines and other cooked dishes that will not overpower their delicate flavor.

Raisins are dried grapes and are a good source of fiber, boron, calcium, phosphorus, iron, potassium and vitamin A. They add natural sweetness to recipes. Add $\frac{1}{4}$ cup (50 mL) to salads, baked goods and grain recipes. Golden sultanas are a very good cooking variety because they are light in color and plump. Use only sulphur-free raisins that have not been sprayed with mineral oils.

Recipe:
• Spinach and Whole-Grain Salad with Kiwi Dressing (v) (page 207)

Honeydew Melon

See Melons

Kiwifruits

Actinidia chinensis

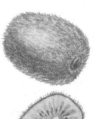

Actions: Antioxidant, anticancer, aid digestion.

Uses: Kiwifruits are often used as part of a cleansing regimen or to aid digestion. They are high in vitamins C and E (one of few fruits that contain vitamin E) that both act as antioxidants, protecting cells from damage. Kiwifruits are also high in potassium and contain some calcium.

Buying and Storing: Choose ripe kiwifruit that yield to gentle pressure. Kiwifruit will ripen at room temperature in a brown paper bag after 2 or 3 days. Ripe kiwifruit keep for at least 1 week in the produce drawer of the refrigerator.

Culinary Use: Use fresh in salads, jams, cakes and desserts. They make an attractive garnish for cooked sweet or savory dishes.

Recipes:
- Chickpeas with Kiwi and Avocado Salsa (page 208)
- Fruited Rice Spring Rolls (page 351)
- Kiwi and Avocado Salsa with Pomegranate and Red Onion (page 189)
- Kiwi Dressing (page 204)
- Spinach and Whole-Grain Salad with Kiwi Dressing (page 207)

Lemons

See Citrus Fruits

Limes

See Citrus Fruits

Mangoes

Mangifera indica

Actions: Antioxidant, anticancer.

Uses: High in vitamins A (there are 8,000 IU of beta-carotene in one mango) and C, potassium, B_3 (niacin) and fiber, mangoes help protect against cancer and atherosclerosis. They help the body fight infection and maintain bowel regularity.

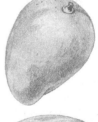

Buying and Storing: Choose large, firm, yellow to yellow-red, unblemished fruit with flesh that gives slightly when gently squeezed. Store ripe fresh mangoes in the produce drawer of refrigerator for 3 or 4 days.

Culinary Use: Mangoes are fibrous with a sweet, banana-pineapple flavor. They combine well with peaches, apricots, nectarines and plums. Use fresh mangoes in salads, grain dishes, desserts and beverages.

Handle mangoes carefully because the peel contains a skin irritating sap. To separate the flesh from the fibrous seed, cut the fruit lengthwise on one side, close to the seed. Repeat on the other side of the seed. With the tip of a paring knife, separate the two halves from the seed. Using a large spoon, scoop the flesh out of the skin. Dried mangoes are available, but use them sparingly due to their extra sweetness and look for ones that are dried naturally (and not treated with sulphur).

Recipes:
- Fruited Rice Spring Rolls (page 351)
- Green Tea Mocktail (page 336)
- Mango Pineapple Mocktail (page 335)
- Tropical Fruit with Orange Liqueur (page 355)
- Tropical Nog (page 334)

Melons

Cucumis melo
cantaloupe, honeydew, crenshaw, spanish, musk

Actions: Antioxidant, anticancer, anticoagulant (cantaloupe and honeydew).

Uses: Melons are a good source of vitamin A and contain vitamin C and calcium. Adenosine, the anticoagulant chemical found in cantaloupes and honeydews lessens the risk of heart attacks and strokes due to its ability to thin the blood.

Buying and Storing: Ripe melons are heavy and have a full, sweet perfume. Blemished, soft fruit should be avoided.

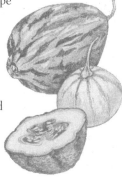

Culinary Use: The low caloric value along with their high water content and delicate sweet flavor make melons a good choice for desserts, smoothies and sweet or savory salads. Melons are often paired with savory spreads or fillings and served as appetizers.

Recipes:
• Strawberries with Balsamic Drizzle (v) (page 351)
• Tropical Nog (page 334)

Musk Melon

See Melons

Nectarines

Prunus persica var. *nectarina*

Actions: Antioxidant, anticancer.

Uses: Nectarines are a good source of vitamins A and C, and potassium. They are an original ancient fruit and not, as many people think, a cross between a peach and a plum.

Buying and Storing: Choose fruit that have some bright red areas and are smooth and tight without soft patches. Nectarines should be heavy (full of juice) and firm when pressed, giving way gently, but not hard.

Culinary Use: Nectarines are usually sweeter than peaches and can be used in place of peaches, plums and apricots in recipes. Peel in the same way as peaches, by pouring boiling water over and allowing them to cool enough to slip the skins off. Lemon juice will prevent browning.

Recipe:
• Tropical Fruit with Orange Liqueur (page 355)

Oranges

See Citrus Fruits

Papayas

Carica papaya

Actions: Antioxidant, anticancer, aid digestion.

Uses: High in vitamins A, E and C, folate and potassium.

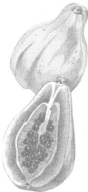

Buying and Storing: Choose large, firm, yellow, unblemished fruit with flesh that gives slightly when gently squeezed. Store in the produce drawer of refrigerator for 3 or 4 days.

Culinary Use: Papayas sweeten and blend well with other fruits in dressings, sauces and desserts. Use fresh papayas with breakfast grain dishes and in smoothies where they add a creamy texture. Dried papaya is usually treated with sulphur and is very sweet, so use sparingly.

Recipe:
• Tropical Fruit with Orange Liqueur (page 355)

Peaches

Prunus persica

Actions: Antioxidant, anticancer.

Uses: Rich in vitamin A and potassium, peaches also contain boron, B_3 (niacin) and some iron and vitamin C. Peaches help protect against cancer, osteoporosis and heart disease. Their sugar content is low (about 9%).

Buying and Storing: Fruit that is full and heavy with fuzzy down and flesh that gives when lightly pressed is preferable. Store peaches in the produce drawer of the refrigerator for up to 4 days. Freestone varieties (such as Loring and Redhaven) are easier to pit than clingstone varieties.

Culinary Use: Use frozen or canned peaches packed in unsweetened juice when the fresh fruit is not in season. Peaches can replace nectarines,

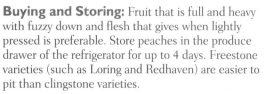

plums and apricots in recipes. They complement blackberries, blueberries and raspberries in salads and fruit desserts. Peel by pouring boiling water over and allowing them to cool enough to slip the skins off. Lemon juice will prevent browning. Dried peaches are added to compotes, chutneys and other long-simmering dessert dishes.

Recipes:
• Baked Rice Pudding with Roasted Peaches (page 348)
• Lentil Tagine (page 229)
• Poached Peaches with Lavender Custard (page 356)

Pears

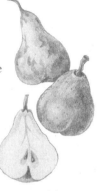

Pyrus communis

Actions: Protect the colon.

Uses: Pears are a good source of fiber, which helps prevent constipation and ensures regularity and protects the colon. Pears' insoluble fiber binds to cancer-causing chemicals in the colon, preventing them from damaging the colon cells.

Perhaps one of the oldest cultivated fruit, pears are a good source of vitamin C, boron and potassium. Healthcare professionals often recommend pears because they are less likely to cause an adverse response. For this reason, they are one of the first fruits introduced to infants.

Buying and Storing: Shop for pears that are lightly firm, unblemished and sweetly "pear smelling." Often available before fully ripe, pears may be ripened in a brown paper bag for 1 to 3 days. Eat pears as soon as they ripen or store in the produce drawer of the refrigerator for up to 3 days.

Culinary Use: Use fresh, frozen or canned pears in sweet and savory dishes. Juicy varieties such as Bartlett, Comice, Seckel and Bosc are great for poached pear desserts. Pears soften in cooking faster than apples so add to stewed fruit compotes 5 to 10 minutes after the apples. Pears team nicely with plums and grapes in recipes.

Recipes:
• Pear and Avocado Pitas (page 344)
• Vanilla Poached Pears with Cinnamon Rice Cream (page 346)
• Warm Pear and Snow Pea Salad with Miso Dressing (page 205)

Pineapples

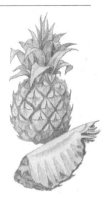

Ananas comosus

Actions: Aid digestion.

Uses: A 1-cup (250 mL) serving of pineapple delivers 128% of the body's daily requirement of manganese and is a good source of potassium and vitamin C. Pineapples also contain vitamin B_1 (thiamin), copper, iron and vitamin B_6 (pyridoxine).

Buying and Storing: Choose large, firm fruits (heaviness in the ripe fruit indicates juiciness), with overall yellow color.

Culinary Use: Pineapples add a fresh sweet taste to smoothies, salads and dessert dishes. The sweetness of pineapples helps soften the tartness of cranberries, blueberries and gooseberries. Pineapple juice is very sweet. Frozen or canned pineapple packed in unsweetened juice may be used in recipes.

To Use Fresh Pineapple: Trim off the base and top leaves. Cut in half and use one half at a time. Slice one half into four wedges. Slice away and discard the skin from each wedge and remove and discard the woody core. One whole, fresh wedge yields about 1 cup (250 mL) chopped fresh pineapple.

Recipes:
• Mango Pineapple Mocktail (page 335)
• Tropical Banana Tahini Smoothie (page 337)
• Tropical Nog (page 334)
• Tropical Tahini Dressing (page 203)

Plums

Prunus species

Actions: Antibacterial, antioxidant.

Uses: Plums contain vitamins A and C, a small amount of vitamin B_2 (riboflavin) and potassium. They have an exceptionally high content of unique phytonutrients called neochlorogenic and chlorogenic acids. These substances, found in both plums and prunes, are classified as phenols, and their function as antioxidants has been well documented.

Buying and Storing: Ripe plums are firm with no soft spots or splits. Look for bright, (yellow, black or red sweet plums), tight skin and heavy, sweet smelling fruit. Keep in the produce drawer of the refrigerator for up to 4 days.

Culinary Use: Wash and peel (if not organic) and remove pit. Dessert plums can be eaten fresh or added to fruit salads. Cooking plums may be stewed in a little water for 10 to 15 minutes or until soft. Canned and frozen plums may be substituted for fresh in some recipes.

For Umeboshi plums, see page 126. Prunes are dried plums and are high in colon cancer-fighting pectin (and other insoluble fiber), low in sugar, and act as a natural laxative. To treat constipation: Take 4 to 6 dried or stewed prunes up to three times a day for 1 or 2 days.

Recipes:
• Roasted Vegetables and Fruit (page 132)
• Roasted Vegetable Salad (page 208)
• Umeboshi Sauce (page 363)

Pomegranates

Punica granatum

Actions: Antidiarrheal, antifever, astringent.

Uses: Used in gargles and thought to reduce fevers, pomegranates are widely used in Indian medicines.

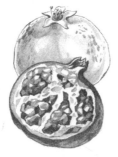

Buying and Storing: Choose firm, even-colored and heavy fruit. Keep in the produce drawer of the refrigerator for up to 4 days.

Culinary Use: The bright red, juicy seeds are eaten fresh and for Middle Eastern recipes are dried and pounded to a powder. Fresh pomegranate seeds are used in salads and as a garnish for dips and desserts and can be pressed for drinks. Crushed dried seeds are sprinkled on hummus and used in Middle Eastern sweet dishes. Pomegranate molasses is available in specialty stores and may be used in place of honey in beverages, dressings, sauces, puddings and other desserts.

Recipes:
• Green Bean, Pecan and Pomegranate Salad (page 206)
• Kiwi and Avocado Salsa with Pomegranate and Red Onion (page 189)

• Pomegranate Molasses (page 146)
• Pomegranate Smoothie (page 337)
• Roasted Beets with Pomegranate Molasses (page 217)

Raspberries

Rubus idaeus

Actions: Support the immune system.

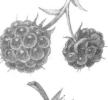

Uses: Raspberries are rich in manganese and vitamin C (supplying over 50% of the daily recommended amounts of each). They contain folate, vitamin B_2 (riboflavin), magnesium, vitamin B_3 (niacin), potassium and copper. See also Red Raspberry leaf (page 120).

Buying and Storing: Buy or pick fresh raspberries in peak season and choose whole, plump berries with bright color. Sort and discard soft or broken berries. Use immediately or store in the produce drawer of refrigerator for 1 day. Wash just before using.

Culinary Use: Raspberries blend with other berries in desserts and salads and the taste is enhanced with a small amount of citrus juice. Substitute frozen, dried or canned raspberries for fresh. Up to $1/4$ cup (50 mL) raspberry jam may also be used in sauces and dressings.

Recipes:
• Açai Mocktail (page 336)
• Berry Chia Smoothie (page 337)
• Minted Raspberry-Marinated Oats (page 327)
• Pomegranate Smoothie (page 337)

Rhubarb

Rheum species

Actions: Laxative.

Uses: Actually a vegetable that is almost always used as a fruit, rhubarb is high in potassium and contains a fair amount of iron. The amount of calcium in 1 cup (250 mL) cooked rhubarb is twice that of milk.

Caution: Never use the leaves of rhubarb, which are toxic and inedible due to the high concentration of oxalic acid in them.

Buying and Storing: If a rhubarb patch is not available, farmers' markets may be the only source in spring. Choose thin, firm stalks with all or 90% red color. Rhubarb should snap when bent. Store in a cool dry place or the produce drawer of refrigerator for 1 or 2 days only.

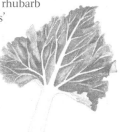

Culinary Use: Cooking mellows the tart taste and softens the laxative effect. To cook fresh rhubarb: Place 1 cup (250 mL) chopped fresh rhubarb in a saucepan. Add 1 cup (250 mL) chopped apple and $\frac{1}{4}$ cup (50 mL) sugar or honey or 2 tsp (10 mL) stevia to sweeten. Cover with water or apple juice and simmer until soft. Frozen or canned rhubarb may also be used in recipes.

Spanish Melon

See Melons

Strawberries

Fragaria species

Actions: Antioxidant, antiviral, anticancer.

Uses: Effective against kidney stones, gout, rheumatism and arthritis, strawberries are also used in cleansing juices and as a mild tonic for the liver. Strawberries are high in the cancer fighting ellagic acid and vitamin C. They are also a good source of vitamin A and potassium and contain iron. Both the leaves and the fruit have been used medicinally. A tea from strawberry leaves is used for diarrhea and dysentery.

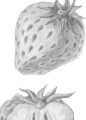

Buying and Storing: Pick your own or choose brightly colored, firm berries with hulls attached. They are best used immediately but may be stored for no more than a couple of days in the refrigerator. Wash just before using.

Caution: Strawberries are heavily sprayed; choose organic when possible.

Culinary Use: Strawberries add a sweet and powerful flavor to salads, desserts, sauces, dressings and drinks. They blend well with bananas and other berries and the taste is enhanced with a small amount of lemon or lime juice.

Recipes:
• Strawberries with Balsamic Drizzle (page 351)
• Strawberry Pecan Crisp (page 352)
• Strawberry Sauce (page 362)

Tangerines

See Citrus Fruits

Watermelon

Citrullus vulgaris

Actions: Antibacterial, anticancer.

Uses: Watermelons contain vitamins C and A, iron and potassium. Their high water content makes them a refreshing summer ingredient.

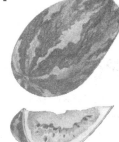

Buying and Storing: A watermelon should be bright green with firm flesh (no blemishes or soft spots) and feel heavy for its size.

Culinary Use: Watermelon is a refreshing summer fruit that combines well with other fruits as a sweet thirst quencher. To use in salads and smoothies, cut in half lengthwise and use half at a time. Use a slice whole as a garnish or remove and discard rind and seeds, and chop the flesh. One slice (from half a watermelon) yields approximately 1 cup (250 mL) chopped fruit. Wrap tightly and keep cut watermelon in the refrigerator.

Recipe:
• Strawberries with Balsamic Drizzle (v) (page 351)

Artichokes (Globe)

Cynara scolymus

Actions: Antioxidant, anticancer, heart protective.

Uses: Artichokes are high in flavanones, phytochemicals that offer protection against heart disease. They also contain phosphorus, iron, zinc and calcium.

Buying and Storing: Artichokes are the flower of a thistle plant and as such, have tough outer leaves and hairy, inedible centers or chokes. Choose bright green-purple artichokes with no signs of browning and tightly closed leaves.

Culinary Use: Fresh artichokes have a delicate flavor. Trim the thick stems and remove the tough outer leaves. Simmer in a saucepan half filled with boiling water for 30 to 40 minutes or until the outer leaves pull away easily. Cut in half and remove the hairy, inedible center. Serve fresh artichokes with any of the mayonnaise recipes (pages 178 and 179) for a starter dish. Canned artichoke hearts are usually marinated and are more flavorful than fresh. Artichoke hearts are used in salads, pasta and in baked legume and grain dishes.

Recipes:
- Jerusalem Artichoke Stew (page 251)
- Pan-Seared Artichokes with Pomegranate Molasses (page 166)
- Penne with Spinach-Artichoke Cream Sauce (page 300)
- Roasted Eggplant and Artichoke Dip (page 186)
- Roasted Garlic and Artichoke Spread (page 180)

Asparagus

Asparagus officinalis

Actions: Antioxidant, anticancer, promotes healing, prevent cataracts, diuretic.

Uses: Asparagus is an excellent source of vitamin K (supplying over 100% of the Recommended Daily Amount) and folate, needed for the production of red blood cells and the release of energy from food.

It is also a good source of vitamins C and A. It contains B vitamins, tryptophan, manganese, copper, protein, potassium, iron, zinc and some calcium.

Buying and Storing: Look for tight buds at the tips and smooth green stalks with some white at the very end. Fresh asparagus will snap at the point where the tender stalk meets the tougher end. Store stalks upright in $\frac{1}{2}$ inch (1 cm) of water in the refrigerator for up to 2 days.

Culinary Use: Wash grit from flower ends by soaking and swishing in cool water. Snap off and discard the tough stem bottoms. Roasting caramelizes the sugars and brings out the nutty, slightly smoky flavor of asparagus. Steam tender tips by standing whole stalks upright in a tall, narrow pot so that only the lower two-thirds of the stems are immersed in boiling water. Cover and gently simmer for 3 to 5 minutes. Frozen or canned asparagus may be substituted in recipes when fresh is not available.

Recipes:
- Baked Cranberry Tofu with Creamed Asparagus and Leeks (page 270)
- Bulgur Asparagus Salad (page 212)
- Cream of Leek and Asparagus on Toast Points (page 171)
- Creamy Asparagus Soup (page 195)
- Green Pea and Asparagus Curry (page 259)
- Portobello Pot-au-Feu (page 280)
- Spring Dolmades (page 162)
- Vegetable Stock (page 137)

Avocados

Persea americana

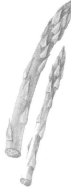

Actions: Antioxidant, anticancer, heart protective.

Uses: Avocados contain more potassium than many other fruits and vegetables (banana is just slightly higher). While high in essential fatty acids, they contain 17 vitamins and minerals including vitamins K, C, A, E and B_6 (pyridoxine), iron, calcium, copper, phosphorus, zinc, B_3 (niacin), magnesium, selenium, folate as well as the highest amount of protein of any fruit. Not only are avocados a rich source of monounsaturated fatty acids including oleic acid, they are also a concentrated dietary source of the carotenoid lutein.

Buying and Storing: Look for ripe, heavy avocados with dull dark green skin. When held in the hand, ripe avocados give gently. Don't press the flesh and avoid avocados with dents in the skin. Ripen in a paper bag and store in the refrigerator for just over 1 week once ripe.

Culinary Use: One avocado added to salads adds a creamy texture and exceptional nutrients. Brush with lemon juice to keep avocado flesh from turning brown once peeled. Avocados thicken uncooked sauces, dips and smoothies (in much the same way as bananas) due to their lower water content. Up to 30% of the fruit's weight may be oil and for this reason, avocados should be used sparingly.

Recipes:
- Avocado Sauce (page 148)
- Avocado Vichyssoise (page 199)
- Kiwi and Avocado Salsa with Pomegranate and Red Onion (page 189)
- Pear and Avocado Pitas (page 344)
- Roasted Corn Salsa (page 190)

Beans

Phaseolus vulgaris
fresh green runner, yellow wax runner, broad, flat, Italian, snap, string, green peas

Pisum sativum
snow peas

For Legumes (dried peas and beans), see page 87.

Actions: Help memory, antioxidant.

Uses: Green beans and peas are leguminous plants — the same botanically as dried beans and peas because they all produce their seeds in pods. However, fresh beans and peas have a lower nutrient level than dried legumes. A good source of choline, which improves mental functioning beans, beans and peas contain vitamin A and potassium along with some protein, iron, calcium and vitamins B and C. The amino acids in beans and peas make them a valuable food for vegetarians.

Buying and Storing: Buy fresh peas and beans with firm pods showing no signs of wilting. The bigger the size of the pea or bean inside the pod the older the vegetable. Fresh yellow or green beans are pliant but still snap when bent. Store unwashed fresh peas (in their pods) and beans in a vented plastic bag in the refrigerator for 2 or 3 days. Parboiled fresh beans and peas freeze well.

Culinary Use: Fresh, frozen, canned or cooked dried peas and beans (legumes) can all be used in recipes. Fresh summer beans are exceptional as a dish on their own or in salads or baked vegetable dishes and they complement grains.

Recipes:
- Corn, Beans and Squash Bake with Oat Nut Topping (page 275)
- Green Bean, Pecan and Pomegranate Salad (page 206)
- Green Pea and Asparagus Curry (page 259)
- Okra and Broad Beans with Tomato Sauce (page 213)
- Portobello Pot-au-Feu (page 280)

Beets

Beta vulgaris

Actions: Antibacterial, antioxidant, tonic, cleansing, laxative, fight colon cancer.

Uses: Beets (the roots of the beet plant) are high in folate, manganese, potassium and the enzyme betaine, which nourishes and strengthens the liver and gall bladder. With 8% chlorine, beets are cleansing for the liver, kidney and gall bladder. The pigment that gives beets their rich, purple-crimson color — betacyanin — is also a powerful cancer-fighting agent. Beets are also a good source of vitamin C, magnesium, tryptophan, iron, copper and phosphorus.

Buying and Storing: Bright glossy, crisp green beet tops or leaves indicate fresh beets. Buy firm, unblemished, small beets with greens intact, if possible. For storing, cut off the tops and treat as leafy greens. Store unwashed beets in a vented plastic bag in the refrigerator. Beets will keep for up to $1\frac{1}{2}$ weeks.

Culinary Use: Grate fresh, raw beets into salads. Roast, steam or boil fresh beets in water for a vegetable side dish. Use cooked canned or frozen beets when fresh are not available. For using beet tops as a leafy vegetable, see page 78.

Recipes:
- Borscht (page 202)
- Citrus Beets (page 221)
- Quinoa Beet Potato Salad (page 325)
- Roasted Beets with Pomegranate Molasses (page 217)

Broccoli

Brassica oleracea var.
italica

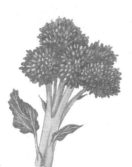

Actions: Antioxidant,
anticancer, promotes
healing, prevents
cataracts.

Uses: Like other
cruciferous vegetables,
broccoli contains cancer-
fighting indoles, glucosinolates
and dithiolthiones. A 1-cup (250 mL) serving of
broccoli packs over 200% of the body's daily
requirement of vitamin C and over 190% of vitamin
K. It is high in vitamin A and is one of only four
vegetables with vitamin E. It has a fair amount of
folate, manganese, tryptophan and potassium.
Vitamin B_6 (pyridoxine), B_2 (riboflavin),
phosphorus, magnesium, protein, omega-3 fatty
acids, vitamin B_5, iron, calcium, vitamins B_1
(thiamin) and B_3 (niacin) and zinc are also present
in broccoli. Purple sprouting broccoli is an excellent
source of lignans, believed to help protect against
hormone-related cancers and may help relieve
symptoms associated with menopause.

Buying and Storing: Broccoli yellows as it ages.
Deep green color and firm tight buds are a sign of
freshness. Thin stalks are more tender than thick,
woody stems that tend to be hollow. Store in a
vented plastic bag in the produce drawer of the
refrigerator for up to 3 days.

Culinary Use: Raw broccoli is eaten with dips
and sauces. Fresh broccoli may be boiled, steamed
or stir-fried. Cooked broccoli should retain some
crunch and bright green color. Use frozen broccoli
when fresh is not available.

Recipes:
- Almond and Curry Broccoli Stir-Fry (page 264)
- Broccoli Lemon Rice (page 317)
- Chickpeas and Potatoes in Cashew Cream
  (page 240)
- Lentil and Broccoli Casserole (page 231)
- Spiced Winter Vegetables (page 263)
- Udon Noodles with Tofu and Gingered Peanut
  Sauce (page 304)
- Vegetable Stock (page 137)

Brussels Sprouts

See Cabbage

Cabbage

Brassica oleracea var.
capitata
green, red, Savoy,
bok choy, Chinese,
kohlrabi, Brussels
sprouts

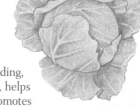

Actions: Immune building,
antibacterial, anticancer, helps
memory, antioxidant, promotes
healing, prevents cataracts, detoxifying, diuretic,
anti-inflammatory, tonic, antiseptic, restorative,
prevents ulcers.

Uses: Cruciferous vegetables, of which cabbage
is one, appear to lower our risk of cancer more
effectively than any other vegetable or fruit.
Cabbage is high in cancer-fighting indoles and a
good source of choline, which improves mental
functioning. It is also an excellent source of vitamins
K and C. A very good remedy for anemia, cabbage
has also been used as a nutritive tonic to restore
strength in debility and convalescence. Of benefit
to the liver, cabbage is also effective in preventing
colon cancer and may help diabetics by reducing
blood sugar. Cabbage juice is significant in
preventing and healing ulcers. Cabbage contains
manganese, vitamins B_1 (thiamin), B_2 (riboflavin),
B_6 (pyridoxine), folate, omega-3 fatty acids,
calcium, potassium, vitamin A, tryptophan, protein
and magnesium.

Buying and Storing: Fresh cabbage has loose
outer leaves around a firm center head. Older,
stored cabbage does not have the outer wrapper
leaves and tends to be paler in color. Cabbage will
keep for up to 2 weeks in a vented plastic bag in the
refrigerator. Wash and cut or slice just before using.

Culinary Use: Fresh cabbage is available year-
round and is an excellent vegetable to have on hand
at all times. It is an essential ingredient in vegetable
stock. Steam, broil or stir-fry cabbage with other
vegetables, legumes and grains or slice thin and
serve raw in salads.

Recipes:
- Baked Winter Greens (page 276)
- Bok Choy, Mushroom and Black Bean Stir-Fry
  (page 288)
- Curried Chestnut–Stuffed Cabbage (page 261)
- Curried Green Sauté (page 226)
- Fennel and Cucumber Salad with Ginger Dressing
  (page 204)
- Jerusalem Artichoke Stew (page 251)

- Leek, Kohlrabi, Garlic and Onion Tart (page 273)
- Maple-Glazed Cabbage Greens with Pecans (page 217)
- Pad Thai (page 291)
- Rainbow Tempeh Lettuce Cups (page 294)
- Roast Potatoes, Fennel and Leeks (page 286)
- Sweet Potato Ragoût (page 246)
- Vegetable Stock (page 137)
- West African Mafé (page 250)

Carrots

Daucus carota ssp. *sativus*

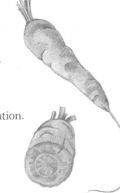

Actions: Antioxidant, anticancer, artery protecting, expectorant, antiseptic, diuretic, immune boosting, antibacterial, lower blood cholesterol, prevent constipation.

Uses: Carrots have a cleansing effect on the liver and digestive system, help counter the formation of kidney stones and relieve arthritis and gout. Their antioxidant properties from carotenoids (including beta-carotene) have been shown to cut cancer risk, protect against arterial and heart disease and lower blood cholesterol. Carrots enhance mental functioning, decrease the risk of cataracts and promote good vision. Carrots are extremely nutritious and rich in vitamins A (1 cup/250 mL supplies over 600% of our daily requirement), K and C. Potassium, some B vitamins, manganese and folate are also present.

Buying and Storing: The inedible green tops continue to draw nutrients out of the carrot so choose fresh carrots that are sold loose with the tops removed or remove and discard the tops immediately. Choose firm, well-shaped carrots with no cracks. The deeper the the carrot's color, the higher the concentration of carotene. If stored unwashed in a cold but moist place, carrots should not shrivel. Keep for up to 2 weeks in a vented plastic bag in the produce drawer of the refrigerator.

Culinary Use: Carrots are a versatile vegetable with natural sweetness that can be used in almost any vegetable recipe. Cooking frees up carotenes (precursors to vitamin A), the anticancer agents in carrots. Steam, roast, stir-fry or simmer carrots just until tender. Grated carrots are used raw in salads and grain and pasta dishes.

Recipes:
- Borscht (page 202)
- Gingered Carrot-Turnip Purée (page 218)
- Herbed Carrot and Turnip Fritters (page 177)
- Mini Mushroom Burgers with Apricot Tamarind Marmalade (page 168)
- Portobello Pot-au-Feu (page 280)
- Roasted Corn Salsa (page 190)
- Roasted Spice-Glazed Root Vegetables (page 215)
- Roasted Vegetable Hummus (page 185)
- Tomato Sauce (page 151)
- Vegetable and Tempeh Pie (page 236)
- Vegetable Pancakes (page 160)
- Vegetable Raita (page 187)
- Vegetable Stock (page 137)
- Vietnamese Spring Rolls with Peanut Sauce (page 172)
- Winter Vegetable Bake with Coconut Nut Topping (page 277)

Cauliflower

Brassica oleracea var. *botrytis*

Actions: Antioxidant, anticancer.

Uses: As are all cruciferous vegetables (cabbage, Brussels sprouts, broccoli, collard greens, kohlrabi), cauliflower is rich in indoles, the cancer preventing phytonutrients. Cauliflower is an excellent source of vitamin C. It is a good source of vitamin K, folate and vitamin B$_6$ (pyridoxine). Potassium and some protein and iron are also present.

Buying and Storing: Fresh cauliflower has dense, tightly packed florets and crisp, green leaves surround the head. Keep loosely covered in the refrigerator for no longer than 1 week.

Culinary Use: Wash and cut away outer leaves, save and use them as you would any leafy green vegetable. Cut the head into florets, discarding the woody core and stems. Use cauliflower raw in salads and appetizers with dips and sauces. Cauliflower is very good in soups, curries, stir-fries and chutneys. Steam or boil cauliflower or bake with other ingredients.

Recipes:
- Baked Cauliflower (page 176)
- Cauliflower Gratin (page 272)
- Chickpea and Swiss Chard Ragoût (page 245)

- Chickpeas and Potatoes in Cashew Cream (page 240)
- Coconut Rice with Cauliflower (page 316)
- Madras Cauliflower (page 225)
- Red Curry Cauliflower (page 258)
- Roasted Vegetable Salad (page 208)
- Spiced Winter Vegetables (page 263)
- Sweet Potato Curried Cauliflower Soup (page 192)

Celery

Apium graveolens var. *dulce* and *Celeriac Apium graveolens* var. *rapaceum*

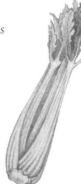

Actions: Mild diuretic, anticancer.

Uses: Sometimes used as a treatment for high blood pressure (two to four stalks per day). The coumarins in celery help prevent free radicals from damaging cells, thus helping to prevent cell mutation, a pre-cancer condition. Coumarins also boost immune responses. The acetylenic compounds in celery have been found to stop the growth of tumorous cells. For the healing properties of celery seeds, see page 108.

Buying and Storing: Fresh celery has some crisp green leaves and firm crisp ribs. Older stalks have had the leaves removed. Celery varieties range in color from very light to dark green and as the color darkens, the taste gets stronger. Store for up to 2 weeks in a vented plastic bag in the refrigerator.

Culinary Use: Use celery (stalks and leaves) when making salads, appetizers and vegetable cocktails to add a natural saltiness. Celery combines well with eggs, apples and walnuts. The light, almost white inner stalks are tender and serve well with dips. Pan-fry, include in stir-fries, braise or chop and include celery in baked dishes.

Celeriac is the root of a different variety of celery than the common table celery. It adds a stronger celery flavor to dishes. Scrub and cut celeriac into wedges. Peel the tough outer skin of celeriac and slice or chop. To prevent browning, drop the pieces into a bowl of water with a squeeze of lemon juice added. Steam, broil, stir-fry or cook celeriac au gratin with other vegetables.

Recipe:
- Jerusalem Artichoke Stew (page 251)

Celeriac

See Celery

Chile Peppers

Capsicum annuum

Actions: Stimulant, tonic, diaphoretic, stimulates blood flow to the skin, antiseptic, antibacterial, expectorant, prevents bronchitis, prevents emphysema, decongestant, blood thinner, carminative.

Uses: Chiles are hot peppers (including cayenne, jalapeño, ancho/poblano, habanero, serrano and pasilla to name only a few) that contain the active element capsaicin. They are high in vitamin A and contain some vitamin C, iron, magnesium, phosphorus and potassium. Chile peppers help people with bronchitis and related problems by irritating the bronchial tubes and sinuses by causing the secretion of a fluid that thins the constricting mucus and helps move it out of the body. Capsaicin also blocks the pain message from the brain, making it an effective pain reliever. In addition, it also has clot-dissolving properties that make it useful if taken on a consistent basis. See also Cayenne Pepper (page 108).

Buying and Storing: Look for firm, crisp peppers with smooth skin and no blemishes. Store peppers in a paper bag in the produce drawer of the refrigerator for up to 4 days. Peppers freeze easily and may be added to sauces, soups and stews without thawing. Buy clean, fully dried chile peppers and store in a cool dry place.

Culinary Use: Wash and handle chile peppers carefully and wash hands thoroughly after handling because capsaicin will irritate skin and eyes. Remove the stem and inside pulp including seeds (seeds do not contain the fire). When first using chile peppers add half of the recommended amount to the recipe. Taste and add more, if desired.

Use fresh, reconstituted dried or canned chiles in recipes. Whisk in a drop of hot or jerk sauce or a quarter teaspoon (1 mL) of powdered cayenne to sauces, dips, dressings, soups or smoothies to substitute for fresh chiles.

Recipes:
- Baked Plantain and Peanut Stew (page 249)
- Black Bean and Four-Pepper Stew (page 242)
- Green Curry Paste (page 256)
- Red Hot Hummus (page 184)
- Stir-Fried Chipotle Chili (page 296)
- Succotash and Corn Dumplings (page 238)
- Tomato Sauce (page 151)
- West African Mafé (page 250)

Collard Greens

See Leafy Greens

Corn

Zea mays

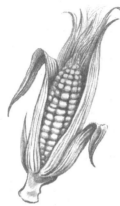

Actions: Anticancer, antiviral, raises estrogen level, neutralizes stomach acid, high fiber helps with kidney stones and water retention.

Uses: Corn is a good source of B_1 (thiamin) and B_6 (pyridoxine). Corn adds roughage to the diet.

Caution: Corn and corn products (cereals, corn chips or foods with cornstarch) may trigger food intolerances that lead to chronic conditions, including rheumatoid arthritis, headaches and irritable bowel syndrome.

Buying and Storing: Fresh corn is best if cooked within minutes of picking. When that is not possible, buy fresh corn that has been kept cold and use as soon as possible.

Culinary Use: Corn is sweet and blends with most vegetables. It is added to soups, risottos, egg dishes, salads, grains and baked vegetable dishes. Use leftover cooked fresh corn by slicing kernels off the cob with a sharp knife. Frozen or canned whole-kernel corn packed in water can be used when fresh is not available.

Recipes:
- Corn, Beans and Squash Bake with Oat Nut Topping (page 275)
- Roasted Corn Salsa (page 190)
- Spinach Cream Gazpacho (page 200)
- Succotash and Corn Dumplings (page 238)
- Vegetable Pancakes (page 160)

Cucumbers

Cucumis sativus

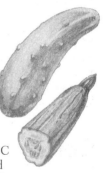

Actions: Diuretic, anti-inflammatory.

Uses: The ascorbic and caffeic acids in cucumbers help soothe skin irritations and reduce swelling. Cucumbers are moderate sources of vitamins C and A, potassium, manganese and folate. They are high in water, making cucumbers refreshing vegetables for summer salads. Cucumbers contain sterols, which may help the heart by reducing cholesterol.

Buying and Storing: Choose bright shiny green-skinned, firm cucumbers. Avoid yellow spots (although this is a sign of ripeness, the seeds will be bitter and the flesh too soft) and wax on the skin. Store in the produce drawer of the refrigerator for 4 to 5 days.

Culinary Use: Wash before using, peel (especially if skin has been waxed or if not organic), cut into cubes and leave seeds intact. Shred into salads and sauces. Use thinly sliced fresh cucumbers to replace greens in some salads.

Recipes:
- Fennel and Cucumber Salad with Ginger Dressing (page 204)
- Grilled Mediterranean Vegetable and Lentil Salad (page 210)
- Vegetable Raita (page 187)

Eggplant

Solanum melongena

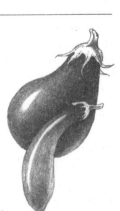

Actions: Antibacterial, diuretic, may lower blood cholesterol, may prevent cancerous growths.

Uses: Now used topically to treat skin cancer, eggplant's terpenes may also work internally to deactivate steroidal hormones that promote certain cancers. A fair amount of potassium in eggplant normalizes blood pressure. They are a good source of folate, vitamin B_6 (pyridoxine) and vitamin C. Eggplant is low in fat and calories.

Buying and Storing: Choose small, heavy, deep purple eggplants with firm, smooth skin that have no scrapes, cuts or bruises. Use immediately or keep for 1 to 2 days in the produce drawer of the refrigerator.

Culinary Use: Wash before using, peel (if not organic), cut into cubes and leave seeds intact. Salting is not as important now because the varieties sold today are not as bitter, but it can prevent the absorption of oil in recipes in which they are fried. The meaty texture and subtle, earthy flavor are what makes eggplant popular in vegetarian dishes. Eggplants are used in dips, appetizers and baked vegetable dishes such as moussaka, ratatouille and curries. Garlic, onions, tomato sauce and mozzarella cheese enhance eggplant in baked dishes.

Recipes:
- Country-Style Eggplant (page 170)
- Creamy White Sauce (page 149)
- Eggplant and Lentil Stew (page 241)
- Eggplant Curry (page 260)
- Eggplant, Lettuce and Tomato Sandwiches (page 344)
- Eggplant Wraps (page 274)
- Garlic White Sauce (page 150)
- Grilled Mediterranean Vegetable and Lentil Salad (page 210)
- Maple and Orange–Glazed Eggplant (page 214)
- Moroccan Roasted Vegetables with Garlic Mashed Potatoes (page 283)
- Roasted Eggplant and Artichoke Dip (page 186)
- Roasted Vegetable Lasagna (page 232)
- Roasted Vegetables with Garlic White Sauce (page 282)
- Sweet and Sour Tempeh and Eggplant Stir-Fry (page 289)

Fennel

Foeniculum vulgare

Actions: Antioxidant, anti-inflammatory, anticancer. For the medicinal benefits of fennel seeds, see page 112.

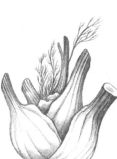

Uses: A bulb-like vegetable similar to celery, but with a distinctly sweet anise taste, fennel is a good source of vitamin C. Fennel also contains potassium, manganese, folate, phosphorus and calcium.

Buying and Storing: Avoid bulbs with wilted or browning stalks or leaves. The bulb should be firm and white with a light green tinge. Remove leaves and keep for up to 1 week in the refrigerator.

Culinary Use: Use the leaves in recipes if they are still attached to the stalks. Use raw fennel with vegetables for dipping or in a salad. Soups and stews and all baked vegetable dishes are enhanced by fennel. One-quarter fennel bulb measures about 1 cup (250 mL) when chopped.

Recipes:
- Fennel and Cucumber Salad with Ginger Dressing (page 204)
- Mushroom-Stuffed Fennel and Red Peppers (page 228)
- Red Curry Cauliflower (page 258)
- Roast Potatoes, Fennel and Leeks (page 286)

Garlic

See Herbs

Kale

See Leafy Greens

Kohlrabi

See Cabbage

Leafy Greens

kale, Swiss chard, collard greens, mustard greens, turnip greens, lettuce

Actions: Antioxidant, anticancer.

Uses: Although the nutrient amounts change with each green, in general it can be said that leafy greens are excellent sources of vitamin A and chlorophyll, and good sources of vitamin C, with some calcium, iron, folic acid and potassium.

Buying and Storing: Buy bright green, crisp (not wilted) greens and store them unwashed in a vented plastic bag in a cold spot in the refrigerator. Leafy greens are very tender and will go limp and turn yellow (or brown) when not stored or handled properly. Store away from fruits and wash just before using.

Culinary Use: Remove tough spine and stem, and shred or chop leafy greens or tear the tender greens for salads. The stronger-tasting greens (kale, Swiss chard, collard, mustard, turnip) work well in hearty dishes like curries, legumes and spicy Indian and Moroccan dishes. Use the milder flavored greens in salads, with grains and as garnishes.

Recipes:
- Baked Winter Greens (page 276)
- Braised Greens with Cherries and Pine Nuts (page 223)
- Chickpea and Swiss Chard Ragoût (page 245)
- Citrus Greens with Fig Dressing (page 209)
- Citrus Wheat Berries and Greens (page 323)
- Maple-Glazed Cabbage Greens with Pecans (page 217)
- Mushroom and Sweet Potato Cocktail Quesadillas (page 161)
- Potato, Leek and Kale Curry (page 265)
- Spinach-Stuffed Red Pepper Rolls (page 174)
- Vietnamese Spring Rolls with Peanut Sauce (page 172)

Leeks

Allium ampeloprasum

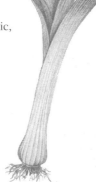

Actions: Expectorant, diuretic, relaxant, laxative, antiseptic, digestive, hypotensive.

Uses: Leeks are easily digested and often used in tonics, especially during convalescence from illness. They can be blended in toddies for relief from sore throats due to their warming, expectorant and stimulating qualities. Leeks are good sources of folate and contain some vitamin C, B$_2$ (riboflavin), allicin, quercetin and magnesium.

Buying and Storing: Choose leeks with firm white bulbs with white roots still intact and crisp, bright green tops. Leeks with the base removed will deteriorate quickly. Unwashed and kept in a plastic bag in the refrigerator, leeks should last from 1 to 2 weeks.

Culinary Use: Trim white roots and outer dark green leaves, split and wash under running water to remove grit or soil trapped between the layers. Slice, chop or cut into chunks. Leeks may be used raw but mellow and soften when cooked. Savory tarts, casseroles, soups, stuffing, egg dishes, pasta and baked vegetable dishes make good use of the milder onion-like taste of leeks.

Recipes:
- Baked Cranberry Tofu with Creamed Asparagus and Leeks (page 270)
- Cauliflower Gratin (page 272)
- Cream of Leek and Asparagus on Toast Points (page 171)
- French Canadian Onion Soup (page 201)
- Herbed Tomato-Leek Sauce (page 285)
- Leek, Kohlrabi, Garlic and Onion Tart (page 273)
- Moroccan Pumpkin Soup (page 193)
- Mushroom Broth (page 138)
- Potato, Leek and Kale Curry (page 265)
- Roast Potatoes, Fennel and Leeks (page 286)
- Roasted Squash and Parsnip Stew (page 244)
- Vegetable Stock (page 137)

Lettuce

See Leafy Greens

Mushrooms

Actions: see Maitake and Shiitake, page 80.

Uses: Used and thought of as a vegetable, mushrooms are actually fungi living off other host organisms. Mushrooms reproduce by spores and have no roots, leaves, flowers or seeds, as do plants.

Buying and Storing: Look for mushrooms that are firm, plump and clean. Mushrooms should be free of any signs of softness, deterioration or mold. Common button mushrooms are widely available. Fresh mushroom varieties such as portobello, oyster, cremini, shiitake and maitake, and dried whole or cut mushrooms are available in Oriental markets, whole or natural food stores and some supermarkets. Store fresh mushrooms, loosely covered, in a paper bag for up to 5 days. Dried mushrooms keep for up to 6 months if stored in a cool dry place.

Caution: Always purchase mushrooms from reliable sources such as supermarkets and food markets. Many mushroom varieties are toxic and eating varieties from the wild may be fatal.

Raw mushrooms contain hydrazines, potentially toxic substances that are destroyed in cooking or drying. Do not eat fresh, raw mushrooms — always cook them.

Culinary Use: Clean mushrooms using a minimum amount of water or wipe with a clean, damp cloth. Cooking with shiitake and maitake mushrooms at least three times per week (more if possible) will contribute to overall immune and cardiovascular health and may lower your risk of cancer.

Whole, fresh mushrooms are roasted or grilled. Halved or chopped mushrooms are used in stews, broths and soups. Sliced mushrooms for rice (risotto) and grain dishes, stir-fries and roasted vegetable dishes. Shredded mushrooms complement cooked salads and sandwich fillings.

Dried mushrooms are added to soups and stews or reconstituted by soaking them in water or other liquids. Save the soaking water and use it in soups, stews, gravies and sauces or add to other cooking liquids in recipes.

Recipes:
- Bok Choy, Mushroom and Black Bean Stir-Fry (page 288)
- Creamy Asparagus Soup (page 195)
- Maple Baked Beans (page 269)
- Mini Mushroom Burgers with Apricot Tamarind Marmalade (page 168)
- Mushroom and Sweet Potato Cocktail Quesadillas (page 161)
- Mushroom Bean Loaf with Herbed Tomato-Leek Sauce (page 284)
- Mushroom Broth (page 138)
- Mushroom Lasagna (page 299)
- Mushroom Sauce (page 154)
- Mushroom-Stuffed Fennel and Red Peppers (page 228)
- Portobello Mushrooms With Olive Tapenade (page 167)
- Portobello Pot-au-Feu (page 280)
- Potato Cake (page 276)
- Roasted Mushroom and Wild Rice Soup (page 196)
- Roasted Vegetable Lasagna (page 232)
- Steamed Rice and Mushroom Pockets (page 164)
- Summer Vegetable Ragoût (page 248)
- Sweet Potato and Black-Eyed Pea Curry (page 266)
- Sweet Potato Ragoût (page 246)
- Tomato Sauce (page 151)

Maitake Mushroom

Grifola frondosa

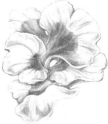

Maitake means dancing mushroom in Japan because it is made up of many overlapping, fan-shaped fruit bodies that resemble butterflies dancing. In North America, maitake mushrooms are referred to as "hen of the woods" because they grow at the base of trees or stumps in big clusters resembling a hen's tail feathers.

Actions: Liver protective, lowers blood pressure, protect against breast and colorectal cancers, antioxidant.

Uses: In the late 1980s, Japanese scientists identified the maitake mushroom as being more potent than any mushroom previously studied. Maitake has remarkable tonic effects, especially on the immune system. It is used in the prevention of some cancers and may help protect against high blood pressure, constipation, diabetes and HIV.

Maitake's polysaccharide compound, known as beta 1,6 glucan (or D-fraction) is recognized by researchers as the most effective active agent stimulating cellular immune responses and inhibiting tumors.

Shiitake Mushroom

Lentinula edodes

Amber to brown, medium in size and traditional mushroom shaped. Shiitake have a flat, leathery cap, with a tough, woody stem.

Actions: Recognized as a symbol of longevity in Asia, shiitake mushrooms have long been used in traditional Chinese medicine. They have proven immune-boosting, antitumor, anticancer, antiviral, anti-AIDS, antibacterial, cholesterol lowering, hepato-protective and liver-protective properties.

Uses: A strengthened immune response due to the action of shiitake mushrooms means increased body resistance to bacterial, viral, fungal and parasitic infections. Shiitake is beneficial in soothing bronchial inflammation, regulating urinary incontinence, reducing chronic high cholesterol and inhibiting cancer metastasis. It is used to treat arthritis and chronic fatigue syndrome.

Lentinan in shiitake mushrooms has been shown to enhance immunity cells in clearing the body of tumor cells and in fighting HIV and hepatitis B viruses. Lentinan is one of three different anticancer drugs extracted from mushrooms approved by Japan's Health and Welfare Ministry. According to Dr. Moss, an expert in cancer treatment, incorporating fresh or dried shiitake into a diet rich in whole grains, vegetables and fruits is a low-cost cancer prevention strategy.

One 8 oz (250 g) serving yields 20% of the body's daily requirement of iron. Shiitake mushrooms are high in vitamin C, protein, dietary fiber and calcium.

Caution: Shiitake mushrooms contain uric acid forming purines and individuals with kidney problems or gout may wish to limit or avoid them.

Mustard Greens

See Leafy Greens

Onions

Allium species

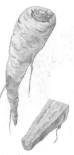

Actions: Antibacterial, anticancer, antioxidant, circulatory and digestive stimulant, antiseptic, lower cholesterol, hypotensive, hypoglycemic, diuretic, heart protective.

Uses: Onions help prevent thrombosis, reduce high blood pressure, lower blood sugar, prevent inflammatory responses and prohibit the growth of cancer cells. Shallots and yellow or red onions are the richest dietary source of quercetin, a potent antioxidant and cancer-inhibiting phytochemical. Onions are good sources of vitamin B_1 (thiamin), vitamin B_6 (pyridoxine) and vitamin C.

Buying and Storing: Choose onions that feel firm and have dry, tight skins. Avoid onions with woody centers in the neck and black powdery patches. If stored in a cool dry place with good air circulation, onions will keep for up to 1 month or more.

Culinary Use: Vidalia, red and Spanish onions are milder in flavor than yellow cooking onions. Shallots have a mild delicate flavor and are used whole in some dishes. Use onions raw in salads, sandwich fillings and for toppings. Include onions in stir-fries, salsas and other sauces, pasta, stuffing,

baked vegetable dishes, soups and stews. They caramelize and sweeten when roasted.

Recipes:
- Caramelized Red Onions (page 158)
- Cashew Curry Sauce (page 156)
- Country-Style Eggplant (page 170)
- Creamy White Sauce (page 149)
- French Canadian Onion Soup (page 201)
- Garlic White Sauce (page 150)
- Green Pea and Asparagus Curry (page 259)
- Hearty Potato and Leek Soup (page 194)
- Leek, Kohlrabi, Garlic and Onion Tart (page 273)
- Maple–Roasted Garlic Glaze (page 148)
- Mushroom Broth (page 138)
- Roasted Fingerling Potatoes with Shallots and Rosemary (page 221)
- Roasted Spice-Glazed Root Vegetables (page 215)
- Roasted Squash and Parsnip Stew (page 244)
- Roasted Vegetable Hummus (page 185)
- Tofu Aïoli (page 178)
- Tomato Grilling Sauce (page 152)
- Tomato Sauce (page 151)
- Vegetable Stock (page 137)

Parsnips

Pastinaca sativa

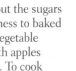

Actions: Anti-inflammatory, anticancer.

Uses: Parsnips are best fresh, after frost has concentrated the carbohydrate into sugar, making them sweeter. They are a good source of vitamin C and E, as well as potassium with some protein, iron and calcium. Like other root vegetables, parsnips store well and are an excellent fresh winter vegetable.

Buying and Storing: Look for firm flesh with no shriveling, soft spots or cuts. Parsnips should snap when bent. Small thin parsnips with tops still intact are best (remove and discard the tops before storing). Keep in a vented plastic bag in the refrigerator for up to $1\frac{1}{2}$ weeks.

Culinary Use: Small, fresh parsnips are surprisingly sweet and roasting brings out the sugars even more. Parsnips add natural sweetness to baked goods, soups, sauces, stir-fries, baked vegetable dishes and jams. Pair older parsnips with apples and/or carrots for a more pleasant taste. To cook parsnips, wash and peel if not organic, roughly chop, place in a small saucepan, cover with water and simmer until soft.

Recipes:
- Parsnip Carrot Cake (page 360)
- Roast Vegetable and Polenta Pie (page 287)
- Roasted Spice-Glazed Root Vegetables (page 215)
- Roasted Squash and Parsnip Stew (page 244)
- Roasted Vegetables with Garlic White Sauce (page 282)
- Spiced Winter Vegetables (page 263)
- Tomato Sauce (page 151)
- Vegetable and Tempeh Pie (page 236)
- Winter Vegetable Bake with Coconut Nut Topping (page 277)

Peas

See Beans

Peppers

Capsicum annuum
green, red, yellow, orange
and purple bell peppers

Actions: Antioxidant, anticancer, heart protective.

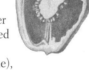

Uses: Red peppers are high in vitamins C and A (supplying over 100% of the Daily Recommended Amounts of each) and are good sources of vitamin B_6 (pyridoxine), with some manganese, folate and potassium.

Buying and Storing: Look for firm, crisp peppers with smooth skin and no blemishes. Avoid waxed peppers because the wax can accelerate bacteria growth. Store peppers in a paper bag in the crisper drawer of the refrigerator for up to 4 days. Peppers freeze easily and may be added to soups and stews without thawing.

Culinary Use: Peppers are versatile vegetables, used raw in appetizers, salads and fillings. Mediterranean cooking relies on peppers for vegetable dishes. Orange, red and yellow varieties are sweeter in flavor than the green and purple types. For directions on roasting red peppers, see page 132.

Recipes:
- Black Bean and Four-Pepper Stew (page 242)
- Grilled Mediterranean Vegetable and Lentil Salad (page 210)
- Mushroom-Stuffed Fennel and Red Peppers (page 228)

- Red Pepper Sauce (page 150)
- Roasted Corn Salsa (page 190)
- Roasted Red Peppers with Moroccan Couscous (page 220)
- Roasted Tomato and Red Pepper Soup (page 198)
- Roasted Vegetable Hummus (page 185)
- Roasted Vegetable Lasagna (page 232)
- Roasted Vegetable Salad (page 208)
- Roasted Zucchini Shells with Almond Filling and Red Pepper Sauce (page 281)
- Romesco Tomato Tapenade (page 189)
- Spinach-Stuffed Red Pepper Rolls (page 174)
- Vegetable Pancakes (page 160)
- Vietnamese Spring Rolls with Peanut Sauce (page 172)

Potatoes

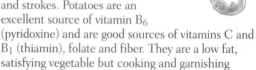

Solanum tuberosum
white, yellow, red, purple

Actions: Anticancer, heart protective.

Uses: Potatoes are high in potassium, which may help prevent high blood pressure and strokes. Potatoes are an excellent source of vitamin B_6 (pyridoxine) and are good sources of vitamins C and B_1 (thiamin), folate and fiber. They are a low fat, satisfying vegetable but cooking and garnishing methods determines how nutritious they are.

Buying and Storing: Select clean, smooth, well-shaped potatoes. Wrinkled skin, soft spots and bruises should be avoided. One medium potato weighs about 8 oz (250 g) and dices into about 1 cup (250 mL). If kept in a dry cool and frost-free place (cellar or porch), potatoes will last for 2 to 3 weeks. Keep covered with a brown paper or burlap bag because light causes potatoes to form chlorophyll and turn green. The green itself is not harmful but it is a sign that there is an increase in solanine, a glycoalkaloid that can cause allergic reactions and illness.

Culinary Use: Fresh potatoes are a versatile staple, cooked in gratins, soups, stews, and salads and baked vegetable dishes. They are mashed, boiled, roasted, sautéed, baked or deep-fried. Always use fresh potatoes.

Recipes:
- Almond Garlic Spread (page 179)
- Avocado Vichyssoise (page 199)
- Cauliflower Gratin (page 272)

- Chickpeas and Potatoes in Cashew Cream (page 240)
- Garlic Mashed Potatoes (page 224)
- Hearty Potato and Leek Soup (page 194)
- Moroccan Roasted Vegetables with Garlic Mashed Potatoes (page 283)
- Potato Cake (page 276)
- Potato, Leek and Kale Curry (page 265)
- Quinoa Beet Potato Salad (page 325)
- Roast Potatoes, Fennel and Leeks (page 286)
- Roasted Fingerling Potatoes with Shallots and Rosemary (page 221)
- Shredded Vegetable Bake (page 222)
- Winter Vegetable Bake with Coconut Nut Topping (page 277)
- Zucchini Moussaka (page 268)

Pumpkin

See Squash

Rutabagas

Brassica napo brassica
See Turnips

Spinach

Spinacea oleracea

Actions: Anticancer, helps memory, antioxidant, promotes healing, prevents cataracts, anti-anemia.

Uses: A good source of choline, which improves mental functioning, and folic acid (a heart protector), spinach is one of only four vegetables high in vitamin E. It is also high in cancer-fighting lutein, as well as chlorophyll and vitamins C and A. Spinach is a good source of calcium, iron, protein and potassium.

Buying and Storing: Choose loose spinach instead of packaged whenever available. Look for broad, crisp leaves with deep green color and no signs of yellow, wilting or softness. Spinach keeps for up to 3 days in a vented plastic bag in the produce drawer of the refrigerator. Pick over and remove yellow or wilted leaves of pre-packaged spinach and rewrap in a vented plastic bag for storing.

Culinary Use: Wash fresh leaves well, remove tough spine and stem and shred or coarsely chop the leaves. Spinach is served raw in salads and appetizers. It may be added to soups, sauces, stuffing, risottos, vegetable dishes and pasta. To measure, tightly pack torn or chopped spinach into a dry measuring cup. Use frozen, or canned spinach when fresh is not available.

Recipes:
- Citrus Wheat Berries and Greens (page 323)
- Curried Green Sauté (page 226)
- Garlic Greens with Chickpeas and Cumin (page 219)
- Madras Frites (page 225)
- Penne with Spinach-Artichoke Cream Sauce (page 300)
- Portobello Pot-au-Feu (page 280)
- Potato and Vegetable Scallop (page 234)
- Potato Rösti (page 224)
- Spiced Winter Vegetables (page 263)
- Spinach and Whole-Grain Salad with Kiwi Dressing (page 207)
- Spinach Cream Gazpacho (page 200)
- Spinach-Stuffed Red Pepper Rolls (page 174)
- Vietnamese Spring Rolls with Peanut Sauce (page 172)

Squash

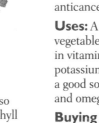

Cucurbita species
acorn, butternut, hubbard, pumpkin, turban

Actions: Antioxidant, anticancer.

Uses: A good winter vegetable, squash is high in vitamins A and C and potassium. Squash is also a good source of manganese, folate and omega-3 fatty acids.

Buying and Storing: Summer squash, such as zucchini, pattypan, cocozelle and the marrows, are small and tender with pliable skin and seeds. Winter squash, such as acorn, spaghetti, butternut, hubbard and pumpkin, have matured on the vine and their rind and seeds are tough and woody. Keep whole squash in a cold moist place or in the produce drawer of the refrigerator. Winter squash may keep as long as 1 month if stored properly. Cooked squash freezes well for use in recipes.

Culinary Use: Squash is often baked whole or split, seeded and baked. Acorn squash is often stuffed with a variety of savory fillings and baked. Use squash in soups, stews, pasta sauces and some baked goods. To bake, wash and prick with a sharp knife. Arrange whole squash on a baking dish and bake at 375°F (190°C) for 40 to 45 minutes or until tender.

Recipes:
- Black Bean and Four-Pepper Stew (page 242)
- Corn, Beans and Squash Bake with Oat Nut Topping (page 275)
- Creamy White Sauce (page 149)
- Herbed Millet and Spaghetti Squash (page 320)
- Moroccan Pumpkin Soup (page 193)
- Red Curry Cauliflower (page 258)
- Roasted Butternut Squash with Spiced Lima Beans (page 279)
- Roasted Mushroom and Wild Rice Soup (page 196)
- Roasted Squash and Parsnip Stew (page 244)
- Roasted Squash Gnocchi (page 302)
- Roasted Squash in Cashew Curry Sauce (page 278)
- Succotash and Corn Dumplings (page 238)
- West African Mafé (page 250)
- Yellow Barley Risotto (page 311)

Sweet Potatoes

Ipomoea batatas

Actions: Antioxidant, anticancer, heart protective.

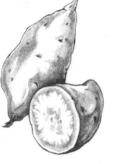

Uses: Sweet potatoes are high in vitamin A (retinol), beta-carotene, vitamin C and fiber. They are a good source of copper and potassium and they also contain some calcium, iron, magnesium and zinc.

Buying and Storing: Select clean, smooth, well-shaped and firm sweet potatoes. Wrinkled skin, soft spots and bruises should be avoided. If kept in a cool dry and frost-free place (cellar or porch), sweet potatoes will last for up to 1 month.

Culinary Use: Although not related to the ordinary potato, sweet potatoes are often prepared in the same way, with baking as the most common method. Mashed sweet potatoes make a good topping for baked vegetable dishes. One medium sweet potato weighs about 10 ounces (300 grams) and dices into about 1 cup (250 mL).

Recipes:
- Moroccan Chickpea Tagine (page 230)

- Mushroom and Sweet Potato Cocktail Quesadillas (page 161)
- Roasted Mushroom and Wild Rice Soup (page 196)
- Sweet Potato and Black-Eyed Pea Curry (page 266)
- Sweet Potato, Bean and Wild Rice Quesadillas (page 292)
- Sweet Potato Crackers (page 177)
- Sweet Potato Curried Cauliflower Soup (page 192)
- Sweet Potato Ragoût (page 246)
- Sweet Potato Spread (page 182)
- Sweet Potato Wild Rice Cakes (page 308)
- Vegetable Paella (page 295)
- West African Mafé (page 250)

Swiss Chard

See Leafy Greens

Tomatoes

Lycopersicon esculentum

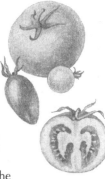

Actions: Antioxidant, anticancer.

Uses: High in lycopene and glutathione, two powerful antioxidants, raw tomatoes reduce the risk of many cancers. Lycopene is also thought to help maintain mental and physical functioning and is absorbed by the body more efficiently when tomatoes are juiced. Tomatoes also contain glutamic acid that is converted in the human system to gamma-amino butyric acid (GABA), a calming agent, known to be effective for kidney hypertension. Drink tomato juice or smoothies made with tomatoes to relax after a stressful day. Tomatoes are also good sources of vitamins B_6 (pyrodoxine) and C.

Buying and Storing: Vine-ripened heritage varieties have the best flavor. Tomatoes are best bought fresh only when in season (use canned or reconstituted dried at other times). Local tomatoes are not treated with ethylene gas to force reddening. Plump, heavy, firm skinned, bright red tomatoes keep for 2 to 3 days at room temperature. When almost over-ripe, store tomatoes in the refrigerator for 1 or 2 more days only.

Culinary Use: Raw fresh tomatoes are used in salads, sandwiches and as a side dish in the summertime. Fresh tomatoes are stuffed and eaten raw or baked. To remove the skin, cut a cross in the skin of each tomato using a paring knife. Place in a heatproof bowl and cover with boiling water. Leave for 30 seconds and drain. The skins will easily slip off. To remove the seeds, cut tomatoes in half and gently squeeze the seeds out. Use canned tomatoes in sauces, soups, stews and baked vegetable dishes.

Recipes:
- Chickpea and Swiss Chard Ragoût (page 245)
- Eggplant and Lentil Stew (page 241)
- Eggplant, Lettuce and Tomato Sandwiches (page 344)
- Hearty Potato and Leek Soup (page 194)
- Herbed Tomato-Leek Sauce (page 285)
- Lentil and Broccoli Casserole (page 231)
- Mini Mushroom Burgers with Apricot Tamarind Marmalade (page 168)
- Moroccan Roasted Vegetables with Garlic Mashed Potatoes (page 283)
- Okra and Broad Beans with Tomato Sauce (page 213)
- Red Hot Hummus (page 184)
- Roasted Garlic and Lentil Soup (page 197)
- Roasted Spice-Glazed Root Vegetables (page 215)
- Roasted Squash and Parsnip Stew (page 244)
- Roasted Tomato and Red Pepper Soup (page 198)
- Roasted Vegetable Lasagna (page 232)
- Romesco Tomato Tapenade (page 189)
- Spinach Cream Gazpacho (page 200)
- Tomato and Zucchini Bulgur (page 332)
- Tomato Grilling Sauce (page 152)
- Tomato Sauce (page 151)
- Zucchini Moussaka (page 268)

Turnips

Brassica rapa

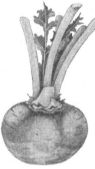

Actions: Tonic, decongestant, antibacterial, anticancer, diuretic.

Uses: Turnips have a beneficial effect on the urinary system. They purify the blood and aid in the elimination of toxins. For this reason, they make a good addition to recipes. Both the root and the green tops are high in glucosinolates, which are thought to block the development of cancer. Good sources of calcium, iron and protein, small fresh tender turnips are available in the spring and sometimes in the fall.

Buying and Storing: Small, firm turnips with dark green leaves showing no signs of wilting or yellow are best. Rutabagas (similar to turnips but a different species in the cabbage family) may be waxed to hold in their moisture and are generally a lot bigger than the young fresh turnip. Turnips keep for up to 1 week in a vented plastic bag in the refrigerator. Rutabagas will keep longer.

Culinary Use: Fresh turnips can be hot and peppery in taste. They may be steamed, boiled or shredded and added raw to salads. Treat young turnips as you would parsnips — add to soups, stews and baked vegetable dishes. For using the green leafy turnip tops, see Leafy Greens, page 78.

Recipes:
- Fruited Rutabaga Purée (page 216)
- Gingered Carrot-Turnip Purée (page 218)
- Herbed Carrot and Turnip Fritters (page 177)
- Jerusalem Artichoke Stew (page 251)
- Pad Thai (page 291)
- Portobello Pot-au-Feu (page 280)
- Roasted Spice-Glazed Root Vegetables (page 215)
- Shredded Vegetable Bake (page 222)
- West African Mafé (page 250)

Watercress

Rorippa nasturtium-aquaticum

Actions: Antioxidant, diuretic, anticancer, tonic, antibiotic, cleansing.

Uses: High in fiber and vitamin C, and a good source of vitamin A. Purchase from farmers' markets in spring. Watercress grows wild around streams and wet areas, but be careful not to harvest in areas where fields drain directly into streams.

Buying and Storing: Pick watercress just before using. If purchasing, choose bright green, crisp sprigs with leaves intact. Sort through and remove any yellow or wilted stems. Watercress is fragile and should be used immediately or wrapped in a towel in the produce drawer of the refrigerator for 1 or 2 days.

Culinary Use: Watercress adds a hot and peppery bite to salads and baked dishes. Use watercress to replace spinach, parsley or other greens in sauces, soups, fillings and egg dishes.

Recipe:
- Portobello Pot-au-Feu (page 280)

Wild Greens

dandelion leaves, mustard, sorrel, turnip,
wild garlic mustard, wild leeks or ramps

See Leafy Greens

Zucchini

Cucurbita pepo
Italian, yellow straightneck,
yellow crookneck

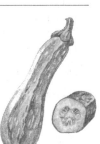

Actions: Antioxidant.

Uses: A good source of
vitamins A and C, folate,
potassium and B$_3$ (niacin),
zucchini is mild tasting and blends
well with stronger vegetables.

Buying and Storing: Although zucchini grows
quite large, the smaller fruit are tender and less
woody. Look for soft thin skin with no cuts or
bruises and stem end intact.

Culinary Use: The fresh flowers may be stuffed
and baked. Zucchini are eaten raw in salads, often
mixed with carrot. They are steamed, stir-fried
or added to soups, sauces, stews and baked
vegetable dishes.

Recipes:
- Cauliflower Gratin (page 272)
- Grilled Mediterranean Vegetable and Lentil Salad
  (page 210)
- Rice Noodles with Roasted Mediterranean
  Vegetables (page 298)
- Roasted Zucchini Shells with Almond Filling and
  Red Pepper Sauce (page 281)
- Steamed Rice and Mushroom Pockets (page 164)
- Stir-Fried Chipotle Chili (page 296)
- Summer Vegetable Ragoût (page 248)
- Tomato and Zucchini Bulgur (page 332)
- Vegetable and Tempeh Pie (page 236)
- Vietnamese Spring Rolls with Peanut Sauce
  (page 172)
- Zucchini Moussaka (page 268)

Legumes

Definition: Leguminous plants include 10,000 plant species. Peas and beans, along with clover, alfalfa, wisteria and lupines all produce their seeds in pods. The term "legume" is applied to the plant, the pods or the seeds. "Pulse" is a common term in Asia that means fresh or dry edible leguminous seeds. The words "pulse" and "legume" may be interchanged. "Dal" is a Middle Eastern term applied to lentils, mung beans and split peas. The word "dal" also refers to a puréed dish made from lentils, mung beans or split peas.

Actions/Uses: The high levels of fiber in legumes work to lower cholesterol in the body and prevent blood sugar levels from rising too rapidly after a meal. This makes legumes a good choice for individuals with diabetes, insulin resistance or hypoglycemia.

Legumes help to control weight by retaining water in the digestive tract, giving the feeling of fullness. Legumes flush fats rather than allowing the body to store them. The oils in legumes are rich in linoleic and linolenic acids, two of the three essential fatty acids, which help the immune system. The fiber in legumes is a valuable tool for preventing colon cancer.

The amino acids (protein) in beans and peas make them a valuable food for vegetarians. Legumes are low in the amino acid methionine and high in lysine. Cereals are high in methionine and low in lysine. When legumes are combined with cereals in a dish (for example Red Beans and Rice), the combined amino acids make up complete, high-quality protein, an important issue for vegetarians.

A 1-cup (250 mL) serving of most legumes delivers 100% or more of the Recommended Daily Amounts of molybdenum, a trace mineral responsible for detoxifying damaging sulfites in the body.

Legumes are high in most B vitamins — 1 cup/ 250 mL cooked beans yields 40% of the daily requirement of B_1 (thiamin) and B_6 (pyridoxine). A good source of iron and choline, which improves mental functioning, legumes also contain vitamin A and potassium as well as calcium and vitamin C.

Buying and Storing: Whole or natural food stores and ethnic (Middle Eastern, Indian, Caribbean) stores carry a wide selection of legumes both prepackaged and in bulk. Look for clean dried peas and beans with no signs of wrinkling or mildew. Dried legumes will keep for a very long time if kept in a clean glass container away from heat and light.

Culinary Use: Grain and legume dishes are especially important for vegetarians, who benefit from the complete proteins formed when grains and legumes are combined. Lentils and split peas may be added to soups and stews without soaking but all other legumes must be soaked to soften and rehydrate them. Soaking reduces the cooking time by half. Cooked canned peas, beans and lentils are an excellent and easy way to use legumes when time does not permit soaking and cooking the dried beans. When using canned legumes, if the recipe calls for them to be drained, reserve the liquid and use it in soups and stock recipes because it retains many of the water-soluble nutrients.

To Soak Legumes: Place washed beans in a large saucepan and cover with 2 inches (5 cm) of water. Bring to a boil over high heat. Reduce heat and gently simmer for 2 minutes. Leave the pan on the element and turn off the heat. Let stand 1 hour or overnight. Discard the soaking water and rinse the beans. Legumes have now been rehydrated and are ready to cook.

To Cook Legumes: Place soaked, drained, rinsed beans in a large saucepan. Cover with 2 inches (5 cm) of fresh water. Cover the pan and bring to a boil. Reduce heat and simmer for 45 minutes to 2 hours (cooking times differ for the varieties), or cook until tender. Add salt or other seasonings after legumes have been cooked because if added before, salt toughens the beans.

Adzuki Beans

Phaseolus angularis

Native of Asia, the small, oval, dark red adzuki beans grow on bushes rather than vines, as do most legumes. They are eaten fresh, dried or sprouted and ground into flour. The taste is mild, slightly nutty. Adzuki beans have a thick skin and take up to 2 hours to cook.

Black Beans

Phaseolus vulgaris

Large, shiny black, kidney-shaped beans from South America, black beans are a staple in South and Central American and Caribbean dishes. In traditional dishes, they are boiled and fried and often paired with rice for complete protein. The taste is earthy, with overtones of mushroom. Cook black beans for 1 hour.

Recipes:
- Black Bean and Four-Pepper Stew (page 242)
- Bok Choy, Mushroom and Black Bean Stir-Fry (page 288)
- Open-Face Black Bean Tostadas (page 343)
- Refried Rice and Beans (page 318)
- Roasted Eggplant and Artichoke Dip (page 186)
- Stir-Fried Chipotle Chili (page 296)
- Sweet Potato, Bean and Wild Rice Quesadillas (page 292)

Black-Eyed Peas

Vigna unguiculata

Originating in China, black-eyed peas traveled the Silk Route to Arabia and from there to Africa. Slaves carried them to America where they became an important part of "soul food" dishes.
Kidney-shaped and smooth, with thin skin, black-eyed peas are cream-colored with a definite black or brown spot or eye. They are smooth and buttery in texture and the taste is subtle. Black-eyed peas may be cooked in soups or stews without soaking. Check for doneness after 30 minutes and do not overcook, which will cause them to loose their texture.
Substitute black-eyed peas for flageolets in any recipe.

Recipes:
- Mushroom Bean Loaf with Herbed Tomato-Leek Sauce (page 284)
- Sweet Potato and Black-Eyed Pea Curry (page 266)

Cannellini Beans

Phaseolus vulgaris

See also Haricot Beans

Cannellini beans are a member of the haricot bean family and are used extensively in Italian cooking. Cannellini beans are white, oval and medium size. Their tough skin means that cannellini beans will take 1 to $1\frac{1}{2}$ hours to soften. Their texture is smooth and buttery and the taste is subtle, making them a good bean for soups and spreads.

Recipe:
- Jerusalem Artichoke Stew (page 251)

Chickpeas

Cicer arietinum

(also known as Garbanzo)

The Roman word, arietinum means "like a ram." Arietinum is an apt name for chickpeas because they resemble a ram's head with horns curling around the sides. Large, round and tan-colored, chickpeas are nutty in flavor and firm in texture. Chickpeas require up to $1\frac{1}{2}$ hours to cook. They are very versatile, used in salads, soups, stews, sauces, spreads and dips.

Recipes:
- Chickpea and Swiss Chard Ragoût (page 245)
- Chickpea Stuffing (page 158)
- Chickpeas and Potatoes in Cashew Cream (page 240)
- Chickpeas with Kiwi and Avocado Salsa (page 208)
- Garlic Greens with Chickpeas and Cumin (page 219)
- Moroccan Chickpea Tagine (page 230)
- Moroccan Roasted Vegetables with Garlic Mashed Potatoes (page 283)
- Potato Rösti (page 224)
- Red Hot Hummus (page 184)
- Roasted Vegetable Hummus (page 185)
- Seasoned Chickpeas and Almonds (page 338)
- Shredded Vegetable Bake (page 222)
- Vegetable Pancakes (page 160)

Fava Beans

Vicia faba

(also known as broad beans)

Used in European soups and stews since before medieval times, the fava bean has been an important staple throughout history. Fava beans are large, light brown or taupe in color with wrinkled skin and a strong, earthy flavor. They are usually tender after 1 hour of cooking. Fava beans can overwhelm some dishes and are at their best in hearty soups and stews.

Recipe:
- Lima Bean and Wheat Berry Stew (page 247)

Flageolets

Phaseolus vulgaris

See also Haricot Beans

Popular in French and Mediterranean dishes, flageolets are immature kidney beans, picked before they ripen and considered a delicacy. Smaller than mature kidney beans, flageolets are pale green, tender and very mild tasting. Salads are the best way to feature the subtle taste and texture of flageolets.

Recipe:
• Jerusalem Artichoke Stew (page 251)

Haricot Beans

Phaseolus vulgaris

The Haricot family of beans includes cannellini beans, great Northern beans, white kidney, navy beans, flageolets and small whites. They are the mature (except in the case of flageolets), dried white, small round or oval seeds of the green bean (string bean), known as *haricot vert* in France. These beans are common beans, easily found in most supermarkets and in dried soup packets. Haricot beans take about 1 hour to cook but stand up to long, slow simmering. They are the beans used in the fabulous French cassoulet and the popular Boston Baked Bean dish that originated in the city still known as Beantown.

Recipe:
• Roasted Butternut Squash with Spiced Lima Beans (page 279)

Red Kidney Beans

Phaseolus vulgaris

Native to Mexico, red kidney beans (sometimes called kidney) are now used throughout the world in ethnic dishes such as Chile con Carne and Three-Bean Salad. Also known as red beans, they have evolved into many different varieties. Kidney-shaped and usually deep red in color, kidney beans also come in brown, black and white varieties. The texture is mealy and the taste is rich and unique. Check for doneness after 1 hour of simmering because red kidney beans will start to loose their texture if cooked too long.

Recipes:
• Cranberry Baked Beans (page 235)
• Open-Face Black Bean Tostadas (page 343)
• Red Rice and Lentil Curry (page 262)
• Stir-Fried Chipotle Chili (page 296)

Lentils

Lens esculenta and *L. culinaris*

Dating from about 8000 BC, lentils are believed to be the first legumes to be cultivated. They originated in Asia and spread to India and the Middle East and are still very popular in dishes from those areas, where they play an important role in providing protein to the diet.

Lentils range in color from a tan and gray-brown, to dark brown, green, red, yellow and blue. They are small flat disks that can be very small ($1/8$ inch/0.25 cm) or larger ($1/4$ inch/0.5 cm). Lentils do not need to be presoaked and cook in 10 to 15 minutes. They should not be overcooked because they will loose their texture and turn to mush. Lentils are used in soups, baked vegetable dishes, stews and purées.

Recipes:
• How to Cook Lentils (page 309)
• Grilled Mediterranean Vegetable and Lentil Salad (page 210)
• Lentil and Broccoli Casserole (page 231)
• Lentil and Rice Bowl (page 309)
• Lentil Tagine (page 229)
• Potato and Vegetable Scallop (page 234)
• Red Lentil and Buckwheat Waffles (page 322)
• Red Rice and Lentil Curry (page 262)
• Roasted Garlic and Lentil Soup (page 197)
• Sweet Potato Ragoût (page 246)
• Yellow Curry Dal (page 216)

Lima Beans

Phaseolus lunatus

There are two main species of lima bean, the large lima from Central America and the smaller variety originating in Mexico. The name actually comes from the capital city of Peru. American Indians used lima beans as part of their three sisters dishes. Corn and squash were the other sisters. They have traveled around the world and are now the most important bean in Africa.

Lima beans are flat, white to pale green seeds with a mealy texture when cooked. Cook lima beans for 1 to $1/2$ hours. They are available fresh, dried, canned and frozen and can be added to soups and stews and baked grain and vegetable dishes.

Recipes:
• Lima Bean and Wheat Berry Stew (page 247)
• Roasted Butternut Squash with Spiced Lima Beans (page 279)
• Roasted Vegetable Lasagna (page 232)
• Succotash and Corn Dumplings (page 238)
• Vegetable Paella (page 295)

Mung Beans

Vigna radiata

Mung beans are sold with or without their husk. They can be whole or split. Native to India, they are known as *moong dal*. Mung beans are the variety of legume that the Chinese sprout (they are five times richer in vitamins A and B and contain vitamins C and B_{12} when sprouted). Each of the many varieties of mung beans are small, round and most often yellow inside a dull green skin. There are brown and black varieties but the green or yellow (when hulled) mung beans are the most common. Cook mung beans for less than 1 hour or add directly to soups and other dishes that will simmer for at least that long.

Recipe:
• How to Cook Lentils (v) (page 309)

Peas

Pisum sativum

Peas originated in the Middle East and spread to China, the Mediterranean, India and Europe. A staple in Greece, Rome and ultimately Great Britain, peas were the perfect food to grow in earlier times because they would keep all winter. Small, round, bright green when fresh, dried peas are usually split. Dried split peas are green or yellow. Use fresh, dried, canned or frozen peas. Fresh peas have a fresh, sweet taste. All dried split peas cook quickly without soaking and have a deeper, richer flavor than their fresh counterparts.

Recipes:
• Asian Primavera (page 306)
• Green Pea and Asparagus Curry (page 259)
• Spring Dolmades (page 162)
• Summer Vegetable Ragoût (page 248)
• Vegetable Pancakes (page 160)
• Warm Pear and Snow Pea Salad with Miso Dressing (page 205)

Soybeans

Glycine max

See Soy Foods (page 102)

Whole and Ancient Grains

Definition: Cereal grains are part of the grass family of plants. Whole grains have not been refined and stripped of their outer bran and inner germ. Whole grains supply complex carbohydrates and nutrients to the body because the whole seed package, with its three major sections and their nutrients, is intact.

Ancient is a term that is often used to describe grains (spelt, kamut) and herb seeds (quinoa, amaranth, teff) that have survived thousands of years without hybridization or significant genetic modification. They are much the same now as when prehistoric man gathered them. Ancient grains have largely been introduced to the Western world within the last half of the twentieth century and enjoy limited availability.

The outer layer, called bran, protects the life force and nourishment of all grains. Bran contains fiber, some minerals and protein. It is always removed when grains are refined. The largest part of grain is the endosperm, which provides a storehouse of food in the form of carbohydrate intended for the growing seed. The third, perhaps most important section of whole grains, the germ, is the life-spark of the grain. It is a rich source of protein, antioxidant vitamin E, phytate, iron, zinc and magnesium.

Actions/Uses: Whole grains supply fiber, which helps prevent against colon cancer. They are rich in phytoestrogens that halt the early stages of breast cancer and protect against cancer of the large intestine. The vitamin E in grains has an antioxidant effect. Whole grains protect against heart disease, fight obesity and lower blood sugar levels. Whole grains supply selenium, potassium and magnesium to the body. Each grain or seed listed below has its own nutrient quota.

Buying and Storing: Whole or natural food stores carry a wide selection of whole and ancient grains both packaged and in bulk. Purchase small quantities of ground grain and a wide variety of whole grains. Use them often, and store in glass containers below 65°F (18°C) or in the refrigerator.

Flavor: The presence of the outer bran makes whole grains chewier and more flavorful. A nutty flavor is evident, yet each grain species has its own characteristic flavor.

Culinary Use: Whole grains are sprouted, toasted, used with dried fruit as a breakfast cereal or casserole topping, cooked and added as an ingredient in baked products, soups, salads and stir-fries and baked with custard and fruit for desserts.

To Wash Whole Grains: Place whole grains in a sieve and swish in cool water. Whole grains benefit from presoaking for up to several hours before cooking. Whole grains double their bulk when cooked.

To Cook Whole-Grain Berries: Measure berries into a medium-size pot. Cover with twice the amount of water, place over medium-high heat and bring to a boil. Cover pot with a lid, turn heat off and set aside overnight or for a minimum of 2 to 3 hours. Most of the liquid will be absorbed. Test to see if the grain is tender. If not, add enough water to cover and simmer until tender (whole grains retain a chewy texture and never get soft like processed grain). Drain and store in a tightly covered glass jar in the refrigerator until ready to use. Cooked whole grains keep 2 to 3 days in the refrigerator.

Amaranth

Amaranthus cruentus

The only seed to provide humans with the most effective balance of protein matched only by milk, amaranth plays an important role in dairy-reduced diets. Lysine is higher in amaranth than any other complex carbohydrate. The ancient Aztecs revered amaranth as a "wonder food," not knowing that science would show it to be lean and high in vitamins and minerals and calcium.

Forms Available: Whole seed, flour and sometimes mixed with other grains in whole-grain blends.

Recipes:
• How to Cook Amaranth (page 329)
• Amaranth Vegetable Pilaf (page 329)

Barley

Hordeum vulgare

Barley is one of the oldest domesticated crops. The gummy fiber in barley is thought to be what is responsible for its ability to reduce high serum cholesterol levels in the body. Barley is a source of potassium, magnesium and B_3 (niacin).

Forms Available: Pot barley is the preferred form because it is milled just enough to remove the inedible hull. Scotch barley is coarsely ground hulled barley and has as many of the nutrients as pot barley. Not really a whole food, pearl barley is whiter than pot barley because more of the hull and bran layers are stripped along with much of the protein, fiber, vitamins and minerals. Rolled barley is pot barley that has been sliced, steamed, and rolled into flakes.

Recipes:
• Chickpea and Swiss Chard Ragoût (page 245)
• Yellow Barley Risotto (page 311)

Buckwheat

Fagopyrum esculentum

Buckwheat is not related to wheat, but is a plant in the same family as rhubarb. Buckwheat is an excellent source of antioxidants and it increases the quality of protein in the diet because it is higher in the amino acid lysine.

Forms Available: Whole kernel, white hulled buckwheat (called groats), kasha (hulled, crushed and toasted white buckwheat), flour and noodles (called soba).

Recipes:
• Red Lentil and Buckwheat Waffles (page 322)
• Spiced Apple Cake with Coconut Pecan Glaze (page 358)
• Spiced Winter Vegetables (page 263)

Bran

Bran is the outer layer of grains and contains fiber, protein and other nutrients. The easiest way to cook with bran is to buy whole grains with the bran still attached. Bran may be purchased at most supermarkets and whole or natural food stores. Store bran in the refrigerator and use it to add fiber and nutrients to most recipes or to enrich milled flour. Use 1 to 2 tbsp (15 to 25 mL) in baked goods, toppings, stir-fries and legume and vegetable dishes.

Forms Available: Oat, wheat and rye bran is available in flakes or buds.

Corn

Zea mays

Commonly called maize, corn is the only widely used grain that is native to the Western hemisphere. It has been proven that corn was grown and used some 80,000 years ago.

Forms Available: Whole corn kernels (see Corn, page 77) are dried and ground into other products. Corn flour is ground from a variety of corn with a soft starch that makes it easy to grind. Hard shell flint corn is ground to a coarse meal called polenta — very deep yellow-orange polenta is highest in beta-carotene. The Algonquin Indians discovered that soaking fresh corn with wood ashes until the kernels burst out of their skins and drying and grinding the inner corn kernels produces hominy and grits. Hominy and grits are not exactly whole foods, but they do deliver fiber and some protein and are usually combined with eggs, vegetables, cheese or legumes for balanced dishes. Cornmeal, polenta, hominy or grits that are processed by the old, traditional stone-ground method retain more of the bran and germ.

Recipes:
• Corn Biscuits (page 342)
• Roast Vegetable and Polenta Pie (page 287)

Kamut

Triticum polonicum

A non-hybrid form of wheat originating in the Fertile Crescent between Egypt and the Tigris-Euphrates region, kamut is truly an ancient grain. It is a good source of calcium, magnesium, phosphorus and potassium and supplies 12% of the body's daily protein requirements. Kamut is a much larger grain than wheat, with a mild, sweet, buttery and nutty flavor. Substitute kamut for wheat or spelt in any recipe.

Forms Available: Whole kernel and flour.

Recipes:
• How to Cook Kamut (page 331)
• Marinated Chickpea and Spelt Salad with Cilantro Dressing (page 330)
• Spiced Apple Cake with Coconut Pecan Glaze (page 358)
• Spinach and Whole-Grain Salad with Kiwi Dressing (page 207)

Millet

Panicum miliaceum

Native to Africa and Asia, millet is the round yellow seed of an annual grass. Millet is not a true cereal but related to sorghum, a type of millet. A good source of protein, millet is an excellent source of the B vitamins, magnesium, zinc, copper and iron.

Combine millet in vegetarian dishes with a good source of vitamin C such as carrots, oranges or broccoli.

Forms Available: Whole seed often mixed with other grains in whole-grain blends.

Recipes:
- How to Cook Millet (page 321)
- Herbed Millet and Spaghetti Squash (page 320)
- Spiced Winter Vegetables (page 263)

Oats

Avena sativa

Oats are higher in protein and essential fatty acids than other cereals because when hulled, the bran and germ remain intact with the groat. Oats are an excellent source of B vitamins and minerals.

Forms Available: Steel-cut oats contain the bran and germ while Scotch-cut (also known as Irish oats) are ground with stones and may be missing some nutrients. Steamed oat groats are sliced and rolled to make rolled oats. Whole rolled oats (also known as old-fashioned oats) are higher in nutrients than quick-cooking oats and the even thinner instant oats, which are partially cooked and may cook faster but are not considered whole foods.

Recipes:
- How to Cook Whole Oats (page 328)
- Corn, Beans and Squash Bake with Oat Nut Topping (page 275)
- Minted Raspberry-Marinated Oats (page 327)
- Oat Nut Topping (page 158)
- Oatmeal Coconut Cookies (page 347)
- Potato Cake (page 276)
- Spiced Apple Cake with Coconut Pecan Glaze (page 358)

Quinoa

Chenopodium quinoa

Actually an herb seed, quinoa is protein rich and extremely high in calcium (1 cup/250 mL of cooked quinoa equals the amount of calcium found in 1 quart/liter of milk). Gluten-free and easily digested, quinoa is classed as an ancient grain. Rinse thoroughly before using to remove the bitter saponin coating.

Forms Available: Whole seed.

Recipes:
- How to Cook Quinoa (page 326)
- Moroccan Chickpea Tagine (page 230)
- Orange-Spiked Power Cereal (page 340)
- Quinoa Beet Potato Salad (page 325)

Rice

Oryza sativa var.

A cereal originating in Asia, rice has been a staple there since about 5000 BC. Brown rice, or rice with the bran intact, is rich in B vitamins, protein, magnesium and fiber and that is why it is considered whole. Eat rice with a fruit or vegetable high in vitamin C.

Forms Available: More than 25 varieties of rice are available — basmati, Wehani, black and red rice are a few — and most can be purchased in the following forms: brown (missing only the hull and the most nutritious); polished white rice, which lacks the protein and other nutrients in brown rice; parboiled rice is steamed white rice; quick-cooking or instant brown rice has been partially cooked and slit to make it cook faster; brown rice farina (stone-ground brown rice); and rice flour, which is usually made by grinding white rice. See also Wild Rice (page 94).

Recipes:
- Baked Rice Pudding with Roasted Peaches (page 348)
- Brazil Nut Rissoles (page 175)
- Broccoli Lemon Rice (page 317)
- Candied Nut Dirty Rice (page 312)
- Candied Nut Fried Rice (page 290)
- Coconut Rice with Cauliflower (page 316)
- Green Risotto (page 310)
- Lentil and Rice Bowl (page 309)
- Lentil Tagine (page 229)
- Herbed Carrot and Turnip Fritters (page 177)
- Mushroom Bean Loaf with Herbed Tomato-Leek Sauce (page 284)
- Red Rice and Lentil Curry (page 262)
- Roasted Garlic and Lentil Soup (page 197)
- Roasted Mushroom and Wild Rice Soup (page 196)
- Roasted Squash in Cashew Curry Sauce (page 278)
- Spiced Lemon Rice (page 315)
- Spring Dolmades (page 162)
- Spring Vegetable Fried Rice (page 313)
- Steamed Rice and Mushroom Pockets (page 164)
- Sweet Potato Wild Rice Cakes (page 308)

Rye

Secale cereale

Rye originated in Southwest Asia and is similar in nutrients to wheat but with more of the lysine amino acid. When rye is crossed with wheat, the hybrid triticale is the result.

Forms Available: Whole kernel called rye berries, rolled, cracked and flour.

Spelt

Triticum aestivum spelta

One of the original natural grains known to man, spelt was grown in Europe more than 9,000 years ago. It contains more protein, fats and crude fiber than wheat, and is high in mucopolysaccharides. Spelt is usually organically grown because it is hardier, resistant to pests and diseases and therefore doesn't require fertilizers, pesticides or insecticides.

Caution: Spelt may be tolerated by people with wheat allergies, but should be avoided by people with celiac disease or gluten intolerance.

Forms Available: Whole kernel called spelt berries, rolled spelt or flakes and flour.

Recipes:
• How to Cook Spelt (page 331)
• Lima Bean and Wheat Berry Stew (page 247)
• Marinated Chickpea and Spelt Salad with Cilantro Dressing (page 330)
• Spinach and Whole-Grain Salad with Kiwi Dressing (page 207)

Teff (or Tef)

Eragrostis abyssinica

Grown by Ethiopians for centuries, teff means "lost" in reference to the tiny seeds that are hard to harvest. Now available in limited supply in the West, teff is a good wheat substitute for some dishes because it does not contain gluten. However, the lack of gluten means that teff will not hold the structure for baked products. The seed is so small it cannot be refined so all the nutrients are intact.

Forms Available: Whole grains.

Recipe:
• Orange-Spiked Power Cereal (page 340)

Wheat

Triticum aestivum

Wheat may have been one of the first cultivated plants 11,000 years ago. There are two main types of wheat — hard (with a higher protein and gluten content) and soft. The berry contains both insoluble and soluble fiber, vitamins, minerals, protein, carbohydrates and phytochemicals. Eating whole wheat with legumes and seeds helps to enrich the incomplete proteins in vegetarian dishes.

Forms Available: Whole kernels called wheat berries are the most nutritious form. Bulgur is wheat that has been steamed, dried and crushed. Couscous is a processed flour product made from cracked wheat that cooks faster than berries but does not have their nutrients. Farina (a fine cracked wheat), rolled wheat or flakes, whole and crushed germ and bran (see page 92) are the other semi-whole wheat forms. Whole unbleached flour is preferred to refined white wheat flour and udon noodles are more nutrient-rich than pasta made from refined white flour. Seitan is a high-protein food made from the gluten in wheat flour (see page 126) and for wheat grass in Cereal Grasses (see page 125).

Recipes:
• How to Cook Wheat Berries (page 324)
• Bulgur Asparagus Salad (page 212)
• Citrus Wheat Berries and Greens (page 323)
• Lima Bean and Wheat Berry Stew (page 247)
• Maple Baked Beans (page 269)
• Moroccan Couscous (page 319)
• Roasted Red Peppers with Moroccan Couscous (page 220)
• Tomato and Zucchini Bulgur (page 332)

Wild Rice

Zizania palustris

Wild rice is not rice at all, but is an aquatic grain harvested from the brown and green reeds of a long-stemmed annual plant that grows primarily in the shallow waters of northern Ontario, Manitoba and Minnesota. It is a sacred plant, central to the Ojibwe religion and the foundation of their belief system. At the same time, it was a staple food, one that can be stored for years against times of famine. The taste of wild rice is nutty and pleasant and the texture is chewy. Wild rice has more protein than wheat and brown or white rice, less fat than corn and is high in B_1 (thiamin), B_2 (riboflavin), B_3 (niacin) and potassium. Substitute wild rice for brown rice in recipes. Use cooked wild rice in soups, salads, breads and cakes and as a breakfast cereal.

Forms Available: Whole grain and mixed with other rice varieties in gourmet blends.

Recipes:
- Candied Nut Dirty Rice (page 312)
- Roasted Mushroom and Wild Rice Soup (page 196)
- Sweet Potato, Bean and Wild Rice Quesadillas (page 292)
- Sweet Potato Wild Rice Cakes (page 308)

Nuts and Seeds

Definition: The term nut describes any seed or fruit of a plant that has an edible kernel and is found in a hard shell. Seeds are found in the fruit of plants or growing on the stalk after the flower dies. Both nuts and seeds are the embryo of the plant — its way of reproducing new life. Unless they are salted, spiced or treated with additives, preservatives or dyes, most raw or dry-roasted nuts are considered whole foods.

Actions/Uses: Because they contain all that is necessary for a plant's new life, nuts and seeds are extremely nutritious, supplying protein, vitamin E and fiber along with essential minerals. Five human epidemiological studies found that nut consumption is linked to a lower risk for heart disease. This is likely due to their monounsaturated fats and the antioxidant action of the vitamin E found in most nuts.

Most nuts (with the exception of coconut and pine nuts) contain linoleic acid and alpha-linolenic acid. These essential fatty acids are associated with decreased risk of tumor formation and heart disease and are also essential for healthy skin, hair, glands, mucus membranes, nerves and arteries. Although their fat is polyunsaturated or monounsaturated, which may actually help decrease blood cholesterol levels, nuts and seeds should be used regularly but in moderation.

Buying and Storing: Whole or natural food stores carry a wide selection of whole raw nuts and seeds that are available packaged and in bulk. Unshelled nuts will keep in a cool place for up to 6 months. Purchase small quantities of shelled whole nuts in the fall when they are harvested and store in a cool place or the refrigerator for up to 2 months. Due to their high oil content, chopped nuts will go rancid quickly and should be stored in the refrigerator for up to 6 weeks.

Flavor: Each nut and seed has its own characteristic flavor and texture. Roasting accentuates and intensifies the "nutty" flavor of nuts and seeds.

Culinary Use: Nuts and seeds are best eaten raw (or lightly toasted). They can be used whole or chopped as snacks, in salads, casseroles, stuffing, cereals and baked goods, as a topping for baked vegetable and fruit dishes, as well as in grain and lentil dishes. Whole shelled nuts may retain their skins, which do not need to be removed unless the taste is just too bitter.

To Blanch Nuts: To remove the skins from almonds, pistachios and walnuts, cover with boiling water, let cool and rub or pinch the skins off. Dry on absorbent towels. To blanch hazelnuts: Place in a single layer in a baking pan in a 350°F (180°C) oven for about 15 minutes or until the skins dry and rub off easily.

To Toast Nuts or Seeds: Preheat the oven to 375°F (190°C). Spread nuts or seeds evenly in one layer on an ungreased baking sheet and bake for 3 minutes. Using a metal lifter, turn the nuts/seeds over and toast for 1 to 3 minutes more, watching closely. Nuts/seeds are done when they color slightly. Remove from the oven and let cool before using. Seeds take much less time to toast than nuts. Store toasted nuts in an airtight container in a cool, dry place for up to 1 week.

Almonds

Prunus amygdalus

Of the two types of almonds — bitter and sweet — only the sweet is edible in the raw state. The poisonous prussic acid in bitter almonds is removed by heating. Bitter almonds are used mainly in the production of almond oil and almond essence and are not readily available to consumers. Jordan and Valencia varieties of sweet almonds from Spain and Portugal are widely available. The flat, medium-size Californian almonds are used mostly for processing but may be available to home cooks in North America.

One-quarter cup (50 mL) of almonds supplies the body with 45% of its daily requirements of manganese and vitamin E. Almonds are high in protein, potassium, magnesium and phosphorus and they have the highest calcium content of all nuts.

Forms Available: Whole unshelled, whole shelled with skin, whole shelled and blanched, blanched halves, blanched slivers, flaked, roasted, chopped and ground (almond meal). Marzipan is a confectionary paste made from ground almonds, sugar and egg whites often used as an icing base for fruitcakes.

Recipes:
- Almond and Curry Broccoli Stir-Fry (page 264)
- Almond Garlic Spread (page 179)
- Almond Milk (page 140)
- Baked Cauliflower (page 176)
- Bulgur Asparagus Salad (page 212)
- Candied Nut Fried Rice (page 290)
- Crumb Nut Topping (page 157)
- Orange-Spiked Power Cereal (page 340)
- Pumpkin Seed Pesto (page 187)
- Roasted Zucchini Shells with Almond Filling and Red Pepper Sauce (page 281)
- Romesco Tomato Tapenade (page 189)
- Seasoned Chickpeas and Almonds (page 338)
- Sweet Potato Spread (page 182)

Brazil Nuts

Bertholettia excelsa

Native to the tropical regions of Brazil, Venezuela and Bolivia, Brazil nuts are rich and sweet tasting. The meat is found inside a coconut-like shell that is larger than most nuts. The taste lends itself to sweet dishes but Brazil nuts may also be used in savory dishes where nuts are called for. Brazil nuts are the best source of selenium, a trace mineral that reduces the risk of cancer and arthritis. They are also high in protein and exceptionally high in potassium, manganese and phosphorus. They are a good source of calcium and sodium, with small amounts of B vitamins.

Forms Available: Whole unshelled, whole shelled with skin, whole shelled and blanched, chopped and roasted.

Recipes:
- Baked Cauliflower (page 176)
- Brazil Nut Rissoles (page 175)
- Candied Nuts (page 157)
- Crumb Nut Topping (page 157)
- Curried Chestnut–Stuffed Cabbage (page 261)
- Mini Mushroom Burgers with Apricot Tamarind Marmalade (page 168)
- Oat Nut Topping (page 158)

Cashews

Anacardium occidentale

Originating in Brazil, cashews now grow in many other tropical areas. Cashews are attached to the outside of pear-shaped fruits (called cashew apples) that grow on small evergreen trees. Often eaten as a snack, the buttery taste of cashews also complements grain and baked vegetable dishes, stuffing and salads. Cashew nuts contain some protein but have high oil content. Cashews are high in copper and have significant amounts of magnesium, tryptophan and phosphorus and they are the only nuts that contain a small amount of vitamin C.

Forms Available: All forms of cashews come shelled. They are available whole raw or roasted, in halves, pieces and chopped, and salted.

Recipes:
- Berry Chia Smoothie (page 337)
- Cashew Butter (page 181)
- Cashew Cream (page 144)
- Cashew Curry Sauce (page 156)
- Cashew Milk (page 141)
- Chickpeas and Potatoes in Cashew Cream (page 240)
- Crumb Nut Topping (page 157)
- Moroccan Pumpkin Soup (page 193)
- Mushroom Bean Loaf with Herbed Tomato-Leek Sauce (page 284)
- Mushroom Sauce (page 154)
- Oat Nut Topping (page 158)
- Spinach Cream Gazpacho (page 200)
- Spinach-Stuffed Red Pepper Rolls (page 174)
- Sweet Potato and Black-Eyed Pea Curry (page 266)
- Teriyaki Sauce (page 154)
- West African Mafé (page 250)

Chestnuts

Castanea sativa

Sweet chestnuts grow on wild trees in Britain, Europe and North America and are cultivated in Italy, France and Spain. Raw chestnuts do not keep long before the flesh deteriorates and so are usually cooked before they are sold. If fresh, chestnuts should be bought in the shell and cooked or used right away. They can be boiled, steamed, roasted or stewed. Chestnuts are low in oils and high in carbohydrates. They are high in potassium, are good sources of calcium, magnesium and phosphorus and have small amounts of the B vitamins.

Forms Available: Cooked whole, usually peeled, dried and ground or canned chestnut purée.

Note: The water chestnut is unrelated to chestnuts. Water chestnuts are the edible fruit from an herbaceous water plant.

Recipes:
• Bok Choy, Mushroom and Black Bean Stir-Fry (page 288)
• Curried Chestnut–Stuffed Cabbage (page 261)
• Mushroom Bean Loaf with Herbed Tomato-Leek Sauce (page 284)
• Steamed Rice and Mushroom Pockets (page 164)

Coconuts

Cocos nucifera

The coconut, largest of all nuts, is the fruit of the coconut palm that grows on tropical islands. Coconuts may be eaten fresh along with their milk or the flesh is dried and usually sweetened. Coconuts are rich in potassium and have significant amounts of phosphorus and magnesium. They are a good source of protein. Both the coconut flesh and milk are used in curries, toppings, fruit dishes, sauces, rice dishes and desserts and baked goods.

Forms Available: Whole (fresh) in the shell and dried, grated, shredded, flaked or desiccated. Canned coconut milk and coconut oil are also available.

Recipes:
• Chilled Chia Chai (page 335)
• Coconut-Carob Milk (page 142)
• Coconut Pecan Glaze (page 358)
• Coconut Rice with Cauliflower (page 316)
• Eggplant Curry (page 260)
• Orange-Spiked Power Cereal (page 340)
• Red Curry Cauliflower (page 258)

• Sweet Potato and Black-Eyed Pea Curry (page 266)
• Winter Vegetable Bake with Coconut Nut Topping (page 277)
• Yellow Coconut Curry Sauce (page 155)

Flaxseeds

Linum usitatissimum

Flaxseed oil is the best vegetable source of essential omega-3 fatty acids, which help lubricate the joints and prevent absorption of toxins by stimulating digestion. They contain 30% of the body's daily requirement of manganese and are high in dietary fiber. Flaxseeds also contain magnesium, folate, copper, phosphorus and vitamin B_6 (pyridoxine).

Flaxseeds must be ground for the body to absorb and benefit from the oils. Once ground, the seeds deteriorate rapidly. It is best to buy in small amounts and store whole, ground seeds and flaxseed oil in the refrigerator.

Forms Available: Whole, ground and flax meal. Flaxseed oil is also available.

Recipes:
• Almond Milk (page 140)
• Brazil Nut Rissoles (page 175)
• Caesar Salad Dressing (page 203)
• Dark Chocolate Pudding (page 353)
• Herbed Carrot and Turnip Fritters (page 177)
• Mini Mushroom Burgers with Apricot Tamarind Marmalade (page 168)
• Oatmeal Coconut Cookies (page 347)
• Pecan Milk (page 141)
• Potato Rösti (page 224)
• Pumpkin Seed Pesto (page 187)
• Walnut Milk (page 142)
• Whole-Grain Power Bars (page 341)

Peanuts

Arachis hypogaea

Widely available and most extensively used, peanuts are an important food staple in some areas, a snack in others. Peanuts are actually legumes encased in a dry, fibrous pod. High in manganese and protein and containing tryptophan, vitamin B_3 (niacin), folate and copper, peanuts also have significant amounts of vitamin E.

Caution: Many individuals experience an allergic reaction when exposed to peanuts and peanut products. Peanuts that have been deep-fried, battered, candied or combined with additives, dyes, fats or sugars have no place in a whole foods diet.

Forms Available: Whole unshelled, shelled raw with skin, shelled and blanched, roasted and salted. Also available chopped.

Recipes:
- Chunky Peanut Sauce (page 153)
- Crumb Nut Topping (page 157)
- Dukkah (page 339)
- Eggplant Curry (page 260)
- Oat Nut Topping (page 158)
- Pad Thai (page 291)
- Smooth Peanut Sauce (page 153)
- Vietnamese Spring Rolls with Peanut Sauce (page 172)
- West African Mafé (page 250)

Pecans

Carya pecan

Native to North America, pecans are sweetly pleasant tasting. Grafting techniques developed thin-shelled varieties in the 19th century. This was crucial to their widespread use. Pecans lend texture and interest to salads, fruit dishes, baked vegetables and grains and can replace most nuts in recipes. They are well used in sweets, pies and fruitcakes. Pecans are high in protein with significant amounts of B vitamins. They have some iron, calcium, potassium and phosphorus.

Forms Available: Whole unshelled, shelled raw with skin, shelled blanched and roasted whole, halves and chopped.

Recipes:
- Candied Nut Fried Rice (page 290)
- Candied Nuts (page 157)
- Coconut Pecan Glaze (page 358)
- Green Bean, Pecan and Pomegranate Salad (page 206)
- Maple-Glazed Cabbage Greens with Pecans (page 217)
- Oat Nut Topping (page 158)
- Pecan Crisp Topping (page 352)
- Pecan Milk (page 141)

Pine Nuts

Pinus pinea

Pine nuts are the edible seed of just over a dozen varieties of pine tree. Pine nuts are probably the most expensive of all the edible nuts. They are small, creamy-colored and buttery in texture. Their oil-rich flesh is what contributes to their taste and texture. High in protein and carbohydrate, they are also good sources of B vitamins. Keep pine nuts in the refrigerator for up to 1 month.

Forms Available: Except when purchased directly from harvesters, pine nuts always come shelled and are usually whole. They may be raw or roasted and salted.

Recipes:
- Basil Pesto (page 188)
- Braised Greens with Cherries and Pine Nuts (page 223)
- Citrus Wheat Berries and Greens (page 323)
- Olive Tapenade (page 188)

Pistachio Nuts

Pistacia vera

Small, green pistachio nuts are native to the Middle East, where they are a symbol of happiness. Pistachio nuts have a soft texture and mild flavor which makes them versatile in cooking. They are used in salads and as a topping for vegetables, grains and legume dishes. Pistachio nuts are also used in sweet dishes and confections.

Forms Available: Whole unshelled raw and salted, shelled raw and salted. Pistachio nuts may be dyed, however, the natural form is preferred.

Recipe:
- Baked Cauliflower (page 176)

Pumpkin Seeds

The pumpkin's small, flat green seeds are used to treat and prevent parasites as well as to nourish and restore the prostate gland. They are high in manganese, magnesium, phosphorus and tryptophan and contain iron, copper, vitamin K, zinc and essential fatty acids. According to nutritionist and naturopathic physician Dr. Paavo Airola, pumpkin seeds contain pacifarin, an antibiotic resistance factor that increases man's natural resistance to disease.

Forms Available: Whole unshelled raw, unsalted and salted, shelled raw, unsalted and salted or toasted and salted.

Recipes:
- Mini Mushroom Burgers with Apricot Tamarind Marmalade (page 168)
- Orange-Spiked Power Cereal (page 340)
- Pumpkin Seed Pesto (page 187)
- Sweet Toasted Pumpkin Seeds (page 339)

Sesame Seeds

Sesamum indicum

Tiny, cream-colored and almond-shaped, sesame seeds are widely available. They originate from Africa, where they are called *benne*. Sesame seeds are high in copper and manganese and are a good source of protein. They work well with legumes or whole grains. They have high levels of tryptophan, calcium, magnesium and iron and some phosphorus, zinc and vitamin B_1 (thiamin). Sesame seeds and sesame oil lend a nutty taste to breads, fruit or vegetable dishes, grains and beans.

Tahini is a thick paste made from ground sesame seeds. It is used in dips, spreads and falafel dishes. Halva is a sweet sesame cake made with honey or cane sugar.

Forms Available: Whole with hulls, raw, hulled and polished, hulled and roasted. Sesame seed oil is available raw and toasted. Tahini paste is available in Middle Eastern stores and some whole or natural food stores.

Recipes:
- Dukkah (page 339)
- Pumpkin Seed Pesto (page 187)
- Sesame Nori Crackers (page 343)
- Whole-Grain Power Bars (page 341)

Sunflower Seeds

Helianthus annuus

Sunflowers most probably originated in Mexico. The long, flat, gray or black-striped seeds are cultivated for oil as well as for eating. One-quarter cup (50 mL) of sunflower seeds supply 90% of the body's daily requirement of vitamin E and almost 55% of vitamin B_1 (thiamin). Sunflower seeds are high in protein, manganese, magnesium, copper, tryptophan and selenium. They also contain significant amounts of phosphorus, vitamin B_5 (pantothenic), folate and potassium. They may be used to replace the more expensive pine nuts in pesto recipes and salads. Sunflower oil is polyunsaturated and has a light, nutty taste, making it a popular salad oil.

Forms Available: Whole and raw with hulls, hulled raw, roasted and salted.

Recipes:
- Basil Pesto (page 188)
- Olive Tapenade (page 188)
- Orange-Spiked Power Cereal (page 340)
- Spinach and Whole-Grain Salad with Kiwi Dressing (page 207)

Walnuts

Juglans regia (English) or *J. nigra* (black)

There are two main varieties of walnut, the English (or Persian) walnut, and the Black walnut (native to North America). Walnuts are widely available and used often in a wide variety of dishes, both savory and sweet. Walnuts are high in oil, protein, potassium and phosphorus. They contain some vitamin B_6 (pyridoxine), and folic acid, which is not found in other nuts. Eaten as a snack or used in stuffing, salads, cakes, vegetable and grain dishes, $1/4$ cup (50 mL) supplies 90% of the body's requirement of omega-3 fatty acids and 40% of manganese. They also contain copper and tryptophan.

Forms Available: Whole unshelled raw, whole shelled raw, halves, pieces, chopped and ground. Walnut oil is available.

Recipes:
- Candied Nut Fried Rice (page 290)
- Citrus Wheat Berries and Greens (page 323)
- Crumb Nut Topping (page 157)
- Mini Mushroom Burgers with Apricot Tamarind Marmalade (page 168)
- Oat Nut Topping (page 158)
- Potato, Leek and Kale Curry (page 265)
- Spinach and Whole-Grain Salad with Kiwi Dressing (page 207)
- Spring Dolmades (page 162)
- Walnut Milk (page 142)
- Whole-Grain Power Bars (page 341)

Sea Vegetables

Definition: Often called seaweeds or sea herbs, sea vegetables are edible, wild plants that grow abundantly in the oceans. They are primitive plants with blades for leaves, stipes for stems and holdfasts for roots. Sea vegetables have been honored by cultures of the Far East and harvested by seaside communities around the world for food, salt, medicine and fertilizer for many thousands of years.

Actions/Uses: Sea vegetables are rich in minerals and trace elements, particularly iodine, calcium, potassium and iron. They contain small amounts of protein, but their protein includes essential amino acids, unlike most plants that only contain incomplete amino acids. They have a significant amount of vitamins A, B, C and D, including vitamin B_{12}, which is only found in three other plant foods (alfalfa, comfrey and fermented soybean products). Most sea vegetables have anticancer properties.

Caution: Do not consume sea vegetables if you have a hyperthyroid condition.

Buying and Storing: Whole or natural food stores carry a selection of packaged dried sea vegetables. Some supermarkets offer a few dried and prepackaged sea vegetables for sale. Store unopened dried sea vegetables indefinitely and once opened, keep in an airtight container for up to 3 months.

Culinary Use: Most dried sea vegetables require a quick rehydration by soaking in cool water for 10 to 15 minutes. Shredded dried sea vegetables, such as arame, wakame and hijiki, may be added to soups, broths, sauces and stews without soaking but will need to simmer for 20 to 30 minutes to cook and may require slightly more liquid depending on the dish. Finely chopped or powdered dried sea vegetables are almost always used with other herbs as a salt substitute.

Arame

Eisenia bicyclis

Arame appears as short, thin, curled strands. It is dark yellow-brown when growing, black when dried. Arame grows off Japan's northern and southern coasts. It is soft with a slightly resistant texture and sweet, delicate flavor.

Actions/Uses: Alleviates high blood pressure and builds strong bones and teeth. Arame is one of the richest sources of iodine and is highly concentrated in iron and calcium.

Culinary Use: Add to curries, salads, soups, stews, and tomato sauce and baked vegetable and grain dishes. Soak in water for 3 to 5 minutes, then cook as directed in recipe or add to long-simmering soups and stews directly.

Agar (or Agar-Agar)

See Whole Food Ingredients (page 127)

Dulse

Palmaria palmata

Dulse has large, dark red fronds. Found off North Atlantic waters, it has a chewy texture that is salty and nutlike.

Actions/Uses: Prevents scurvy, induces sweating, is a remedy for seasickness and treats symptoms of the herpes virus. Dulse is exceptionally concentrated in iodine, which is important to the thyroid gland. It is rich in manganese, which activates the enzyme system. Dulse is a good source of phosphorus, B vitamins, vitamins E and C, bromine, potassium, magnesium, sulfur, calcium, sodium, radium, boron, rubidium, manganese, titanium and other trace elements.

Culinary Use: Use dulse in the same way as spinach — chopped, in stuffing, relishes, salad dressings, grain and vegetable bakes. Toast and eat dulse as a snack. It thickens gravies and sauces. Soak in water for 20 minutes, then cook as directed in recipe, or add to long-simmering soups and stews directly.

Recipe:
• Cashew Milk (page 141)

Hijiki

Hizikia fusiforme

Brown when fresh and black when dried, hijiki has short, thin, curled strands. It is harvested off the northern and southern coasts of Japan, Korea and China. The sweet, delicate flavor and crisp texture of hijiki make it very popular in vegetarian dishes.

Actions/Uses: Diuretic, resolves heat-induced phlegm, helps remove toxins, benefits thyroid, helps normalize blood sugar levels, aids weight loss, soothes nerves, supports hormone functions, builds bones and teeth. Hijiki is an excellent source of calcium, iron and iodine, and is abundant in vitamin B_2 (riboflavin) and B_3 (niacin).

Caution: Canadian, Hong Kong, UK and New Zealand government food safety agencies advise consumers to avoid consumption of hijiki seaweed. Test results have indicated that levels of inorganic arsenic were significantly higher in hijiki than in other types of seaweed. Inorganic arsenic, which can occur naturally in some foods, is known to add to the risk of people developing cancer.

Culinary Use: Hijiki adds interest and texture to salads and rice dishes, soups, stews, stuffing and stir-fries. Soak in water for 15 to 20 minutes, then cook as directed in recipe, or add to long-simmering soups and stews directly.

Kelp

Pleurophycus gardneri

Kelp's broad light brown to light olive-brown leaf-like fronds are found off the Pacific coast of North America. The fresh or dried frond has a delicate, mild taste when cooked. Kelp is usually available in granular, powdered or tablet form. However, the dried and shredded or long strips may be available in whole or natural food stores.

Actions/Uses: Antibacterial, antiviral (herpes), may lower blood pressure and cholesterol, high in calcium, phosphorus and iodine.

Culinary Use: Wrap fresh kelp fronds (if you can find them) around rice or other fillings, or steam, chop and add to stir-fries, salads or stuffing. Use the dried whole or strips of kelp in the same way as fresh but rehydrate first. Sprinkle the powder or granules into soups, stews, salads and stir-fries, or mix with dry ingredients in breads, pancakes and muffins. Granular kelp is added to most vegetable and grain dishes, sauces, gravy, dips and spreads. No soaking is needed if the granular or powdered forms are used but rehydrate if using dried whole or strips.

Kombu

Laminaria japonica

Fresh kombu (called sashimi) is a long, thick, dark green frond. Most often kombu is sold dried whole or in strips or shredded. Used for centuries, kombu

is found mainly off the coastal waters of China, Korea and Japan, where it's cultivated. Kombu's taste is sweet and yet robust.

Actions/Uses: Rich in protein, calcium, iodine, magnesium, iron and folate.

Caution: Kombu contains significant amounts of glutamic acid, a forerunner of monosodium glutamate (MSG) and so should be used in small quantities.

Culinary Use: Kombu is used to flavor soups, broths, sauces and stews. The Japanese make a soup broth called Dashi using kombu. Kombu is removed and discarded before the soup is served. Soak dried kombu for 10 minutes and simmer for 15 to 20 minutes to soften it.

Nori

Porphyra tenera

Both coasts of North America and the middle and lower tidal zones of Europe's seacoasts grow nori. Called "laver" in Britain, nori is bright pink when young, turning to dark purple as the plant ages. To get a consistent size and thickness that works for rolling rice, the leaves are pressed into thin sheets. Nori tastes like mild, salty corn. The sheets are often toasted before being used in sushi or other dishes.

Actions/Uses: Antibacterial, diuretic, treats painful urination, goiter, edema, high blood pressure, beriberi, appears to heal ulcers, is high in protein and rich in vitamins A, C, B_1 (thiamin), B_3 (niacin) and phosphorus.

Culinary Use: Use green, black or toasted nori sheets to wrap vegetables and rice for sushi. Chopped or crumbled, nori adds interest and texture to salads, stir-fries and vegetable dishes. Toast nori sheets lightly over a low flame or element on high until black and crisp.

Recipe:
• Sesame Nori Crackers (page 343)

Wakame

Undaria pinnatifida

The thin black fronds of the wild wakame grow in Japan's northern seas. Wakame has a softly resistant texture and a strong, sweet flavor.

Actions/Uses: Boosts immune functioning, promotes healthy hair and skin. Wakame is used in Japanese tradition to purify mother's blood after childbirth. It is rich in calcium, B₃ (niacin) and B₁ (thiamin).

Culinary Use: Chop whole fresh wakame and use as any leafy green vegetable in soups, stews, salads, sandwiches, vegetable and stir-fry dishes. The shredded dried wakame strips may be added to most vegetarian dishes. Soak dried wakame in water for 5 minutes, drain and simmer for 45 minutes.

Soy Foods

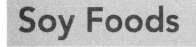

Definition: Soybeans are legumes that are generally classed as oilseeds. They are native to China where they have been cultivated for 13,000 years although they no longer resemble their wild progenitors. Their smooth texture and bland taste make soybeans adaptable to processing into other forms. Foods made from soybeans are called "soy foods."

Soybeans

Glycine max

Actions/Uses: Soybeans are the only known vegetable source of complete protein, meaning they contain all of the essential amino acids in the appropriate proportions essential for the growth and maintenance of body cells. In addition to being an excellent source of fiber, the fat in soybeans (34%) is polyunsaturated, lower than animal fat in calories and rich in linolenic fatty acids.

Caution: A large percentage of soybeans grown today are genetically modified and are produced using high amounts of pesticides. Fresh soybeans contain enzyme inhibitors that block protein digestion and may cause serious gastric distress and organ damage. The inhibitors are not present in such high amounts in the fermented bean products of tofu, tempeh or soy sauce. The high amounts of phytic acid in soybeans and soy foods may block the uptake of essential minerals and cause deficiencies. Isoflavones, once thought to minimize cell damage from free radicals, block the damaging effects of hormonal or synthetic estrogens, and inhibit tumor cell growth, may in fact, be toxic.

Soybeans and soy foods contain goitrogens, naturally occurring substances in certain foods that can interfere with the functioning of the thyroid gland. Individuals with already existing and untreated thyroid problems may want to avoid soy foods.

Textured vegetable protein (TVP) made from soybeans is produced using chemicals and harmful techniques and is not considered a whole food.

Excessive soy intake should be avoided during pregnancy and soy-based baby formulas should not be used.

Forms Available: Dried organic soybeans are available in whole or natural food stores.

Buying and Storing: Keep dried soybeans as you would other legumes in a dry, dark and cool place for up to 1 year. Processed soybeans in the forms of tofu and tempeh are available in most supermarkets. Follow package directions for storing these foods. Canned soybeans are sometimes available along with other canned legumes.

Culinary Use: Use fresh or dried whole organic soybeans infrequently in cooking and add fermented soy products (tofu, tempeh, tamari and soy sauce) on an occasional basis only. Soak and cook dried soybeans as you would other dried legumes. Fresh, canned or frozen beans are added to soups, stews and baked vegetable dishes.

Whole dried soybeans must be rehydrated in the same way that other legumes are soaked, then cooked.

To Soak: Place washed beans in a large saucepan and cover with 2 inches (5 cm) water. Bring to a boil over high heat. Reduce heat and simmer for 2 minutes. Leave the pan on the element and turn off the heat. Let stand for 1 hour or overnight. Discard soaking water and rinse beans. Soybeans have now been rehydrated and are ready to cook. Never use salt or other seasonings at the soaking stage.

To Cook: Place soaked, drained and rinsed beans in a large saucepan and cover with 2 inches (5 cm) fresh water. Cover pan and bring to boil over high heat. Reduce heat and simmer for about 3 hours or until tender. Using a pressure cooker reduces the soaking and cooking time significantly (check manufacturer's instructions).

Using cooked canned soybeans is a convenient way to use these legumes without any significant loss of nutrients.

Edamame

Edamame is the Japanese name for fresh green soybeans in the pod. They can be cooked and eaten as a green vegetable. The beans are round, smooth and green with firm, unbruised pods.

Forms Available: Edamame is usually frozen but the fresh can be found in some urban supermarkets as well as in whole or natural food stores and Asian markets.

Caution: It is wise to eat small amounts of fresh soybeans and not often (see Caution, left).

Recipe:
• Green Pea and Asparagus Curry (v) (page 259)

Miso

See Whole Food Ingredients (page 125).

Natto

See Whole Food Ingredients (page 125).

Soy Milk

Soy milk is made from ground soybeans that are mixed with water to form a milk-like liquid. Soy milk is an excellent source of protein, B vitamins and iron, and if fortified, provides adequate calcium. It has low levels of saturated fat and no cholesterol.

Caution: Use moderate amounts in cooking and do not consume large amounts on a daily basis (see Caution, page 102).

Forms Available: Non-flavored, called natural or original, or with flavors added.

Recipes:
• Avocado Sauce (page 148)
• Avocado Vichyssoise (page 199)
• Baked Rice Pudding with Roasted Peaches (page 348)
• Berry Chia Smoothie (page 337)
• Black Blondies (page 350)
• Cashew Cream (page 144)
• Cashew Curry Sauce (page 156)
• Cauliflower Gratin (page 268)
• Choco-Cappuccino (page 334)
• Corn Biscuits (page 342)
• Cream of Leek and Asparagus on Toast Points (page 171)
• Creamy White Sauce (page 149)
• Dark Chocolate Pudding (page 353)
• Kamut Spaghetti with Creamy Mushroom and Leek Sauce (page 307)
• Lavender Custard (page 356)
• Lentil and Broccoli Casserole (page 231)
• Mango Pineapple Mocktail (page 335)
• Oatmeal Coconut Cookies (page 347)
• Orange Creamsicle (page 336)
• Soy Ice Cream (page 346)
• Soy Sour Cream (page 145)
• Spinach Cream Gazpacho (page 200)
• Spinach Stuffing (page 174)
• Tropical Banana Tahini Smoothie (page 337)
• Tropical Nog (page 334)
• Vegetable Pancakes (page 160)

Soy Sauce

See Whole Food Ingredients (Tamari Sauce, page 126).

Tamari Sauce

See Whole Food Ingredients (page 126).

Tempeh

Pronounced tem-PAY, this soy food is mild and meaty-tasting. The firm white cake is made from fermenting cooked soybeans. Tempeh gives a chewy texture to vegetarian dishes and is a good substitute for ground beef in pasta sauce or chili. It can be fried, baked, broiled, grilled or simmered with vegetables in other dishes.

Forms Available: Usually frozen in a solid cake form.

Recipes:
• Pad Thai (page 291)
• Rainbow Tempeh Lettuce Cups (page 294)
• Sweet and Sour Tempeh and Eggplant Stir-Fry (page 289)
• Tomato Grilling Sauce (page 152)
• Vegetable and Tempeh Pie (page 236)

Tofu

Also called bean curd or soy cheese, tofu is one of the most versatile of all the soy foods. Tofu is a custard-like product made from heating soymilk with either calcium sulfate (the preferred method) or magnesium sulfate and pressing the curds into "cakes." Tofu can be frozen (the color turns yellow and the texture is more chewy), marinated, stir-fried, used as cottage cheese, as sandwich spreads, or mixed with salads, soups and pastas.

Forms Available: Tofu can be purchased as silky, soft and firm, with the harder forms having more water pressed from them.

Recipes:
- Baked Cranberry Tofu with Creamed Asparagus and Leeks (page 270)
- Chocolate Cake with Lemon Cream (page 354)
- Dark Chocolate Pudding (page 353)
- Lavender Custard (page 356)
- Mushroom Lasagna (page 299)
- Soy Ice Cream (page 346)
- Soy Sour Cream (page 145)
- Tofu Aïoli (page 178)
- Tofu Mayonnaise (page 178)
- Udon Noodles with Tofu and Gingered Peanut Sauce (page 304)
- Vietnamese Spring Rolls with Peanut Sauce (page 172)

Herbs

Definition: Herbs are defined as plants whose parts are used to enhance our lives. Strictly speaking, an herb (pronounced *herb* or *erb*) is a plant that is used for culinary, medicinal, cosmetic or ornamental purposes. That definition is broad enough to encompass some trees, spices and flowers that we otherwise might not think of as herbs.

Actions/Uses: The vitamins, minerals and phytochemicals found in herbs can make a significant contribution to our health through diet. Generally, most herbs are antioxidant and the green parts supply chlorophyll, which enhances the body's ability to produce hemoglobin and thus to increase the delivery of oxygen to cells. (See the individual herbs for their specific actions.)

Caution: Avoid medicinal doses of all herbs while pregnant unless following advice by a medical herbalist or midwife.

Buying and Storing: As with fruits and vegetables, the whole fresh herb is the best form to use in cooking. Grow your own or look for fresh organic herbs in supermarkets and farmers' markets. Store fresh herbs rolled in a damp tea towel in the produce drawer of the refrigerator.

For teas, beverages and medicinal applications, dried herbs are used. Dry fresh herbs for use over the winter or purchase small quantities of organic dried herbs from a farm or whole or natural food stores. Replace all dried herbs after 8 to 10 months. Use dark-colored glass or ceramic containers with tight-fitting lids to store herbs individually. Label and date and keep in a cool, dark place for no longer than 1 year.

Culinary Use: Herbs are used in both savory and sweet dishes. They enliven and are an integral part of vegetarian recipes. When a smooth texture is desired in sauces, beverages or dressings, it is advantageous to make an herb tea. Strain off the herbs and use the infused liquid to flavor the dish. The recipes in this book call for the use of fresh herbs except where dried are indicated. (See the individual herbs for the specific flavors and combinations that they complement.)

To substitute dried herbs in recipes: Use one-half to one-third less dried herbs than the quantity of fresh called for in the recipe. Crush or grind the dried herb to a powder then add to the recipe.

To Make Herbal Infusion (Tea or Tissane): Bring 1 cup (250 mL) of pure or filtered water to a boil. Measure 1 tsp (5 mL) dried herb into a teapot. Pour boiled water over top. Place a lid on the teapot and a cork in the spout (to prevent steam from escaping). Steep the tea for 10 to 15 minutes. Let the infusion cool before adding to recipes. Strain and discard solids. For convenience, make 1 to 2 cups (250 to 500 mL) medicinal tea and store in a covered jar in refrigerator for use throughout the day.

To Dry Herbs: Most herbs dry well, except for parsley, chives and basil, which are better frozen. To dry well, herbs require a warm, dry, dark atmosphere where air circulates freely, such as an attic, dark corner of a room, basement or a barn.

For long-stemmed herbs (mints, yarrow, sage), gather in small bunches, tie the stems and hang upside down in a warm, dry, dark place. Paper bags may be used to catch the falling bits and to keep the light away. For leaves on short stems (thyme) and flowers (calendula, violets and all others), strip leaves off the stems and the petals off the center of the flower (or dry the flower head whole). Scatter leaves or petals in a single layer on a nylon net or screen. The faster the plant parts dry, the more color and fragrance they will retain. Scrub roots, cut into $1/2$-inch (1 cm) pieces, and place in one layer on a drying rack, screen or suspended fabric to dry. Leave in pieces for longer storage. Grind small amounts to a powder just before using. Bottle and store in dark-colored bottles in a cool, dark place.

Alfalfa

Medicago sativa

A hardy perennial that is easily grown in most parts of North America.

Parts Used: Leaves, flowers and sprouted seeds.

Actions: Tonic, nutritive, lower blood cholesterol, anti-anemia.

Uses: Alfalfa is a cell nutritive and overall tonic for the body. It promotes strong teeth, bones and connective tissue. Alfalfa is one of the best sources of chlorophyll, which has the ability to stimulate new skin growth, heal wounds and burns, diminish the symptoms of arthritis, gout and rheumatism, lower cholesterol levels, reduce inflammation and improve the body's resistance to cancer.

The mature tops and seeds are high in amino acids and chlorophyll, as well as minerals such as calcium, magnesium, phosphorus and potassium and vitamins K, B and P, which the body uses to repair and build musculoskeletal system structures and tissues.

Sprouted seeds have an enhanced concentration of vitamins. Alfalfa shoots (per 100 g) have 3,410 I.U. of beta-carotene and 162 mg of vitamin C.

Caution: Alfalfa seeds and sprouts are rich in the amino acid canavanine, which can contribute to inflammation in rheumatoid arthritis, systemic lupus erythematosus and other rheumatoid and inflammatory conditions. Alfalfa leaf is NOT a source of canavanine and can be used in inflammatory and rheumatic conditions.

Availability: Whole or cut dried leaf is available in whole or natural food stores. Sprouted seeds are readily available.

Culinary Use: Alfalfa has a light, grassy taste to the fresh flowers and leaves and a stronger, also grassy taste to the dried aerial parts. Add fresh or dried whole sprigs to soups and stews during the last hour of cooking, then remove. Fresh leaves are perfect in salads, rice and vegetable dishes. Use a generous handful of fresh or dried alfalfa in vegetable stock. Add the chopped fresh leaf to soups and stews during the last 10 minutes of cooking.

Fresh flowers and sprouts work well in salads, stir-fries and sandwiches. Add them when juicing vegetables and include alfalfa tea with liquids in breads.

Astragalus

Astragalus membranaceus

Astragalus is a hardy, shrub-like perennial native to eastern Asia but grown in temperate regions including Canada and the United States.

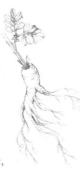

Parts Used: Root.

Actions: Immune stimulant, antimicrobial, heart tonic, diuretic, promotes tissue regeneration.

Uses: Used throughout the Orient as a tonic, astragalus is a safe and powerful immune system stimulator for virtually every phase of immune system activity. It also has been shown to alleviate the adverse effects of steroids and chemotherapy on the immune system and can be used during traditional cancer treatment.

Availability: While more and more North American herb farms are growing this exceptional medicinal herb, the most reliable sources for the dried, sliced root are Oriental herb stores centered in large urban areas. However, whole or natural food stores do carry cut or powdered astragalus and the tincture form.

Culinary Use: The mild, slightly sweet, earthy taste of astragalus is so subtle it can be used in soups and vegetable stocks without detection. Add one or two pieces of the dried root to soups or vegetable stock or grind and include in root beverages and seasoning blends. Astragalus tincture may be added to smoothies and soups just before serving.

Basil

Oscimum basilicum

A bushy annual with large, waxy, deep green leaves and small tubular flowers that grow in long spikes.

Parts Used: Leaves and flowering tops.

Actions: Antispasmodic, soothing digestive, antibacterial, antidepressant, adrenal stimulant.

Uses: To relieve indigestion, nervous tension, stress and tension headaches.

Availability: Fresh sprigs are sold in season at farmers' markets and supermarkets. Dried, cut and sifted leaves are available in whole or natural food stores.

Culinary Use: Slightly nutmeg and clove with citrus undertones, each variety has a variation of the spicy basil taste. Use about three to six large fresh basil leaves for baked vegetable, legume and grain dishes. Wash, pat dry and strip leaves from stem (discard stem) and roughly chop leaves or cut in chiffonade.

Burdock

Arctium lappa

A hardy biennial that produces fruiting heads covered with hooked burrs that catch on clothing and the fur of animals. Grows wild extensively in North America.

Parts Used: Root, stalk, leaves and seeds.

Actions: Leaves are a mild laxative, diuretic. The root is also a mild laxative, antirheumatic, antibiotic, promotes sweating, diuretic, cleansing, stimulating efficient removal of waste production, a skin and blood cleanser. Burdock also stimulates urine flow. Root and seeds are a soothing demulcent and tonic. They soothe kidneys and relieve lymphatics. The seeds prevent fever, are anti-inflammatory, antibacterial and reduce blood sugar levels.

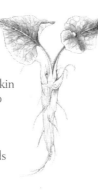

Uses: Leaves may be used in the same way as roots although they are less effective. Burdock root is a cleansing, eliminative remedy. It helps to remove toxins causing skin problems (including eczema, acne, rashes, boils), digestive sluggishness or arthritic pains. It supports the liver, lymphatic glands and digestive system. Burdock seeds relieve lymphatics, are a soothing demulcent tonic, and soothe the kidneys.

For every 1 cup (250 mL) of boiled burdock root, there is 61 mg calcium, 450 mg potassium and 116 mg phosphorus.

Availability: Fresh root is available seasonally at Asian food markets. Due to its extensive growth habit in rural and urban waste areas, burdock can be easily foraged. Dig roots from the wild in the fall. Scrub and chop, then dry for storage. Cut dried leaves and root and tinctures are available in whole or natural food stores.

Culinary Use: Fresh burdock leaves have a taste similar to spinach or Swiss chard. Roots are nutty and pleasant tasting when cooked. Use fresh burdock leaves as you would spinach and other leafy greens. In the summer, use the large fresh leaves to wrap vegetables, fish and meat for grilling. In the spring, use the tender young sprouts and smaller leaves in salads and soups or cooked as a vegetable. The fresh leaf stalks may be peeled and roasted or boiled. They are a delicate vegetable, much like asparagus when cooked.

Use fresh burdock roots and stalks in soups instead of potatoes, roast or grill them as a vegetable, grate and mix with potatoes for latkes. Roasted, dried burdock roots are a good coffee substitute.

Use fresh or dry burdock seeds in tea blends or as seasonings, in the same way you would use sesame seeds.

Calendula

Calendula officinalis

A prolific annual (easily grown from seed) with bright yellow to orange marigold-like flowers, calendula's common name is pot marigold.

Parts Used: Petals.

Actions: Astringent, antiseptic, antifungal, anti-inflammatory, heals wounds, menstrual regulator, stimulates bile production.

Uses: Calendula acts as an aid to digestion and as a general tonic. It is taken to ease menopausal problems, period pain, gastritis, peptic ulcers, gall bladder problems, indigestion, and fungal infections.

Availability: Calendula is widely used in gardens and in vegetable gardens. Whole dried flower heads are available in whole or natural food stores.

Culinary Use: Formerly used to color cheese, calendula adds a soft, flecked yellow color to baked products, rice and sauces. Calendula petals have a delicate floral taste and smell. The flavor and aroma strengthens upon drying, but is still overpowered by other robust ingredients in food. Use calendula as a substitute for saffron and as a natural food coloring. Use fresh petals chopped in salads, soups, stews, rice, egg dishes, custards and puddings. The fresh or dried petals add color as a garnish for all main or dessert dishes, cakes, breads and muffins. They are also used for color in non-alcoholic punches and frozen ices.

Cardamom

Elettaria cardamomum

Originally from Indian rainforests, cardamom is a rhizomatous perennial with large lanceolate leaves. For centuries it has been exported to Europe mainly for its fragrance. When coaxed into blooming, the flowers are white with a dark pink-striped lip.

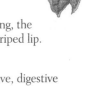

Parts Used: Seeds.

Actions: Antispasmodic, carminative, digestive stimulant, expectorant.

Uses: Cardamom is a pungent herb with stimulating, tonic effects that work best on the digestive system. It relaxes spasms, stimulates appetite and relieves flatulence.

Availability: The whole dried (white or green) pods are preferred because they keep up to 1 year. Whole pods are available at Asian, Indian or Middle Eastern markets. Hulled seeds are widely available in supermarkets and whole or natural food stores. As with all hulled seeds, buy in small quantities and use frequently.

Culinary Use: Used ground or as whole seeds, the lemon and floral taste of cardamom is slightly similar to nutmeg with camphor and smoky notes. Toasting cardamom brings out its complex flavors. It is used in sweet and savory dishes and in many spice blends and some teas. Cardamom is especially good in custards, puddings, with apples and pears, and in rice pilafs. Cardamom combines well with coffee, chiles, coriander, cumin, ginger, pepper, saffron, basil and yogurt.

Cayenne Pepper

Capsicum annum and
Capsicum frutescens

A tropical perennial, grown as an annual in temperate zones. (See also Chile Peppers, page 76)

Parts Used: Fruit

Actions: Stimulant, tonic, carminative, induces perspiration, rubefacient, antiseptic, antibacterial.

Uses: Cayenne stimulates blood circulation, purifies the blood, promotes fluid elimination and sweat, and is most often used as a stimulating nerve tonic. Over-the-counter creams and ointments containing the active capsaicin extract are applied externally and are often effective in relieving the pain of osteoarthritis and rheumatoid arthritis, shingles infection, as well as the burning pain in the toes, feet, and legs of diabetic neuropathy and fibromyalgia. The capsaicin in cayenne works by blocking a protein that normally relays pain messages from nerve endings to the brain.

Cayenne supplies 7.8 mg calcium, 0.4 mg iron, 8 mg magnesium, 15.5 mg phosphorus, 107 mg potassium, 4 mg vitamin C and a whopping 2,205 I.U. vitamin A for every 1 tbsp (15 mL).

Caution: Cayenne has an irritating property that heals unbroken inflammations by bringing the blood to the surface when applied externally. Use on unbroken skin or it will irritate and not be as effective. Natural practitioners often advise that capsaicin should not be used internally in cases of chronic inflammation of the intestinal tract, such as in irritable bowel syndrome, ulcerative colitis and Crohn's disease.

Availability: Fresh, whole chile peppers are available in some ethnic markets, supermarkets and whole or natural food stores. Dried whole chiles and powdered cayenne pepper are widely available.

Culinary Use: To enjoy the health benefits of the hot and biting cayenne, start with small doses. Experts say that virtually everybody can gradually build up a tolerance to the hot taste and learn to love it. Milk, yogurt and ice cream soothe the tongue. Cayenne pepper is the principal ingredient of hot pepper sauce.

Use chopped fresh chiles in tomato sauces, soups and stews, and preserved in chili sauce and in raw or cooked salsas. Roasted, peeled and chopped fresh chiles are excellent in sauces, especially barbecue sauces. Dried, whole chiles complement soups, soup stocks, and may be crushed as a garnish for salads, cooked dishes and blended in teas.

Dried powdered cayenne pepper serves as a garnish for main dish meals and in spice blends and rubs for roasted or grilled vegetables.

Celery Seeds

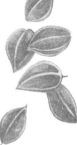

Apium graveolens

The celery plant is a biennial with a bulbous root and thick, fleshy grooved stems. The leaves are pinnately divided. Small gray-brown seeds follow umbels of tiny green-white flowers. Medicinal celery seeds are collected from wild celery.

Parts Used: Seeds (for medicinal purposes). For Celery stalk, see page 76.

Actions: Anti-inflammatory, antioxidant, carminative, reduce blood pressure, sedative, urinary antiseptic.

Uses: Aromatic, tonic, relieve muscle spasms and are used to treat gout, inflammation of the urinary tract, cystitis, osteoarthritis and rheumatoid arthritis.

Caution: Do not use seeds in pregnancy.

Availability: Dried seeds should be purchased from herbalists or whole or natural food stores. The dried seeds found in supermarkets do not have the medicinal value because they are not gathered from the wild plant.

Culinary Use: Medicinal celery seeds have a mild celery taste and can be used in the same ways as other seeds such as sesame or poppy. Crush and add to ingredients in seasonings, soups, baked vegetables, legumes and grain dishes, and use in blended drinks.

Chamomile

See German Chamomile

Cinnamon

Cinnamomum zeylanicum

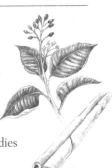

Cinnamon is the dried, smooth inner bark of an evergreen tree indigenous to Sri Lanka and cultivated in hot, wet tropical regions of Mexico, India, Brazil, East and West Indies and Indian Ocean islands.

Parts Used: Bark.

Actions: Carminative, diaphoretic, astringent, stimulant, antimicrobial.

Uses: Cinnamon is a warming carminative used to promote digestion and relieve nausea, vomiting and diarrhea. It is used for upset stomach and irritable bowel syndrome. Recent research has shown that cinnamon helps the body use insulin more efficiently.

Availability: Most of the cinnamon available in supermarkets is *Cinnamomum cassia*, a harder, darker and slightly more bitter-tasting variety of cinnamon. True cinnamon, *C. zeylanicum*, is softer, paler and sweeter in taste. Dried, rolled sticks, called quills may be sold in 2- to 18-inch (5 to 45 cm) lengths in specialty food stores and whole or natural food stores. The ground cinnamon and cinnamon powder widely available is *C. cassia*.

Culinary Use: Fragrant and warm with tones of clove and citrus, cinnamon's sweetly spicy flavor blends well with apples, chile pepper and chocolate. Cinnamon is one of the spices in Garam Masala Spice Blend (see page 254), an Indian seasoning used for savory dishes, rice and curries. Cinnamon is usually used as a carminative with other herbs and spices. It may be used freely to flavor other herbal teas.

Whole quills are used to flavor syrups, sauces, custards, drinks and other liquids. The woody sticks are usually removed after imparting flavor. Crushed sticks are toasted and added to herbal spice and tea blends.

Sweet milk, cream and rice puddings and desserts take advantage of powdered cinnamon and it is widely used in cakes and biscuits, pastries, doughnuts and sweet fritters. Ground cinnamon is mixed with brown or white sugar and sprinkled on porridge, cereal, coffee and toast. Apple crisp, apple pie and pickled dishes are traditional foods that use cinnamon for a dominant flavor.

Cloves

Syzygium aromaticus

Once exotic and only for royalty, cloves are the pink, unopened flower buds of an evergreen tree native to Indonesia, now grown in Zanzibar, Madagascar, West Indies, Brazil, India and Sri Lanka.

Parts Used: Dried buds.

Actions: Antioxidant, anesthetic, antiseptic, anti-inflammatory, anodyne, antispasmodic, carminative, stimulant, prevents vomiting, antihistamine, warming.

Uses: Used for asthma, bronchitis, nausea, vomiting, flatulence, diarrhea and hypothermia. Some studies indicate that cloves may have anticoagulant properties and stimulate the production of enzymes that fight cancer. Clove oil, which is 60 to 90% eugenol, is the active ingredient in some mouthwashes, toothpastes, soaps, insect repellents, perfumes, foods, various veterinary medications and many over-the-counter toothache medications.

Availability: Whole, dried buds and powder widely available.

Culinary Use: Cloves are fragrantly pungent and hot with strong camphor that can leave numbness on the tongue. Their unique flavor is used in spiced or mulled wines, liqueurs, pickles, vegetable stock, sauces and other liquids and studded in fruit and baked goods.

Ground cloves are added to sweet and savory sauces and glazes, fruit dishes, curries, rice, soups and stews, mincemeat, traditional fruit puddings, cakes and stewed fruit dishes. Cloves complement apples, pears, figs and eggplant and they blend well with coriander, cumin, nutmeg, allspice and mace.

Coriander Seeds

Coriandrum sativum

A hardy annual with slender, erect, branched stems that bear pinnate, parsley-like aromatic leaves. Small, flat umbels of tiny white to pale mauve flowers yield round green berries (seeds) that ripen to a brownish yellow.

Parts Used: Seeds.

Actions: Soothing digestive, stimulates appetite, improves digestion and absorption.

Uses: Digestive problems, flatulence.

Availability: Whole dried seeds are readily available in whole or natural food stores and Indian markets. Ground seeds are common at supermarkets.

Culinary Use: Not at all similar in taste to the green leaves (cilantro) that grow on the same plant, coriander seeds are warm, sweet and mild with citrus and floral notes. Coriander seeds are used in most curry seasonings and they are often added to coffee and dessert dishes. Sweet-and-sour dishes and pickles make use of coriander's sweet floral flavors. Coriander complements mushrooms, onions, cinnamon, fennel, nutmeg, plums, apples and pears.

Cumin Seeds

Cuminum cyminum

Cumin seeds are taken from a slender annual plant with dark green leaves that is found wild from the Mediterranean to the Sudan and central Asia. Bristly oval seeds follow umbels of tiny white or pink flowers.

Parts Used: Seeds.

Actions: Stimulant, soothing digestive, antispasmodic, diuretic, increase milk in breastfeeding.

Uses: Indigestion, flatulence.

Availability: Whole dried seeds are readily available in whole or natural food stores and Indian markets. Usually supermarkets only carry the ground seeds.

Culinary Use: Toasting the seeds in a dry skillet brings out a nutty sweetness to the seeds that, without toasting, are pungent, sharp and bitter with earthy spice. Cumin seeds are combined with coriander, cardamom, allspice and anise in spice blends. They are one of the main spice flavors in chili con carne.

Dandelion

Taraxacum officinalis

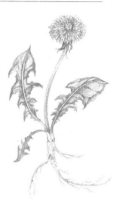

A low-growing, common, hardy and herbaceous perennial, dandelion develops from a long, thick, dark brown taproot with white and milky flesh. One brilliant yellow round flower head sits atop a smooth, hollow stem. Oblong, bright green, deeply toothed leaves grow in a basal rosette directly from the root.

Parts Used: Roots, stems, leaves and flowers.

Actions: Dandelion leaves are diuretic and a tonic for the liver and digestive system. The root is a liver tonic, promotes bile flow, diuretic, mildly laxative and antirheumatic.

Dandelion is highest in lecithin (29,700 ppm) of any of the plant sources. Lecithin is important for cell membrane protection and replacement, reducing cholesterol, converting fat into energy, prevention of strokes and heart attacks and is used in treating Alzheimer's disease.

Uses: Leaves are used specifically to support the kidney. The root works to support the liver. Dandelion is used for gall bladder, kidney and bladder ailments. It is used for liver ailments, including hepatitis and jaundice to promote the liver's processing of toxins for elimination. It also provides important nutrients for storage or release into the system. It's used in skin problems and rheumatism and increases the flow of urine. As a diuretic, dandelion is important for its high potassium content since many other diuretics deplete the body's supply of potassium. Related disorders of digestion, such as dyspepsia, have also been shown to benefit from the ingestion of dandelion.

Dandelion is high in inulin, a form of carbohydrate easily assimilated by diabetics and hence is a potential source of nutritional support for diabetics. It is one of the best food sources of vitamin A (8,400 I.U. beta-carotene per 100 g). The greens yield 187 mg calcium, 66 mg phosphorous, 3 mg iron, 397 mg potassium and 35 mg vitamin C per 100 grams.

Availability: The whole plant is easily foraged spring through fall. Fresh leaves are found in some supermarkets, farmers' markets and whole or natural food stores. The chopped, dried leaf is available in whole or natural food stores.

Culinary Use: Dandelion leaves are tart, bitter and somewhat lemon-like in taste. The fresh root is similar to parsnip but not as strong and the roasted, dried root has a nutty, earthy flavor. Treat the fresh, peeled root in the same way as any root vegetable. Chop and use the fresh root to make a decoction for spring tonic or grate it into salads to help the transition from winter to spring. The dried root is excellent in teas, broths, soups, sauces, stews or any other long-simmering dish. Roasted roots are used as a coffee substitute, often blended with roasted chicory and/or burdock roots.

The fresh, young spring leaves are used as a salad staple or steamed, braised or sautéed as greens, with pasta, in soups and stocks.

Dandelion flower has traditionally been used to flavor wine. The fresh or dried leaves add color to sauces, butter, dips and cheese mixtures. They may be added to baked products, rice dishes or chopped in salads, soups, egg dishes, custards and puddings. Dandelion flowers make a healthy substitute for saffron and may be used as a garnish for all main or dessert dishes, in cakes, breads and muffins. The unopened buds are steamed or sautéed with vegetables. Dried leaves and flowers are combined with other herbs, such as nettles, burdock and yellow dock, to make herb beer or a healing tea blend.

Dill Seeds

Anethum graveolens

Dill is a tall top-heavy, annual plant with a long hollow stem growing out of a spindly taproot. Terminal flowers appear in a wide, flat umbel with numerous yellow flowers. Branches along the stem support feathery blue-green leaflets.

Parts Used: Seeds.

Actions: Soothing digestive, antispasmodic, increase milk in breastfeeding.

Uses: Flatulence, infant's colic, bad breath.

Availability: Dill is easy to grow. Harvest seeds in late summer, early fall. Dried seeds are readily available in whole or natural food stores and supermarkets.

Culinary Use: Dill seeds combine well with potatoes, rye, squash and sweet potatoes, cabbage, onion and vinegar, lending a warm, pleasantly anise and citrus flavor. Salad dressings, sauces and some seasonings use dill seeds.

Echinacea

Echinacea angustifolia or *E. purpurea*

The bright purple petals surrounding a brown cone make echinacea a top choice for perennial beds. A hardy perennial native to North America, its common name is purple coneflower.

Parts Used: Root, leaves and flowers with the root being the most potent.

Actions: Immune stimulating, anti-inflammatory, antibiotic, antimicrobial, antiseptic, analgesic, antiallergenic, lymphatic tonic.

Uses: Studies have shown that echinacea works best at the first sign of cold or flu, taken in 4 to 6 doses daily for not more than 10 days. It has interferon-like actions, helping to prevent and control viral infections. It hastens the healing of tissue and also fights viruses and candida. Echinacea root is more potent than the leaves.

Availability: Dried root, dried stems and leaves are available whole or cut in whole or natural food stores. Echinacea is also available in tincture and tablet form.

Culinary Use: The root is sweet and pleasantly aromatic while the flowers and stems are faintly aromatic. Using echinacea in cooking may aid in general well being and help head off minor illnesses if taken in a soup for 2 or 3 days following bouts of stress or excessive fatigue. Echinacea root combines well with garlic for fighting colds and flu.

Petals and leaves enliven salads, vegetable

dishes and stir-fries, as garnish. Dried petals are used in seasonings.

Whole, fresh or dried echinacea root is added to long-simmering soups and stews. Fresh roots are grated into salads and vegetable and grain dishes. Ground root is dried and combined with other spices or added to sauces, dips, puddings and desserts.

Dried echinacea leaves, petals and finely chopped dried root may be blended with other herbs, such as hyssop, peppermint and thyme, for an effective cold remedy tea blend.

Add 1 tsp (5 mL) echinacea tincture to stocks, soups and stews when colds and flu threaten.

Fennel Seeds

Foeniculum vulgare

Fennel grows wild in Mediterranean Europe and Asia and has naturalized in many other parts of the world where the fleshy bulb is harvested and used as a vegetable. Fennel looks like a larger version of the dill plant. Stout, solid stems support bright yellow, large umbel clusters of flowers. Thread-like and feathery green leaves alternately branch out from joints of the stem. Flowers appear in summer, followed by gray-brown seeds.

Parts Used: Seeds. For the fennel bulb, see page 78.

Actions: Soothing diuretic, anti-inflammatory, antispasmodic, soothing digestive, promote milk flow, mild expectorant.

Uses: Indigestion, flatulence, increase milk flow in breastfeeding, relieve colic in babies when taken by the nursing mother and used directly for colic and coughs.

Caution: Avoid high doses in pregnancy, as it is a uterine stimulant.

Availability: Harvest fennel seeds in late summer, early fall. Dried seeds are readily available in whole or natural food stores and supermarkets.

Culinary Use: Fennel seeds are lightly anise-flavored, with astringent citrus tones. They are often combined with cinnamon, cumin, allspice, fenugreek, thyme and cumin for spice blends. The anise flavor complements both sweet and savory dishes, especially custards, rice and egg dishes. Cabbage, lentils, beets and potatoes go well with fennel seeds.

Fenugreek

Trigonella foenum-graecum

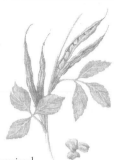

Grown as a fodder crop in southern and central Europe, fenugreek is widely naturalized from the Mediterranean to southern Africa and Australia. This annual legume has aromatic trifoliate leaves and solitary or paired yellow-white flowers, followed by beaked pods with yellow-brown seeds shaped like a pyramid.

Parts Used: Aerial parts and seeds.

Actions: Expectorant, soothing digestive, protects intestinal surfaces, reduces blood sugar and increases milk in breastfeeding.

Uses: Bronchitis, coughs, diabetes, diverticular disease, ulcerative colitis, Crohn's disease, menstrual pain, peptic ulcer, stomach upsets.

Availability: Dried seeds are found in whole or natural food stores and some supermarkets. The dried (and rarely fresh) leaves may be found in Indian markets when in season.

Culinary Use: Fresh fenugreek leaves are mildly pungent with a hint of lemon. Dried seeds are pungent, bitter and give the "curry" aroma to spice blends. Toasting the seeds brings out a slightly sweeter, nutty taste with maple overtones. For a nutritious soup stock, simmer 1 to 2 tsp (5 to 10 mL) lightly crushed seeds and 1 cup (250 mL) water for 10 minutes. Let cool. Strain and discard seeds. Add to the liquid in the recipe. Fenugreek seeds are combined with cumin, cinnamon, coriander, allspice, fennel, chiles and garlic in seasonings. Toasted fenugreek works well with other sweet spices (cinnamon and nutmeg) in sweet custards and desserts.

Garlic

Allium sativum

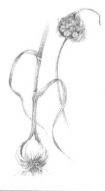

A hardy perennial plant with an edible root bulb made up of four to 15 cloves enclosed in a white, tan or pinkish papery skin. At the tip of the round, hollow and sturdy stem, white flowers appear encased in a teardrop-like membrane that tapers to a sharp, green point. Just before the flowers open, the bud causes the stem to curl and the flower stalk forms a twisted shape. The edible green flower stalks with unopened buds are called "scapes." Flowers form a round ball when in full bloom.

Parts Used: Bulb or head, sometimes called "bud" at the root of the plant. Fresh scapes (the green tops) are eaten as green vegetables.

Actions: Antimicrobial, antibiotic, cardioprotective, hypotensive, anticarcinogen, promotes sweating, reduces blood pressure, anticoagulant, lowers blood sugar levels, expectorant, digestive stimulant, diuretic, antihistaminic, antiparasitic.

Uses: Research has shown that garlic inhibits cancer cell formation and proliferation. It lowers serum total and low-density lipoprotein cholesterol in humans and reduces the tendency of the blood to clot, thereby reducing the risk of blocked arteries and heart disease. Garlic is an antioxidant and helps stimulate the immune system. It has strong antibiotic and anti-inflammatory properties that make it a good wound medicine. Garlic protects organs from damage induced by synthetic drugs, chemical pollutants and the effects of radiation.

One raw garlic clove provides 6 g protein, 29 mg calcium, 202 mg phosphorus, 529 mg potassium and 15 mg vitamin C.

Caution: Dried garlic salt has no medicinal value.

Availability: Fresh whole organic bulbs are found at farmers' markets, food stores and supermarkets. Scapes are found at farmers' markets and Asian markets in mid to late summer.

Culinary Use: Garlic's hot, sharp and strong unique taste is due to the active compound *allicin*. Fresh cloves have the highest medicinal value. It is beneficial to add half to 1 whole fresh raw clove to ingredients in dips and spreads.

To get reliable medicinal benefit from garlic, it is recommended that about two medium-size whole garlic bulbs (about 2 oz/60 g) be taken per week. That requires that almost every main dish you consume contain a minimum of two cloves each. Start to increase your fresh garlic consumption by blending minced fresh garlic into prepared sauces, dips and salad dressings and adding a minimum of one garlic clove to every main dish you make.

The whole head or bulb is often roasted to caramelize the sugars for use in spreads, dips, sauces, vegetable and pasta dishes and spreads. (For Roasted Garlic, see page 132.) Whole, blanched (boiled 30 seconds in water) cloves add subtle flavor to dressings or stir-fries, spiced oils and vinegars. Puréed blanched cloves are used to thicken sauces. Slivered whole garlic works in stir-fries, rice, legume and grain dishes. Chopped, fresh, raw cloves are combined with other herbs and spices for salad dressings, aïoli, pesto, hummus, salsas and seasonings.

Fresh, chopped scapes are mixed into dips, salads, sauces, salad dressing, used as a garnish, stir-fried with butter and lemon or added to grilled or baked vegetable and rice dishes.

Garlic's flower is a beautiful garnish and enlivens vinegars and oils, salads, stir-fries and other main dishes.

German Chamomile

Matricaria recutita

A low-growing hardy annual easily grown in North America. Flowers have daisy-like petals surrounding rounded yellow centers.

Parts Used: Flower heads and petals.

Actions: Gentle sedative, anti-inflammatory, mild antiseptic, prevents vomiting, antispasmodic, carminative, nervine, emmenagogue, mild pain reliever.

Uses: Anxiety, insomnia, indigestion, peptic ulcer, travel sickness and inflammations (such as gastritis) and menstrual cramps are often eased with chamomile. Chamomile also reduces flatulence and pain caused by gas.

Phytonutrients: To date, more than 120 chemical components have been identified from chamomile's clear blue essential oil. Chamazulene, alpha-bisabolol and matricinare have been evaluated individually and found to reduce inflammation. Alpha-bisabolol is also strongly antispasmodic, antimicrobial and mildly sedative.

Availability: Whole dried flower heads and chamomile tincture are available in whole or natural food stores.

Culinary Use: Use fragrant, apple-tasting chamomile to flavor jams, jellies, syrups and sauces. Fresh or dried petals may be used in salads and as an edible garnish, in baked goods and other desserts such as puddings. To relieve an acute upset stomach, take chamomile tea between meals on an empty stomach so the tea will have direct contact with the mucous lining.

Ginger

Zingeber officinalis

The fleshy root we use in cooking is the edible rhizome of a tender perennial plant that is native to Southeast Asia.

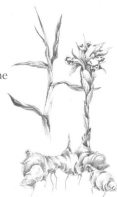

Parts Used: Root.

Actions: Antinausea, relieves headaches and arthritis, anti-inflammatory, circulatory stimulant, expectorant, antispasmodic, antiseptic, diaphoretic, guards against blood clots, peripheral vasodilator, prevents vomiting, carminative, antioxidant.

Uses: Ginger root calms nausea and morning sickness and prevents vomiting. Take ¼ to ½ tsp (1 to 2 mL) ground ginger in water every 3 to 4 hours to relieve nausea and motion sickness. It is a cleansing herb with warming effects. Ginger is used to stimulate blood flow to the digestive system and to increase absorption of nutrients and increases the action of the gall bladder, while protecting the liver against toxins and preventing the formation of ulcers. Studies show that ginger offers some relief from the pain and swelling of arthritis without side effects. Ginger is also used in flatulence, circulation problems, impotence, and to prevent nausea after chemotherapy.

Caution: Ginger can be irritating to the intestinal mucosa, and should be taken with or after meals. Ginger is contraindicated in kidney disease.

Availability: Fresh gingerroot and dried powdered ginger are widely available in supermarkets, Asian and Indian markets and whole or natural food stores.

Culinary Use: Fresh gingerroot is hot and pungent with a sweet, spicy-citrus bite. The dried powder has a stronger, more bitter taste. Both fresh and dried ginger possess therapeutic properties, so use fresh or dried, ground ginger liberally in cooking, as a general tonic (hormone balancer) and to ward off colds and flu. Cook with fresh and dried ginger daily if you or someone in your family suffers from migraine headaches, influenza threatens, rheumatoid arthritis is diagnosed, joint stiffness is a problem, or embarking on a weight loss program.

Fresh and clean tasting with a hot bite, fresh ginger blends well with most fruits and many vegetables. Add sliced fresh ginger to vinegars, oils or stocks. Use julienned ginger in stir-fries and vegetable dishes. Chop or grate raw ginger into salad dressings, marinades, Asian sauces and spreads. Ginger enhances all main dishes, stir-fries, cakes, baked goods, preserves and pickles. Use ginger juice to flavor salad dressings, marinades or sauces and candied ginger in fruit salads, desserts, salad dressings and sauces. Peel and chop fresh ginger, dry and blend with other herbs for teas.

To store fresh gingerroot: If left in a cool, dry place, fresh ginger will only keep for several days. Wrap fresh root in a paper towel and set in an open plastic bag to keep for several weeks in the refrigerator or seal in a plastic bag, freeze and cut off as needed. Fresh ginger keeps indefinitely when peeled, sliced, placed in a glass jar, covered with vodka, sealed and refrigerated.

Use candied or preserved ginger where fresh ginger is called for, especially in desserts and drinks. Candied ginger keeps for a year or longer, and is easy to use in cooking.

If fresh leaves are available, use them as a decorative plate liner, to wrap fish for the grill or to serve finger foods and hors d'oeuvres. If fresh flowers are available, use for salads and as an edible garnish.

Dried ground or powdered ginger is used in cooking as you would fresh.

Ginseng

Siberian *Eleutherococcus senticosis,* North American *Panax quinquefolius,* Asian *Panax ginseng*

A hardy perennial, native to cool, wooded areas of Eastern and Central North America.

Parts Used: Root (from plants older than 4 years) and leaves if organic.

Actions: Antioxidant, adaptogen, tonic, stimulant, regulates blood sugar and cholesterol levels, stimulates immune system.

Uses: Ginseng helps the body resist and adapt to stress. It is a mild stimulant and as a tonic, it promotes long-term overall health. Along with increasing the body's resistance to diabetes, cancer, heart disease and various infections, the medical literature claims that ginseng can improve memory, increase fertility, protect the liver against many toxins and protect the body from radiation. It is also used in impotence and depression.

Caution: Avoid ginseng if you have a fever, asthma, bronchitis, emphysema, high blood pressure or cardiac arrhythmia. Avoid in pregnancy and with hyperactivity in children. Do not take with coffee. Do not take continuously for periods of longer than one month.

Availability: Dried root (whole or chopped), tea, powder and tincture are all found in whole or natural food stores and Asian markets. Fresh ginseng is sometimes found in Chinese and Asian markets. While native to North American woodlands, ginseng has been harvested to near extinction. Please do not collect from the wild or purchase wild crafted North American ginseng.

Culinary Use: The flavor of ginseng is pungent, bitter and astringent with notes of lime but when cooked in dishes, ginseng imparts only a slight flavor to the food. Use in the same way as ginger. Dried ginseng root is very hard and brittle. A good grater, such as those used for nutmeg, will shred the root fine. Whole fresh or dried root is excellent in soups, stocks and stews. Dried whole, grated or flaked ginseng is used in long-simmering soups and stews, and strained off.

Chopped fresh or dried ginseng is added to muesli and granola and dessert bars, whole-grain toppings for desserts and mixed with other herbs for tea blends.

Ground dried ginseng is more bitter than the fresh and works best in milkshakes and smoothies, salad dressings, puddings and other cooked desserts, as part of an antibiotic herbal seasoning, chili pastes and roux. The dried organic leaves are brewed into teas, then added to soups, broths, stews and puddings.

Hemp

Cannabis sativa

A tall woody plant that grows on multi-cellular stalks. Leaves consist of five, deeply cut lobes.

Parts Used: Leaves, stalks, seeds, flowering tops and fruit.

Actions: Promotes healthy menstruation, carminative, treats glaucoma, anti-emetic, aids breathing and inhibits lung tumor growth.

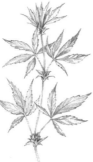

Uses: Hemp has been used to treat digestive disorders, neuralgia, insomnia, depression, migraines, asthma and inflammation.

Tetrahydrocannabinol (THC), cannabinol (CBN) and cannabidiol (CBD) are the active compounds in hemp. Hemp seed contains 26 to 31% pure protein with the essential amino acids and fatty acids.

Availability: Seeds low in THC and hemp oil are available in Canada and Europe. Medicinal use of marijuana is still controversial, but available with prescription in some Canadian provinces, and is legislated in 12 states in the United States.

Culinary Use: Hemp oil is thick and green with a rich, pleasant earthy taste. Hemp oil is rich in linoleic and linolenic fatty acids. It is used without heating, in dressings, sauces, dips and spreads. Hemp seeds are used in commercial snacks and a tahini-like paste and may be used in desserts, soups, baked vegetable and grain dishes and stews. In the Middle East a nutritious drink called *Bhang* is made using hemp leaves, black pepper, cloves, nutmeg and mace as the seasoning base. Water, watermelon juice or cucumber juice is added to the spices for a refreshing drink.

Hyssop

Hyssopus officinalis

An evergreen, bushy, woody perennial, hyssop is native to central and southern Europe, western Asia and northern Africa. The square, upright stem bears linear, opposite leaves and purple flowers in whorls from the dense spikes at the top of the stems.

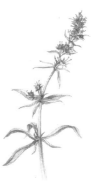

Parts Used: Leaves and flowering tops.

Actions: Antispasmodic, expectorant, promotes sweating, mild painkiller, diuretic, antiviral against herpes simplex, reduces phlegm, soothing digestive.

Uses: Relieves asthma, bronchitis, colds, coughs, influenza, fevers and flatulence. The green tops, boiled in soup, have actually been used in the treatment of asthma. Caffeic acid and unspecified tannins in extracts of hyssop have been shown to have strong anti-HIV activity.

Availability: Hyssop is easy to grow and is harvested from May through fall. Dried leaves are available from whole or natural food stores.

Culinary Use: A fresh, minty, peppery, slightly bitter and pungent taste makes the fresh leaves and flowers excellent additions to salads, fruit cocktails and wraps. The fresh or dried leaves and/or flowers are added to baked goods (especially brownies and date squares), fruit flans and pies, dessert and cough syrups, jams, jellies, sauces, dessert dishes, soups, stews, stocks and stuffing. Hyssop is also dried and mixed with green tea and other herbs for beverages.

Lavender

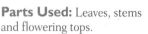

Lavandula spp

A shrub-like plant with dense, woody stems from which linear, pine-like, gray-green leaves grow. The flowers grow in whorls of tiny flowers on spikes from long stems.

Parts Used: Leaves, stems and flowering tops.

Actions: Relaxant, antispasmodic, antidepressive, nervous system tonic, circulatory stimulant, antibacterial, antiseptic, carminative, promotes bile flow.

Uses: Lavender relieves colic, depression, exhaustion, indigestion, insomnia, and stress and tension headaches.

Laboratory research on the anticancer activity of perillyl alcohol distilled from lavender shows promise in the fight against cancer of the breast, pancreas, colon and prostate.

Caution: Avoid high doses in pregnancy because it is a uterine stimulant.

Availability: Easily grown in temperate climates, harvest lavender from June through fall. Organic, food grade dried flower buds are available in whole or natural food stores.

Culinary Use: Lavender is fragrant and distinctly floral. It can overwhelm the flavors of any dish if over used, so it is best to start with small amounts and increase in very small increments. Dried lavender is three times as potent as the fresh. Fresh or dried flowers are best in baked goods such as cookies, cakes, scones, quick breads, sauces, jellies, sorbets and vinegars. They can also be used as a garnish, to flavor honey and vinegar and in jams, jellies and candies. Dried flowers and leaves are often included in Herbes de Provence spice blend and in sugar substitutes or blended with other herbs

and green tea. Lavender teams nicely with lemon in tarts and other desserts and was used to flavor condiments.

Lemon Balm

Melissa officinalis

Opposite, oval, strongly lemon-scented leaves grow on thin, square stems. Flowers are tubular, white or yellow, growing in clusters, at the base of the leaves.

Parts Used: Leaves and flowering tops.

Actions: Antioxidant, antihistamine, carminative, antispasmodic, antiviral, antibacterial, nerve relaxant, antidepressive, stimulates bile flow, lowers blood pressure.

Uses: Lemon balm eases anxiety, depression, stress, flatulence, indigestion and insomnia.

Availability: An easily grown perennial, harvest leaves and flowers from June through autumn. Organic dried leaves are available in whole or natural food stores.

Culinary Use: Lemon balm is distinctly lemon flavored but it can have a slightly soapy taste. For this reason, it is usually blended with other lemon herbs such as lemon thyme and lemon verbena. Dried lemon balm blends are used in teas or the teas are used in sauces, custards and puddings. The fresh leaves are added to salads and dressings, puddings, egg dishes and rice pilafs. Lemon balm may be added in small amounts to recipes whenever lemon juice is an ingredient but it does not replace the lemon juice.

Lemon Verbena

Aloysia triphylla

A fast-growing, deciduous shrub, and native to South America, lemon verbena grows to over 6 feet (1.8 m) in zones 8 to 10. Long, pointed green leaves grow on erect stems with green to brown bark that turn woody with maturity. Lavender-colored flowers are tiny and grow in spikes.

Parts Used: Leaves.

Actions: Antispasmodic, digestive.

Uses: Indigestion, flatulence.

Availability: Dried leaves may be available in whole or natural food stores.

Culinary Use: Lemon verbena imparts a clear, strong, sweetly lemon taste to foods. Dried lemon verbena leaves are combined with fennel seeds for a refreshing pre- or after dinner tonic beverage that aids digestion and helps to reduce gas. Fresh or dried leaves are blended with thyme, basil, mint and chives for seasoning. Lemon verbena leaves are used with whole grains, baked vegetables and desserts.

Licorice

Glycyrrhiza glabra

A tender perennial, hardy in zones 7 to 9, native to the Mediterranean region and southwest Asia.

Parts Used: Root.

Actions: Gentle laxative, tonic, anti-inflammatory, antibacterial, anti-arthritic, soothes gastric and intestinal mucous membranes, expectorant.

Uses: Licorice root is considered to be one of the best tonic herbs because it provides nutrients to almost all body systems. It detoxifies, regulates blood sugar levels and recharges depleted adrenal glands. It has also been shown to heal peptic ulcers and is used to soothe irritated membranes and loosen and expel phlegm in the upper respiratory tract. It is also used to treat sore throat, urinary tract infections, coughs, bronchitis, gastritis and constipation.

Caution: Large amounts taken over long periods of time may cause fluid retention and a reduction in blood potassium levels. Avoid or use sparingly if you have high blood pressure. Extracts lack the tonic action.

Availability: Whole or powdered dried root available in whole or natural food stores.

Culinary Use: Licorice has a sweet, earthy flavor. Although we think of licorice as a flavor, the taste most people associate with licorice is actually anise. The terms anise and licorice are commonly interchangeable now, however, the medicinal qualities are not. Licorice root is 50 times as sweet as table sugar. Brewers use licorice because it gives port and stout their characteristic black color and thick consistency. It can also be used in cooking for the same purpose in sauces, puddings and gravies.

To use licorice in desserts and sauces, make a tea by simmering 1 tsp (5 mL) of the cut and sifted dried root in a cup of boiling water for 5 minutes. Strain the tea and use for sauces and in baked goods such as cookies and puddings.

Linden Flower

Tilia x *europaea*

Found throughout northern temperate regions, common linden is a deciduous tree with dark green, shiny, heart-shaped leaves and yellow-white flowers that appear in mid-summer. It is often grown as an ornamental in North American cities.

Parts Used: Flowering tops.

Actions: Antispasmodic, promotes sweating when taken as a hot tea, diuretic when taken as a warm tea, lowers blood pressure, relaxant, mild astringent.

Uses: Linden flower tea is a pleasant-tasting, relaxing remedy for stress, anxiety, tension headache and insomnia. It relaxes and nourishes blood vessels, making it useful in high blood pressure and heart disease. In promoting sweating, it is useful in colds, flu and fevers. The tea can be given to children as a calming remedy or to reduce fevers.

Availability: Harvest leaves and flowers in mid-June and leaves from early summer through autumn. Dried aerial parts are available in whole or natural food stores. Linden tea bags are often found in supermarkets.

Culinary Use: The actions in linden is partially due to its essential oils, which are only released with heat. For this reason, dried or fresh linden is not added to raw dishes. The easiest method to incorporate the pleasant and mildly lime taste of linden into recipes is by making a tea with the fresh or dried leaves. Use the strained infusion to replace some or all of the liquid in grains, sauces, puddings and desserts.

Mustard

Brassica spp

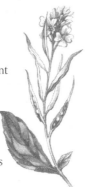

A hearty annual indigenous to North America, the mustard plant is tall with bright green oval leaves. Yellow flowers appear in mid-summer and seedpods develop late summer to early fall.

Parts Used: Seeds (and leaves for cooking) (see Leafy Greens, page 78).

Actions: Blood cholesterol regulator, blood sugar regulator, heartbeat regulator, reduces flatulence.

Uses: Mustard seeds are a good source of magnesium (1 tbsp/15 mL ground mustard seed contains 33 mg magnesium) which helps regulate cholesterol, blood sugar and heartbeat. Native Americans used it to treat asthma, bronchitis, congestion, constipation, dropsy, fever, indigestion, sore muscles and toothache. It has been found to boost energy levels of people with chronic fatigue syndrome.

Availability: Yellow, white, black or brown dried mustard seeds are widely available in food stores. Easily grown from seed.

Culinary Use: Dried mustard seeds are sharp, hot and biting. They are ground into a paste and combined with other spices, vinegar and liquids to make a pungent and hot paste. Mustard seeds or paste may be added to soups, stews, legume and baked vegetable dishes. Use mustard leaves as you would other green leafy vegetables.

Nutmeg

Myristica fragrans

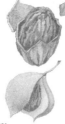

Native to tropical rainforest in the Moluccas and the Banda Islands, the bushy evergreen nutmeg tree is now grown for commercial production in Asia, Australia, Indonesia and Sri Lanka. Pale yellow flowers are followed by fleshy, yellow, round or pear-shaped fruits (generally called seeds).

Parts Used: Dried kernel of the nutmeg fruit.

Actions: Anti-inflammatory, antispasmodic, carminative, digestive stimulant, sedative.

Uses: Nutmeg relieves colic, diarrhea, flatulence, nausea, vomiting and muscle tension.

Caution: Do not use in pregnancy.

Availability: Whole, dried nutmeg seeds are available in whole or natural food stores. Ground nutmeg is widely available.

Culinary Use: Sweetly aromatic with a woodsy clove tone, nutmeg adds depth to savory dishes such as soups, stews, sauces and grain and pasta dishes. It is equally good in desserts and milk puddings. Nutmeg combines well with cinnamon, cloves, allspice, cardamom, coriander, fennel and ginger.

Parsley

Petroselinum crispum

A hardy biennial, native to the Mediterranean and grown as an annual in colder climates.

Parts Used: Leaves, stems and roots.

Actions: Antioxidant, tonic, digestive, diuretic.

Uses: As a diuretic, parsley helps the body expel excess water and flushes the kidneys. Always look for and treat underlying causes of water retention. As a nutrient, it is one of the richest food sources of vitamin C. Parsley's chlorophyll and myristicin may also inhibit the development of some cancers.

Parsley is an excellent source of vitamin A. One hundred grams of fresh parsley contains 3,200 I.U. beta-carotene along with 390 mg calcium, 281 mg vitamin C, 200 mg phosphorus and 17.9 mg iron.

Caution: Parsley should not be used in high doses during pregnancy because it stimulates the womb. Parsley is contraindicated in kidney inflammation.

Availability: Fresh sprigs are found in most supermarkets year-round.

Culinary Use: Parsley's fresh citrus taste has a hint of anise to it. It has the unique ability to enhance the flavors of other ingredients and so it is widely used in vegetarian cooking. One-third to $1/2$ cup (75 to 125 mL) chopped fresh parsley may be added to soups, stews, legume and grain dishes and baked vegetables.

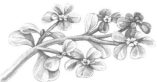

Peppermint

Mentha piperita

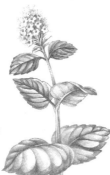

An invasive, hardy perennial, native to Europe and Asia but easily grown in North America, peppermint supports bright green, oval aromatic leaves on purple stems. Small pink, white or purple flowers form elongated conical spikes at the tops of the stems.

Parts Used: Leaves and flowers.

Actions: Antispasmodic, digestive tonic, prevents vomiting, carminative, peripheral vasodilator, promotes sweating, promotes bile flow, analgesic.

Uses: Taking peppermint before eating helps stimulate liver and gall bladder function by increasing bile flow to the liver and intestines. Peppermint is well known for its ability to quell nausea and vomiting. Peppermint is used in ulcerative colitis, Crohn's disease, diverticular disease, travel sickness, fevers, colds, flu and to improve the appetite.

Menthol is the constituent that gives peppermint its antiseptic, decongestant, analgestic and mildly anesthetic (the cooling, numbing sensation) properties.

Caution: Do not use during pregnancy or give to children.

Availability: Fresh sprigs in some markets and supermarkets year-round. Dried leaves are found in whole or natural food stores. Peppermint teas in bulk and bags are widely available.

Culinary Use: Whole fresh sprigs are used in sauces, as a garnish and in teas or drinks. Fresh or dried leaves are great in jellies, sauces, teas, beverages, desserts, salads, marinades, and vegetable and fruit dishes. Fresh flowers enhance salads, stir-fries, and vegetable and fruit dishes. Peppermint tea from fresh or dried leaves and flowers is delicious hot or iced. Blend peppermint with other tea herbs to lend its characteristic fresh and minty flavor.

Purslane

Portulaca oleracea

A wild, low-growing and sprawling perennial that grows throughout much of the world. Leaves are oval, thick (almost succulent) and grow opposite along the horizontal stem. Purslane is considered a weed in North America but eaten as an important food in Europe and the Middle East.

Parts Used: Leaves and tender stems.

Actions: Antioxidant, anti-inflammatory, heart protective.

Uses: Medicinal doses are used to treat heart disease, arthritis and other inflammatory diseases.

Low in saturated fat, purslane is a good source of vitamins B_1 (thiamin), B_3 (niacin) and B_6 (pyridoxine), and a very good source of vitamin A, C, B_2 (riboflavin), calcium, iron, magnesium, phosphorus, potassium, copper and manganese. It is also high in pectin and essential fatty acids.

Caution: Purslane contains oxalic acid and if consumed in very large doses, may be toxic.

Availability: The plant often appears unwanted in gardens and cultivated plots. Fresh leaves may be found in some Greek and Turkish markets but otherwise, must be harvested from the wild.

Culinary Use: Purslane is a very good addition to fresh green salads because of its fresh, astringent citrus taste and juicy leaves that add crunch. Fresh leaves complement beets, zucchini, tomato sauces, beans, and spinach and potato dishes.

Red Clover

Trifolium pratense

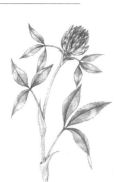

A perennial with tubular pink to red flowers throughout the summer, red clover grows in fields throughout North America. Its three long oval leaflets distinguish it as a clover.

Parts Used: Flowering tops.

Actions: Antispasmodic, expectorant, hormone balancing, nutrient, blood thinning, lymphatic cleanser.

Uses: Coughs, bronchitis, whooping cough, menstrual problems.

Caution: Because it contributes to blood thinning, avoid red clover in times of heavy menstrual flow.

Availability: The flowering tops can be harvested May through September from the wild or cultivated gardens. Dried flowers are available in whole or natural food stores. Dried clover that has turned brown is of little use; be sure that the flowers are still pink.

Culinary Use: Fresh red clover leaves and buds are pleasantly green and woodsy and are added to summer salads. Remove the bitter green centers from the flowers before using. Blend dried red clover with other herbs for a medicinal tea.

Red Raspberry

Rubus idaeus

A deciduous shrub with prickly stems and pinnately divided leaves, widespread in Europe, Asia and North America. Small white flowers appear in clusters with aromatic, juicy red fruit following in early summer.

Parts Used: Leaves (see Fruits for berry information, page 70).

Actions: Antispasmodic, astringent, promotes milk in breastfeeding.

Uses: Red raspberry leaves have long been used to tone the uterus during pregnancy and labor, resulting in less risk of miscarriage, relief of morning sickness and a safer, easier birth. As an astringent, raspberry leaf is useful in sore throat and diarrhea.

Availability: Harvest leaves from early summer through autumn. Dried leaves are available in whole or natural food stores.

Culinary Use: The leaves have a slight raspberry taste but with astringent and lemon tones. Fresh raspberry leaves may be included in fresh green salads or chopped and added to soups and baked vegetable dishes. Dried leaves are blended with thyme or sage for a soothing tea that eases coughs. Red raspberry tea is easy to make and take during pregnancy.

Rose

Rosa

Cultivation of roses dates back thousands of years with *R. rugosa, R. gallica, R. rubra* and *R. damascena* being among the oldest varieties. *Rosa rugosa* is a

deciduous shrub with thorny stems and dark green, oval leaves. Dark pink or white flowers appear in summer and are followed by large, globular, bright red hips (fruit). Wild roses (including the dog rose of North America) grow all over northern temperate regions throughout the world.

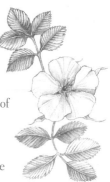

Parts Used: Petals and rose hips.

Actions: Rose hips from *Rosa canina* contain vitamin C and are diuretic, astringent and a mild laxative. Rose petals from *Rosa gallica, R. damascena, R. centifolia, R. rugosa* are antidepressant, anti-inflammatory, astringent, blood tonic.

Uses: Their nutrient value makes rose hips useful in prevention of the common cold and as a tasty addition to herbal teas used to improve immune functioning. As an astringent, they are used in diarrhea. Rose petals can be added to teas for their relaxing and uplifting fragrance. Used in a bath, they have been known to ease the pains of rheumatoid arthritis.

Availability: Harvest fresh petals from organic bushes from mid-summer through autumn and hips in the fall. Dried edible rose petals and rose water are available in Middle Eastern markets. Do not use petals from roses purchased from florist shops.

Culinary Use: Rose petals are perfumed and pleasantly fragrant. Use fresh or dried rose petals to flavor syrups and sauces. Because hips are an important source of vitamin C, use fresh or dried rosehips in teas, syrups and fruit drinks, steep in water, then add to stocks, soups, sauces and gravy. Rose water can replace some of the liquid in desserts and dessert sauces.

Rosemary

Rosmarinus officinalis

An evergreen shrub that grows to 6 feet (180 cm) in warm climates, rosemary is native to the Mediterranean.

Parts Used: Leaves and flowers.

Actions: Antioxidant, anti-inflammatory,

astringent, nervine, carminative, antiseptic, diuretic, diaphoretic, promotes bile flow, antidepressant, circulatory stimulant, antispasmodic, nervous system and cardiac tonic.

Uses: An effective food preservative. Rosemary may be effective in preventing breast cancer, and it fights against the deterioration of brain functions (improves memory). It is also useful in treating migraine and tension headaches, nervous tension, flatulence, depression, chronic fatigue syndrome and joint pain.

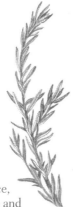

Caution: Avoid large amounts of rosemary during pregnancy.

Availability: Fresh sprigs found in some ethnic markets and supermarkets year-round. Dried whole and powdered leaf found in supermarkets, whole or natural food stores.

Culinary Use: Rosemary is used in smaller amounts than other culinary herbs due to its resinous pine and citrus taste with camphor and spice tones. A combination of rosemary, thyme, garlic and sea salt makes an excellent rub for roasted vegetables and a versatile seasoning for dressings, stuffing and sauces. Rosemary is very good in baked goods such as scones, cookies, focaccia and quick breads. Use a whole sprig the same way you would whole vanilla beans, to impart the spicy essence to egg dishes, syrups and puddings and then remove.

Sage

Salvia officinalis

A hardy, woody perennial evergreen shrub that is native to western United States and Mexico. Tender and hardier varieties of sage grow easily all over Mexico, the United States and southern Canada. Sage has wrinkled, gray-green, oval leaves and purple, pink or white flowers.

Parts Used: Leaves and flowers.

Actions: Antioxidant, antimicrobial, antibiotic, antiseptic, carminative, antispasmodic, anti-inflammatory, circulatory stimulant, estrogenic, peripheral vasodilator, reduces perspiration, uterine stimulant.

Uses: Sage's volatile oil kills bacteria and fungi, even those resistant to penicillin. It is very good as a gargle for sore throat, laryngitis and mouth ulcers. Also used to reduce breast milk production, and to relieve night sweats and hot flashes of menopause.

Caution: Sage can cause convulsions in very high doses. Do not use where high blood pressure or epilepsy is evident, or during pregnancy. Sage should not be consumed during pregnancy. Sage contains steroid-like factors and can encourage miscarriage.

Availability: Fresh sprigs are found at some supermarkets and farmers' markets. Dried, whole, cut, rubbed or ground sage is available at most supermarkets.

Culinary Use: Sage is pungent with balsamic and camphorous notes. Dried sage is often bitter and more potent than the fresh leaves. Small amounts of fresh or dried sage leaves enhance apples, cheese, whole grains, potatoes, tomatoes and legumes. Sage combines well with thyme, garlic, bay, oregano and marjoram, parsley and savory. It is used in stuffing, sauces, and baked vegetable dishes and with legumes and pasta. For a throat-soothing tea, blend sage with thyme, sweet cicely, peppermint and/or licorice. The flower is used chopped fresh in salads, vegetable dishes and as a garnish.

Spearmint

Mentha spicata

Spearmint is a hardy perennial found growing wild in wet soil in most of North America. It is invasive and, like all mints, has a square stem with bright green, lanceolate leaves, lilac, pink, or white flowers borne in a terminal, cylindrical spike.

Parts Used: Leaves and flowering tops.

Actions: Antispasmodic, digestive, induces sweating.

Uses: To relieve the common cold, influenza, indigestion, flatulence and lack of appetite. Spearmint is milder than peppermint, so is often used in treating children's colds and flu.

Availability: The leaves are best harvested just before the flowers open. Dried leaves are available in health food stores.

Culinary Use: Spearmint has a milder, sweeter mint flavor than peppermint and for cooking, fresh spearmint sprigs are preferred. Fresh spearmint leaves are used with potatoes, zucchini and peas. While mint jelly and sauce are usually made with peppermint, salsas are made with the sweeter spearmint. Spearmint combines well with cardamom, coriander, cumin, marjoram and thyme. Spearmint is the mint most often used in Mint Juleps. Lentil and whole grain dishes and some stews can benefit from dried spearmint.

Stevia

Stevia rebaudiana

A small, tender shrub, native to northeastern Paraguay and adjacent sections of Brazil.

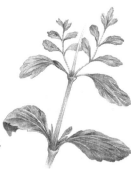

Parts Used: Leaves.

Actions: Energy booster, natural, low caloric sweetener, tonic, digestive, diuretic.

Uses: Stevia's main benefit is in its use as a safe sweetener and sugar alternative. With its powerful sweet, licorice taste (stevia is 200 to 300 times sweeter than sugar), stevia prevents cavities and does not trigger a rise in blood sugar. It increases energy and improves digestion by stimulating the pancreas without feeding yeast or fungi.

Availability: Dried, cut and powdered leaves and liquid extract available in whole or natural food stores.

Culinary Use: Fresh stevia leaves are sweet with a slight citrus taste. They are best used in cooking if made into an infusion. Make a tea from a handful of fresh stevia sprigs and 2 cups (500 mL) boiling water, let steep overnight. Strain and add the liquid to sauces, syrups, dressings, puddings and other desserts.

Substitute 2 tbsp (25 mL) stevia powder for 1 cup (250 mL) sugar in recipes. Add stevia liquid drops to tea, juices, desserts, syrups and other beverages to sweeten.

Note: Some sugar is required for the success of baked goods, so stevia cannot be substituted for sugar in all recipes.

Stinging Nettle

Urtica dioica

Widespread in temperate regions of Europe, North America and Eurasia, this perennial has bristly, stinging hairs on the stem and ovate, toothed leaves that cause minor skin irritation when touched. Minute green flowers appear in clusters during the summer.

Parts Used: Leaves.

Actions: Leaves and flowers are astringent, blood tonic, circulatory stimulant, diuretic, eliminate uric acid from the body, high in iron, chlorophyll and vitamin C, promote milk in breastfeeding. Fresh stinging nettle root is astringent, diuretic.

Uses: A valuable herb, stinging nettle leaves and flowers are useful as a general, daily nourishing tonic, as well as specifically to treat iron-deficiency anemia, gout, arthritis, kidney stones and as a blood tonic in pregnancy, diabetes, poor circulation and chronic skin disease such as eczema.

The fresh root has a strong action on the urinary system. It is useful in water retention, kidney stones, urinary tract infection, cystitis, prostate inflammation and swelling.

Availability: Gather leaves and flowers while flowering in summer, and harvest the root in autumn. Use gloves to protect bare skin from uric acid. Dried leaves and flowers are available in whole or natural food stores.

Culinary Use: Enjoy the peppery and slightly citrus taste of stinging nettle in soups and salads and add to recipes as you would fresh spinach. Cooking and drying neutralizes the uric acid in the hairs on the leaves and stems that causes the sting.

Tea

Camellia sinensis

Green and black tea comes from the shrub or small tree indigenous to the wet forests of Asia and cultivated commercially in Asia, Africa, South America, and North Carolina.

Green tea is heated and dried after harvesting and undergoes no further processing. Black tea is dried, exposed to air (and fermented) before it is heated, causing the antioxidant catechins to oxidize and form equally potent antioxidants called theaflavins.

Parts Used: Leaves.

Actions: Antioxidant, stimulant, astringent, antibacterial, diuretic, antitumor, anti-obesity, prevents gum disease and cavities, lowers blood pressure and blood sugar levels, lowers cholesterol.

Uses: Green tea is a good tonic beverage and can be mixed with other herbs for teas.

Epidemiological studies of Japanese people, heavy consumers of green tea, show that they have lower death rates from cancer of all types, especially cancer of the stomach. A recent Swedish study revealed that women who drank a minimum of two cups of tea daily developed 46% less ovarian cancer than non-tea drinkers.

Catechins in green tea and theaflavins in black tea are strongly antioxidant, protect against cancer, fight viral infection, streptococcus mutans and lower LDL or low-density lipoprotein. The fluoride content in green tea prevents cavities. Vitamins B and C, proanthocyanidins and phenolic compounds are potent antioxidants in green tea.

Caution: Tea (both green and black) contains caffeine — about 3 to 4%, about one-quarter to one-third the amount in coffee and the stronger the tea, the greater the quantity of caffeine in the drink.

Tea interferes with iron intake from foods of plant origin and vegetarians in particular should take tea between meals and not with them.

Availability: Dried green tea in bulk is found in Oriental markets and whole or natural food stores or individually wrapped in supermarkets.

Culinary Use: Green tea is astringent, some are strong tasting while others are refreshingly sweet and mild. Use green tea for syrups, dressings and puddings. Blend dried green tea with other dried herbs for a beverage.

Thyme

Thymus

A bushy, low-growing shrub easily grown in North America.

Parts Used: Leaves.

Actions: Antioxidant, expectorant, antiseptic, antispasmodic, astringent, tonic, antimicrobial, antibiotic, heals wounds, carminative, calms coughs, nervine.

Uses: Thyme is ideal for deep-seated chest infections such as chronic coughs and bronchitis. It is also used for sinusitis, laryngitis, asthma and irritable bowel syndrome.

Thyme is high in calcium (1,890 mg in 100 mg fresh leaves), phosphorus, potassium and beta-carotene (3,800 I.U.).

Caution: Avoid in pregnancy. Children under 2 years of age and people with thyroid problems should not take thyme.

Availability: Fresh sprigs available in farmers' markets in season and most supermarkets year-round. Dried whole leaves in whole or natural food stores.

Culinary Use: The taste of thyme is peppery, pungent, slightly sweet and clove-like. It is extremely versatile and can be added to most dishes. It stands up to long cooking in soups, stews, tomato sauces, gumbos and chowders. Used daily, thyme's antioxidant effect is beneficial. Use thyme in canning and preserving because of its antibacterial, antifungal activity.

Fresh flowering sprigs are great in fruit and vegetable preserves, to flavor vinegar, oils and wine, in long-simmering dishes. Dried sprigs are used in bouquet garni and to release flavor when burned with coals for grilling foods.

Fresh thyme leaves are added to salads, vegetable dishes, soups, casseroles, stuffing, vegetable pâtés, breads, spreads, dips, vinegars, mustards and herb blends. Use lemon thyme with sea vegetables, lemon-flavored baked goods, syrups, puddings and desserts.

The fresh flowers lend a mild taste and rosy color to vinegar, butter and sauces or can be used as a garnish on soups, pasta, rice and desserts. Dried leaves and flowers are blended with other tea herbs.

Turmeric

Curcuma longa

A deciduous tender perennial belonging to the ginger family, hardy to zone 10 and native to southeast Asia. The long rhizome resembles ginger but is thinner and rounder with brilliant orange flesh.

Parts Used: Fleshy root.

Actions: Antioxidant, anti-inflammatory, antimicrobial, antibacterial, antifungal, antiviral, anticoagulant, analgesic, reduces cholesterol, reduces post-exercise pain, heals wounds, antispasmodic, protects liver cells, increases bile production and flow.

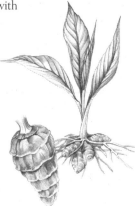

Uses: Turmeric appears to inhibit colon and breast cancer and is used in hepatitis, nausea, digestive disturbances, and where gall bladder has been removed. It boosts insulin activity and reduces the risk of stroke. Turmeric is also used in rheumatoid arthritis, cancer, candida, AIDS, Crohn's disease, eczema and digestive problems.

Availability: Asian stores stock fresh or frozen whole rhizomes at times when it is seasonal in the countries where it grows. Oriental markets or whole or natural food stores offer the dried, whole rhizomes, and supermarkets sell ground turmeric.

Culinary Use: The flavor of turmeric is pungent and charged with a fresh, peppery, camphorous, slightly acrid taste and is at its peak in freshly grated turmeric. Dried, whole rhizomes retain a warm,

sweetish, woody character. Dried, powdered turmeric is weaker and slightly bitter in taste but still gives a yellow color to foods. Turmeric is one of the ingredients in traditional Indian curries. Use the fresh root whenever possible, cutting or grating it as required. Use turmeric to add warmth and a bright yellow hue to rice dishes, cheeses, lentils, pickles, chicken, fish, salsas and liqueurs. The fresh chopped root is also added to stocks, soups, sauces and stews. Fresh sliced root is used to flavor vinegar, oils soups or stocks and the julienne strips are added to stir-fries. Finely chopped or grated, raw fresh turmeric is excellent in salad dressings, marinades, baked vegetable or legume dishes, stir-fries, preserves and pickles. Turmeric juice is used to flavor salad dressings, marinades or sauces. Candied turmeric is used much like candied ginger in fruit salads, salad dressings, syrups and sauces.

Blend fresh or dried turmeric with other spice or herbs such as sweet cinnamon or cloves, hot pepper or mustard, earthy cumin or fenugreek and sharp dill, bay or thyme.

To store fresh root: Wrap the whole fresh root in a dry towel and set in an open plastic bag to keep for several weeks in the refrigerator. To keep longer, seal the fresh root in a plastic bag, freeze and cut off as needed. To keep fresh turmeric indefinitely, peel and slice, place in a glass jar, cover with vodka, seal and refrigerate.

Whole Food Ingredients

Definition: Whole food ingredients are foods used in small amounts to add flavor or to thicken foods. Whole food ingredients are naturally processed. They are products obtained from whole foods without the use of synthetic means. Whole food ingredients retain as many nutrients from their original foods as possible because they have been gently processed, that is, they are not subjected to heat, chemicals or harsh refining methods and do not contain harmful additives or trans fats. Organic whole food ingredients are the very best products we can purchase and use in vegetarian and whole food cooking.

Whole Food Flavorings

Carob

Ceratonia siliqua

Carob beans grow in pods produced by the evergreen carob tree or shrub originating in the Mediterranean region. The beans are ground to a dark powder. Because its taste is similar to cocoa powder or chocolate, carob replaces those ingredients in recipes.

Actions/Uses: Carob does not contain caffeine and is low in saturated fat, cholesterol and sodium. It is a good source of B_2 (riboflavin), calcium, dietary fiber, potassium, copper and manganese.

Forms Available: Powder, flour, chips, chunks, granules.

Culinary Use: Carob is naturally sweeter than cocoa powder and chocolate and may be used in smaller amounts in recipes. Because it does not have the fat, flavor or texture of pure chocolate, carob does not perform the same in baked products. Carob is used in cookies and dessert recipes including puddings, syrups, sauces and fruit bars.

Chocolate

Theobroma cacao

Cocoa and chocolate are derived from the cacao bean, which grows in pods on the tropical cocoa tree. The beans and pulp from the pods are fermented and dried before undergoing a sophisticated process that turns chocolate liquor into the chocolate we eat and use in cooking. For cocoa powder, dried chocolate liquor is ground to a dark powder. Both chocolate and cocoa powders are not naturally sweet, but so bitter, they are inedible.

Actions/Uses: Even though the fats in chocolate are saturated along with the monounsaturated oleic acid, regular consumption of cocoa butter and chocolate has been shown not to raise blood cholesterol levels. This may be due to the relatively high concentrations of stearic acid found in chocolate. Chocolate is rich in magnesium, copper, potassium and manganese. Dark chocolate is rich in flavonoids, which not only act as natural antioxidants (chemicals that combat the damage oxygen does to the body), but that also improve blood vessel flexibility in apparently healthy people. Scientists have found that eating dark chocolate appears to improve the function of important cells lining the wall of blood vessels for at least three hours. Eating dark chocolate seems to make the blood vessels more flexible, which helps prevent the hardening of arteries that leads to heart attacks.

Caution: Chocolate contains caffeine and sugar is usually added in large amounts. Dark, lightly sweetened chocolate is the form to use for health benefits. Check labels and avoid chocolate with wax, vegetable oils or gums as an ingredient or where sugar is listed first.

Forms Available: Unsweetened chocolate with 50 to 58% cocoa butter has no sugar added. To make bittersweet, semisweet and sweet chocolate, cocoa butter, sugar, vanilla and lecithin are added to chocolate liquor in varying degrees. Basically, the sweeter the chocolate, the less cocoa butter and the more sugar it contains. Semisweet chips have a lower cocoa butter content than blocks or squares to keep them from melting when baked in cookies or bars. Milk chocolate is sweetened chocolate with dried milk solids. Milk chocolate is low in cocoa butter (10% minimum by law). White chocolate is made with cocoa butter and not chocolate liquor (so technically it's not a real chocolate) and with milk solids and sugar added. Unsweetened cocoa powder is best for baking. Sweetened cocoa or hot chocolate powders are high in sugar and perhaps milk solids.

Culinary Use: Bittersweet or semisweet dark chocolate (if not too bitter) in block form are the obvious healthy choices for eating chocolate. Generally, expensive dark chocolate has a higher cocoa butter content than the less expensive brands. Unsweetened, bittersweet and semisweet dark chocolate (in squares or blocks) impart a strong chocolate flavor and are all good choices for cooking and baking. However, there must be some sugar in the recipe if these forms of chocolate are used.

Coconut

See Nuts, page 97.

Miso

Miso is a thick, high-protein paste made from soybeans, salt and a fermenting agent. It is similar in taste and color to soy sauce. Sometimes a grain, such as rice and barley, is fermented with the soybeans for additional flavor.

Culinary Use: Small amounts of miso are added to soups, sauces, dressings and stews.

Natto

Natto is made of fermented, cooked whole soybeans, and offers nutritional values similar to those found in miso. It has a sticky, viscous coating and is strong smelling, with a cheese-like texture.

Culinary Use: Natto is used as a spread or in soups.

Sea Salt

Both sea and land salt are the mineral sodium chloride, an essential nutrient that the body requires in small amounts. Sea salt is evaporated from salt water and contains iodine, not naturally found in land-mined salts.

Caution: Excess salt increases the volume of blood in the vessels, causing constriction, which leads to hypertension or high blood pressure.

Culinary Use: Sea salt is added to recipes during the last half hour of cooking or passed at the table for seasoning foods.

Seitan

Made from the gluten in wheat flour, seitan is a high-protein food often used to replace meat in recipes. It has a chewy texture and nutty taste. Purchase seitan in whole or natural food stores.

Caution: The wheat gluten is not appropriate for people with gluten allergies.

Culinary Use: Sold by weight, seitan is broken or crumbled and simmered in liquids.

Tamari Sauce

Similar to soy sauce, tamari is dark brown in color and slightly thicker. Unlike regular soy sauce, which is made by fermenting soybeans with roasted wheat or barley and salt, tamari is fermented naturally. Tamari contains only soybeans, water and sodium and is wheat- and gluten-free.

Actions/Uses: Tamari improve circulation, aid digestion and promote the growth of healthy intestinal bacteria. They are good sources of vitamin B_3 (niacin), manganese and protein.

Culinary Use: Like soy sauce, tamari adds saltiness to foods and should be used in moderation.

Umeboshi

Umeboshi is the name of a Japanese apricot (often called a plum) that is salted or pickled and used as a condiment.

Actions/Uses: Thought to settle an upset and nauseous stomach, umeboshi plums are added to green tea to relieve cold and flu symptoms. Umeboshi is thought to help maintain a low alkaline pH in the blood and this is helpful in neutralizing the acids created by sugars.

Culinary Use: Use umeboshi vinegar as you would rice vinegar. Add small amounts of the salty, pickled umeboshi plums to grains, legumes and baked vegetable dishes. They may be eaten on their own following a meal to improve digestion.

Vanilla

Vanilla planifolia

Vanilla is the edible fruit of a plant that is a member of the orchid family. Bourbon and Tahitian are the two types of vanilla that are used commercially. Pure vanilla extract is an alcohol that has the flavor and fragrance of vanilla. Pure natural vanilla does not contain alcohol; it is made in a glycerin base and contains as much vanilla as the extract.

Actions/Uses: Vanilla has been used medicinally to ease upset stomach and treat asthma, congestion and coughs. A paste made from the vanilla beans is used to treat poisonous bites.

Caution: Beware of inexpensive synthetic vanilla. Pure vanilla extract contains three ingredients — vanilla, alcohol and water.

Forms Available: Liquid extract and whole bean.

Culinary Use: Vanilla may be used to intensify the flavors in both sweet and savory foods. Use vanilla in baked goods, drinks, custards, sauces and syrups. Whole beans are used in sauces to impart flavor, then removed.

Wasabi

Wasabia japonica

Bright green and dangerously hot, wasabi is a Japanese plant that is part of the cabbage family. Known as Japanese horseradish, the green root of the plant is grated and used in ways that are similar to horseradish, that is, in small amounts as a condiment.

Actions: Wasabi's hot taste comes from isothiocyanates that have been known to inhibit microbe growth. The camphor-like vapors burn the nasal passages.

Forms Available: Fresh wasabi is not often seen in North America, but the paste and a powdered wasabi product is found in Japanese food stores, and wasabi-coated peas and peanuts are popular in whole and natural food stores.

Caution: Some products labeled wasabi are actually mixtures of European horseradish, mustard and green food coloring.

Culinary Use: Raw wasabi paste is used in very small amounts and is used most often to accompany sushi or sashimi. It can be used in small amounts in recipes to replace horseradish.

Green Plants

Cereal Grasses

Wheat and barley grass are grown from the seeds or berries of the wheat or barley plant. Harvested when 5 to 6 inches (12.5 to 15 cm) high, the fresh grass is then eaten fresh or juiced. It can also be dried and used in powdered form or pressed into pills.

Actions/Uses: Antioxidant, anti-inflammatory, anticancer, antibiotic, blood cleanser, protective against radiation. High in chlorophyll, which is a powerful healing agent and infection fighter. Also high in beta-carotene and vitamins C and E, these green foods are easily added to juices, blended drinks and uncooked recipes. They have high levels of protein — even higher than soy and legumes — making them the best plant sources of this nutrient.

Culinary Use: Whisk 1 or 2 tsp (5 or 10 mL) powdered wheat or barley grass with 1 or 2 cups (250 to 500 mL) juice, smoothie mixture or other liquids for uncooked spreads, sauces or dips. Chop (or cut with scissors) the fresh green grasses and use as you would parsley in baked vegetable or grain dishes.

Micro-Algae

Chlorella, Spirulina

Rich in carotenoids, protein and chlorophyll, green algae are microscopic single-celled sea vegetables. Ocean or sea algae, including larger sea vegetables (see page 100) are a rich natural source of minerals and trace minerals.

Actions/Uses: Antioxidant, anticancer, immune boosting, reduce heavy-metal toxicity, lower blood pressure. Green algae have been shown to be effective in reducing the effects of radiation and may be helpful in treating HIV infection.

Forms Available: The micro green algae are sold in capsules or bulk loose powder in whole and natural food stores.

Culinary Use: Add up to 1 tbsp (15 mL) to smoothie and other drink recipes. Algae may be added to uncooked foods such as dips, spreads and sauces.

Psyllium Seeds

Plantago ovata

The seed or husk of an annual herb native to Asia and naturalized in the Mediterranean region and North Africa is called psyllium. Psyllium seeds or husks have long been part of traditional and herbal medicine.

Actions/Uses: Psyllium seeds are high in fiber making them an effective natural laxative. By adding bulk to the stool, which causes it to press against the bowel wall, psyllium seeds trigger the contractions leading to a bowel movement. When taking psyllium seeds, you need to drink at least eight glasses of water a day to avoid bowel obstruction. A diet high in whole fresh fruit and vegetables will soon reduce the need for taking psyllium seeds.

Caution: Psyllium can cause an allergic reaction in sensitive individuals, and should be avoided if you have asthma. If you experience an allergic reaction, discontinue immediately. Psyllium must not be taken in cases of bowel obstruction.

Dose: One to 3 tsp (5 to 15 mL) of the seeds mixed in juice or a smoothie, followed by a full glass of water, taken first thing in the morning for 1 week. Another seven glasses of water must be taken during the day.

Plant Thickeners

Agar (or Agar-Agar)

Agar is a substance obtained from some species of red algae (sea vegetable) gathered on the East Indian coast and the Far East. Dissolved in hot water and cooled, agar becomes gelatinous due to its high quantities of mucilage.

Caution: Do not confuse agar with isinglass, which is collagen obtained from the swim or gas bladders of sturgeon and other cold-water ocean fish. Isinglass was extensively used for elaborate molded desserts before gelatin was available. Beer that uses isinglass finings to clarify it is unsuitable for vegetarian diets.

Actions/Uses: Laxative.

Forms Available: Dried granules or flakes are the most common form but whole strips of agar are sometimes available.

Culinary Use: Agar is used as a thickener for sauces, soups, desserts and a clarifying agent in brewing. It is also used to replace gelatin in recipes.

To Use in Recipes: In a saucepan, combine 1 tbsp (15 mL) agar in $2\frac{1}{2}$ cups (625 mL) water, broth or juice. Bring to a boil over medium heat. Reduce heat and simmer for 5 minutes. Let cool and mix with ingredients. Agar sets upon chilling.

Arrowroot

Maranta arundinacea

The root of a tropical rainforest herb that yields a starch that is easily digested, arrowroot is preferred to flour and cornstarch because those ingredients are irritating to people who suffer from food allergies.

Caution: Arrowroot has been known to be adulterated with potato and other vegetable starches.

Culinary Use: Asians use arrowroot in biscuits, puddings, jellies and cakes and in broths and milk puddings. Use arrowroot in place of flour and cornstarch to thicken sauces, custards, puddings and soups. Substitute the same amount of arrowroot as cornstarch in recipes.

Kudzu (or Kuzu)

Pueraria lobata

A cooking starch derived from the roots of a plant belonging to the pea family that is native to Japan. It is used to thicken sauces, custards, puddings and soups. In Japan, along with the roots, which are boiled, the fresh leaves and flowers of the plant are eaten. In southeastern United States, kudzu has taken over large tracts of wasteland along highways and in industrial areas to the point where it is considered a noxious pest.

Actions/Uses: Anti-inflammatory, anticancer, prevents migraines, antimicrobial.

In Japan, kudzu is used to treat cold and flu symptoms, relax muscles and aid digestion. Studies show that it reduces both the ill affects from alcohol consumption and the craving for alcohol itself.

Culinary Use: Kudzu may be used as a substitute for flour or cornstarch to thicken liquids.

Sweeteners

Blackstrap Molasses

Molasses is a thick syrup by-product of the sugar refining process in which the sucrose (sugar) is separated from the liquid and nutrients in the raw cane plant. Several grades of molasses are available, but of the three major types (unsulphured, sulphured and blackstrap), blackstrap contains the least sugar and the most nutrients — iron, six of the B vitamins and calcium, phosphorous and potassium.

In blackstrap molasses, the carbohydrates are quickly assimilated and it is a good source of iron and is totally fat free. Two teaspoons (10 mL) of blackstrap molasses delivers 13.3% of the daily recommended value for iron and 11.8% RDA for calcium. It is also an excellent source of copper and manganese and a very good source of potassium and magnesium.

Sulphured molasses is made by a process that treats green sugarcane with sulphur dioxide fumes during the sugar extraction process.

Culinary Use: Use sparingly in savory dishes or smoothies that require additional sweetening. Molasses adds its own, distinct flavor to baked goods and desserts.

Brown Rice Syrup

When brown rice is cultured with enzymes and the liquid is strained off and cooked, a sweet, dark syrup is the result. Unlike white sugar, brown rice syrup is comprised of about 50% soluble complex carbohydrates that take up to three hours to be digested, providing a steady supply of energy.

Caution: Some rice syrup is produced with the aid of a cereal enzyme that could potentially pose a problem for the gluten intolerant. Look for gluten-free brown rice syrup that uses a fungal enzyme, which produces a superior product safe for people with Celiac disease to consume.

Culinary Use: Brown rice syrup is about half as sweet as table sugar so it cannot be substituted directly. Brown rice syrup and honey may be interchanged in recipes.

Malt Syrup

When barley or other grains are malted, a natural sugar is extracted in the process. The ground, malted grains are heated with water and reduced to syrup. B vitamins and iron are present in malt syrups.

Caution: All malt syrup is produced from grains that could potentially pose a problem for people that are gluten intolerant.

Culinary Use: Barley malt syrup may replace honey or maple syrup in recipes. It sweetens baked products, desserts and drinks.

Maple Syrup

Acer

The clear sap from sugar maples (*Acer saccharum*), red maples (*Acer rubrum*) and silver maples (*Acer saccharinum*) is collected in the spring when it is flowing from the roots into the aerial parts of the tree to provide energy for growth. The sap is 95 to 97% water but when it is boiled down, thick sweet syrup, composed of 65% sucrose, is left behind. The syrup also contains organic acids, minerals (mainly potassium and calcium), and traces of amino compounds and vitamins. One-quarter cup (50 mL) maple syrup provides 6% of the recommended daily intake of calcium and thiamin and 2% of magnesium and riboflavin.

Caution: Avoid maple-flavored syrup because it is primarily corn syrup with artificial flavor.

Culinary Use: Stir 1 to 2 tbsp (15 to 25 mL) pure maple syrup into 1 to 2 cups (250 to 500 mL) of the liquid in sauces, soups, custards or other desserts when a sweetener is required. Fresh maple sap — a thin, watery, clear liquid — may be used as a liquid in soups, stock, syrups, puddings, custards and other desserts, when available in spring.

Organic Cane Syrup Crystals

Cane syrup crystals are produced from the first crystallization of juice pressed from the sugar cane stalk. They are about half as processed as white sugar and contain slightly more molasses and some of the nutrients found in molasses.

Caution: Cane syrup crystals are as high in simple carbohydrates as white or brown sugars.

Culinary Use: Cane syrup crystals lend a mild cane flavor, full sweetness and pale golden color in a fine granulated or powdered form. They may be substituted for white or brown sugar in any recipe.

White Sugar Equivalents

For 1 cup (250 mL) white granulated sugar, substitute any of the following:

- 1⅓ cups (325 mL) unsulphured molasses, minus ⅓ cup (75 mL) liquid specified in recipe, minus baking powder in the recipe, and plus ¾ tsp (4 mL) baking soda
- 1¼ cups (300 mL) honey or rice syrup, minus 2⅔ tbsp (35 mL) liquid in the recipe, plus a pinch of baking soda
- 1¼ cups (300 mL) honey or rice syrup, plus 2⅔ tbsp (35 mL) flour (if no liquid in recipe) plus ½ tsp (2 mL) baking soda

Vinegar

Apple Cider Vinegar

Juice extracted from certified organic apples that is naturally fermented (without heat or the addition of clarifiers, enzymes or preservatives) yields natural vinegar that contains some pectin, trace minerals and beneficial bacteria and enzymes. Organic, natural cider vinegar is usually only available in whole and natural food stores.

Culinary Use: Apple cider vinegar is more robust than the common, non-food distilled white vinegar and should be used in small amounts. It is used in dressings, sauces, soups and other savory or sweet-sour dishes.

Balsamic Vinegar

Called *aceto balsamico* in Italy where it originated in Modena, the production of balsamic vinegar dates back to the Middle Ages. Balsamic vinegar is produced by fermenting and aging white grape juice in wood casks similar to those used in wine making. The longer the grape must ages, the more complex the flavor, texture and sweetness of the resulting vinegar. Balsamic vinegar is priced according to the quality, which is a direct result of the aging process. Labels with the words *tradizionale* and *condimento* indicate vinegars that are made following the ancient methods.

Caution: Some less expensive brands are simply wine vinegar with coloring and sugar added.

Culinary Use: Young balsamic vinegars (3 to 5 years) are used in salad dressing, soups, and sauces and baked dishes. Mid-aged balsamic vinegars (6 to 12 years) enhance sauces, pastas and risottos. Use expensive, long-aged (15 years or older) rich and thick balsamic vinegars in small amounts in simple dishes where the complex aroma, taste and texture will be detected. Good quality, aged balsamic vinegars complement fresh fruit such as strawberries and melon, are brilliant in custards, crème caramel and zabaglione and are sometimes served as a digestive at the end of a meal.

Rice Vinegar

Fermented rice or rice wine is used in China and Japan to produce mild, sweet vinegar that is mellow and light in color. Chinese rice vinegars are slightly darker and stronger than Japanese rice vinegars. Black rice vinegar originated in the eastern Jiangsu province of China and is made with glutinous rice. Black rice vinegar is earthy and smoky in flavor.

Caution: Some inexpensive rice vinegar has salt and sugar added.

Culinary Use: Use rice vinegar in stir-fries, baked vegetable dishes, sweet-and-sour dishes, soups and stews.

Wine Vinegar

Adding some of the vinegar "mother" from organic apple cider vinegar to red or white wine helps the wine to ferment and produce natural wine vinegar. Natural wine vinegars contain a smaller amount of acetic acid than non-food white vinegar, along with smaller amounts of tartaric and citric acids.

Culinary Use: Use wine vinegar in marinades, salad dressings and where a milder taste is preferred for soups, stir-fries, baked vegetable dishes, sweet-and-sour dishes and sauces.

Basics

Roasting Vegetables and Fruit

Roasting is an oven technique that requires a higher heat than baking. This fast-cooking method caramelizes the natural sugars on the outside, concentrating and deepening the flavors. Thick, firm and juicy-fleshed fruit, such as plums, apricots and cherries, and all manner of vegetables, such as beets, onions, squash, turnip, carrots, parsnips, eggplant, sweet potatoes, corn on the cob and asparagus, benefit from roasting.

Roasted Vegetables or Fruit

Serves 4

Roasted fruit and vegetables blacken slightly around the edges and are shriveled in appearance so use them in soups and puréed dishes.

Tip

- For the herbs, use rosemary, sage, thyme, oregano, chives, parsley, basil or savory.

- *Preheat oven to 400°F (200°C)*
- *Baking sheet, lightly oiled*

3 cups	quartered vegetables or pitted fruit	750 mL
2 tbsp	olive oil	25 mL
¼ cup	chopped fresh herbs (see Tip, left)	50 mL

1. On prepared baking sheet, toss vegetables or fruit with oil and herbs. Roast in lower half of preheated oven for 25 to 45 minutes or until browned and tender. Root vegetables will take the full 45 minutes while tender vegetables like asparagus and zucchini will take less time.

Roasted Garlic

Makes 1 head

Whole roasted garlic bulbs morph into a sweet and meltingly tender pulp with a deceptively mellow flavor.

Tip

- Store whole roasted garlic head tightly covered in the refrigerator for up to 5 days. Or squeeze the cloves out of skin, place in resealable freezer bags and freeze for up to 3 months.

- *Preheat oven to 400°F (200°C)*
- *Small heatproof baking dish with lid or foil*

1	whole head garlic	1
1 tsp	olive oil	5 mL

1. Remove loose, papery skin from garlic head. Slice off and discard ¼ inch (0.5 cm) from tops of the cloves in entire head. Place garlic head cut side up in baking dish and drizzle with oil. Cover with a lid or foil. Bake in preheated oven for about 40 minutes or until garlic is quite soft. Transfer to a wire rack and let cool. If using a clay garlic roaster with a lid, roast at 375°F (190°C) for 35 to 40 minutes or until garlic is quite soft.

2. When garlic is cool enough to handle, squeeze cloves from their skins. They are now ready to use in any recipe that calls for roasted garlic.

Seasonings

Experimenting, cooking with and tasting herbs, spices, bark and seeds is what seasoning is all about. In vegan and vegetarian cooking, seasonings are essential tools that take dishes from the ordinary to the extraordinary. When blending seasonings, aim for a balanced mixture that combines woody with fruity; pungent with sweet; or hot and biting with subtle flowery notes.

To make your own herb or spice blends, start with fresh herbs and spices in their whole form. Purchase herbs that are free of sprays (especially check lavender and other flowers) and spices from a seller with a high turnover to guarantee the best quality and freshness. Store whole spices in glass containers in a cool, dry place (never near heat or in sunlight). Roasting the whole seeds before blending and grinding releases the oils and concentrates the flavor. Make only a small amount (1 cup/250 mL or less) of a blend and grind just enough for the recipe at the time of cooking. Store blended or whole spices for a maximum of 6 months. Use the following recipes as a starting point for your own favorite blends.

> Rule of thumb for using herbs in cooking:
> 1 tablespoon (15 mL) fresh herbs = 1 teaspoon (5 mL) dried herbs

Asian Five-Spice Seasoning

Makes ¼ cup (50 mL)

Chinese healers always take into account the five flavors — salty, sour, sweet, pungent and bitter. This seasoning roughly imitates those qualities.

1	piece (2 inches/5 cm) cinnamon stick	1
10	whole cloves	10
8	whole star anise	8
2 tbsp	black peppercorns	25 mL
2 tbsp	whole fennel seeds	25 mL

1. Break cinnamon into small pieces. Using a mortar and pestle or a small electric grinder, pound or grind cinnamon, cloves, star anise, peppercorns and fennel until coarse or finely ground, as desired.

2. Transfer mixture to a small clean jar with lid. Label and store in the refrigerator or a cool, dark place for up to 2 months.

The French herb blend, "fines herbes" is a delicate blend of fresh or dried herbs. It is usually added towards the end of cooking in order to keep the aroma from dissipating with the heat. Here I've given the classic herbs traditionally found in a fines herbes blend but you may wish to add one or two other culinary herbs, such as sage, marjoram or oregano, to the blend.

Fines Herbes Blend

½ cup	coarsely chopped fresh chives	125 mL
¼ cup	fresh tarragon leaves	50 mL
¼ cup	fresh chervil leaves	50 mL
3 tbsp	coarsely chopped fresh parsley or marjoram leaves	45 mL

1. In a bowl, combine chives, tarragon, chervil and parsley. For immediate use, chop herbs and store in an airtight bag in the refrigerator for up to 1 week or in the freezer for up to 2 months.

2. *To dry:* Lay the whole leaves on a clean cloth over a cooling rack and place in a warm, dark place to dry, spreading them out as much as possible to allow for air circulation. This may take 10 to 24 hours, depending on the humidity of the air. When crackling dry, transfer leaves to a clean jar with a lid. Label and store in a cool, dark place for up to 6 months. Crush the herbs just before using in cooking.

Oregano, sometimes called the "pizza herb," is the hero in Italian cooking because it complements tomatoes so well. Basil does not dry well, and that is why I recommend freezing this rich blend that incorporates classic Mediterranean culinary herbs. You may add other favorite herbs to it and, if you omit the basil, the mixture may be dried and stored following the instructions in Fines Herbes Blend (above).

Italian Herb Blend

½ cup	shredded fresh basil leaves	125 mL
¼ cup	coarsely chopped fresh oregano leaves	50 mL
¼ cup	fresh thyme leaves	50 mL
¼ cup	coarsely chopped fresh parsley	50 mL

1. In a bowl, combine basil, oregano, thyme and parsley. Store in an airtight bag in the refrigerator for up to 1 week or in the freezer for up to 2 months.

Herbes de Provence

¼ cup	fresh marjoram leaves	50 mL
¼ cup	fresh thyme leaves	50 mL
¼ cup	fresh rosemary leaves	50 mL
2 tbsp	fresh lavender buds	25 mL
I	fresh or dried bay leaf, cut or crumbled into small pieces	I

Although lavender is a key ingredient in this quintessentially French seasoning, it should not dominate the overall taste and aroma. Be sure to use pesticide-free, food-grade lavender.

1. In a bowl, combine marjoram, thyme, rosemary, lavender and bay leaf. For immediate use, chop herbs and store in an airtight bag in the refrigerator for up to 1 week or in the freezer for up to 2 months.

2. *To dry:* Lay the whole leaves on a clean cloth over a cooling rack and place in a warm, dark place to dry, spreading them out as much as possible to allow for air circulation. This may take 10 to 24 hours, depending on the humidity of the air. When crackling dry, transfer leaves to a clean jar with a lid. Label and store in a cool, dark place for up to 6 months. Crush the herbs just before using in cooking.

Stocks and Broth

The backbone of whole, fresh cooking is often a good vegetable stock. One way to ensure a supply of vegetables for the stockpot is to freeze clean organic trimmings — the tougher parts of asparagus or broccoli stalks, peelings, and leafy tops of celery — and when ready to make stock, they may be tossed directly into the simmering stock. Similarly, freezing homemade stock in 2- or 4-cup (500 mL or 1 L) portions keeps a supply on hand.

Substitutions for Homemade Vegetable Stock

When healing herbs and fresh vegetables are combined and simmered to release their essential qualities, the result has no commercial equivalent. However, to enjoy the goodness of soups when homemade vegetable stock is not on hand, the following may be used in its place:

- Dried organic vegetable bouillon (in powder or pressed cubes) and water (see package directions for mixing with water).

- Organic brown rice milk — generally, the original or plain variety is best for savory soups; the vanilla-flavored version has been used successfully in the mushroom soups in this book, but it does lend a distinctly different flavor.

- Coconut milk — 1 can (14 oz/400 mL) coconut milk plus water can be used especially in chowders and creamy soups.

- Mushroom stock — simmer 8 oz (250 g) mushroom pieces or stems, chopped with 4 cups (1 L) water for 30 minutes. Strain and discard solids.

- Mushroom liquor — when dried mushrooms are reconstituted, save and freeze soaking water to use as a stock or as an ingredient in Vegetable Stock (page 137).

- Vegetable cooking water — when vegetables are cooked in water, save and freeze the cooking water to use as a stock or as an ingredient in Vegetable Stock (page 137).

Tips for Making Vegetable Stock

- Roasting onion, garlic and leek lends a more complex taste and rich color to the stock. An alternative to roasting is to sauté onion, garlic and leek with oil in the stockpot first, then add all other items. Or, for an extremely easy and fat-free stock, omit the oil and toss all the ingredients into the pot, simmer for 1 hour and strain.

- Omit any ingredient in the stock, except onion, garlic and cabbage.

- Potatoes and beets are not ideal for this stock.

- *Other vegetables to use:* Brussels sprouts, parsnips, mushrooms, rutabaga, fennel bulb, zucchini, tomatoes and leafy greens.

- To boost the potassium level of this stock, add sea vegetables (such as dulse, kelp or nori), alfalfa, chamomile, burdock root, dandelion root, stinging nettles or plantain leaves.

- To boost the calcium level of this stock, add sea vegetables (see list above), dandelion greens, kale, Swiss chard or spinach.

Vegetable Stock

The ingredients in this basic vegetable stock are only suggestions. Use vegetables, herbs and spices that you have on hand and omit those you don't have. Cooking with this stock boosts the nutrients in recipes. Use it in every recipe (even baked goods) that calls for water.

- *Preheat oven to 400°F (200°C)*
- *Baking sheet*
- *Large stockpot*

I	onion, quartered	I
4	cloves garlic	4
I	leek, trimmed and cut into large chunks	I
2 tbsp	olive oil	25 mL
8 cups	water	2 L
½	green cabbage, quartered	½
I cup	coarsely chopped broccoli or asparagus stems, optional	250 mL
I	stalk celery, cut into chunks	I
I	carrot, cut into chunks	I
I	apple, cut into chunks	I
I	dried cayenne pepper	I
6	sprigs fresh parsley	6
5	whole allspice berries	5
5	whole cloves	5
5	peppercorns	5
I	bay leaf	I
Few	sprigs fresh thyme	Few
Few	sprigs fresh sage	Few
3	dried astragalus root wafers	3
I	piece (I inch/2.5 cm) gingerroot	I
I	piece (I inch/2.5 cm) burdock root	I
I	piece (I inch/2.5 cm) dandelion root	I

1. On baking sheet, toss onion, garlic and leek with olive oil. Roast in preheated oven, stirring once, for 30 to 40 minutes or until vegetables are soft and brown (some edges may be charred) (see Tips, page 136).

2. In a large stockpot, bring water to a boil over high heat. Add cabbage, broccoli, celery, carrot, apple, cayenne, parsley, allspice, cloves, peppercorns, bay leaf, thyme, sage, astragalus, ginger, burdock, dandelion root and roasted vegetables. Cover, reduce heat and simmer for 1 hour. Remove from heat and let cool slightly. Strain off and discard solids. Let stock cool completely.

3. Store stock in clean jars with lids in the refrigerator for up to 2 days or freeze in 2- or 4-cup (500 mL or l L) portions in freezer containers for up to 2 months.

Mushroom Broth

This broth is brown and rich, full of earthy mushroom essence.

8 oz	shiitake mushrooms	250 g
I	leek, white and light green parts, sliced	I
I cup	chopped onion	250 mL
I	clove garlic, finely chopped	I
2 tbsp	olive oil	25 mL
3 cups	vegetable stock or water, divided	750 mL
I tbsp	pure maple syrup	15 mL
I tsp	salt	5 mL

I. Trim and discard mushroom stems. Slice caps and set aside.

2. In a large saucepan over medium heat, combine leek, onion, garlic and oil. Cook, stirring frequently, for about 10 minutes or until very soft. Add mushrooms and ½ cup (125 mL) of the stock. Bring to a gentle boil. Cover, reduce heat and simmer for 15 minutes.

3. Add remaining 2½ cups (625 mL) of the stock, maple syrup and salt. Bring to a boil. Cover, reduce heat and simmer for 45 minutes.

4. For a clear broth, strain through a sieve and discard vegetables. For a thicker soup, using a slotted spoon, lift out half the vegetables and transfer to a food processor or blender. Process for 30 seconds or until smooth. Pour into a bowl. Repeat with remaining vegetables. Keep remaining broth liquids hot in the saucepan over low heat. Return purée to the saucepan and stir into the liquids.

5. Store stock in clean jars with lids in the refrigerator for up to 2 days or freeze in 2- or 4-cup (500 mL or 1 L) portions in freezer containers for up to 2 months.

Cooking Without Dairy

Preparing plant-based dishes that do not include butter, milk, cream, eggs, cheese and yogurt can be a challenge. For this reason, the glazes, sauce toppings and stuffing recipes found in this section are important because they step in for dairy-based sauces and transform plain vegetables into sophisticated and complex dishes. I prefer to replace only the butter, milk and cream with plant ingredients. Commercial imitations of cheeses are disappointing because in recipes they do not perform like the real thing. (See Sources, page 368, for information on where to obtain commercial non-dairy products.) What follows is a pantry of plant-based substitutions for dairy ingredients and eggs.

Butter

There are many healthy spreads and unsaturated vegetable oils that may be substituted for butter (see Spreads and Dips, pages 178 to 187). Sauté with olive oil and drizzle safflower or sunflower oil over bread and cooked vegetables as a butter alternative. Look for non-hydrogenated solid vegetable fats or use Fruit Purée (recipe below) in place of butter in baked cookies, bars, quick breads and cakes.

Makes 1¾ cups (425 mL)

This purée has the advantage of being lower in fat and cholesterol than butter. I have used 2 tbsp (25 mL) in a 4-cup (1 L) bread stuffing where it replaced both the egg and apple. In the Lemon Sauce recipe (page 362) it stands in for both the eggs and the butter of traditional lemon curd.

Tips

• For a lighter-tasting butter substitute, omit prunes and dates and use 4 apples.

• Lecithin, available in dried granules at natural food stores, is a fatty substance that occurs in both plant and animal tissues.

Fruit Purée (Butter Replacement)

1 cup	water	250 mL
3	apples, peeled and cut into chunks	3
½ cup	pitted prunes	125 mL
¼ cup	chopped dates	50 mL
2 tbsp	organic cane sugar	25 mL
1 tbsp	lecithin granules, optional (see Tips, left)	15 mL
1 tbsp	freshly squeezed lemon juice	15 mL
Pinch	sea salt	Pinch
3 tbsp	olive oil	45 mL

1. In a saucepan over high heat, bring water to a boil. Add apples, prunes, dates, sugar, lecithin, if using, lemon juice and salt. Reduce heat and simmer, stirring occasionally, for 1 hour or until very soft. Let cool.

2. Spoon fruit mixture into a blender or food processor and with the motor running, slowly pour oil through the opening in the lid. Blend until oil is completely incorporated into the mixture. Store purée tightly covered in the refrigerator for up to 4 days.

Milk

Soy milk, rice milk, nut milks (see recipes, pages 140 to 142) and fruit milks (see recipes, page 143) replace cow, sheep and goat's milk in vegan recipes.

Nut Milk

Nuts make a pleasant thick liquid that can be used in some sauces and desserts. Use unsalted organic almonds, pecans, cashews or walnuts (any nut or seed will work) with the skins still on. As you might expect, anyone with an allergy to nuts cannot use nut milks.

Nuts contribute protein, vitamin E and fiber to the diet, but should be taken in small amounts since they have a high fat content (although it's mostly unsaturated and contains essential fatty acids). However, for healthy teens with high energy demands, nut milks can be used regularly in sauces, soups, shakes and baked goods.

Makes 2 cups (500 mL)

Raw, natural almonds give a delicate and sweet almond flavor to the milk.

Tip
- Be sure to bring the water to a boil before making the milk. Boiling destroys many water-bound bacteria.

Almond Milk

1 cup	finely chopped almonds	250 mL
1 tbsp	finely chopped dates	15 mL
1 tbsp	flaxseeds	15 mL
1	piece (1 inch/2.5 cm) vanilla bean	1
2 cups	boiling water (see Tip, left)	500 mL

1. In a clean jar with a lid, combine almonds, dates, flaxseeds, vanilla bean and water. Shake well and let cool in the jar.

2. In a blender or food processor, process until ingredients are liquefied.

3. Store in a clean jar with a lid in the refrigerator for up to 3 days. Shake well before using.

Creamy and somewhat
denser than other nut
milks, this blend is
sweetened slightly by
the addition of raisins.

Cashew Milk

I cup	finely chopped cashews	250 mL
I tbsp	finely chopped dried dulse	15 mL
I tbsp	finely chopped raisins	15 mL
I	piece (I inch/2.5 cm) vanilla bean	I
2 cups	boiling water (see Tip, page 140)	500 mL

1. In a clean jar with a lid, combine cashews, dulse, raisins, vanilla bean and water. Shake well and let cool in the jar.

2. In a blender or food processor, process until ingredients are liquefied.

3. Store in a clean jar with a lid in the refrigerator for up to 3 days. Shake well before using.

The distinctive flavor
of pecans is faintly
discernable in this
nut milk.

Pecan Milk

I cup	finely chopped pecans	250 mL
I tbsp	finely chopped raisins	15 mL
I tbsp	flaxseeds	15 mL
I	piece (I inch/2.5 cm) vanilla bean	I
2 cups	boiling water (see Tip, page 140)	500 mL

1. In a clean jar with a lid, combine pecans, raisins, flaxseeds, vanilla bean and water. Shake well and let cool in the jar.

2. In a blender or food processor, process until ingredients are liquefied.

3. Store in a clean jar with a lid in the refrigerator for up to 3 days. Shake well before using.

Walnut milk is the strongest-tasting of all the nut milks. The dates and vanilla add a sweetness and round out the blend to a pleasant flavor.

Walnut Milk

I cup	finely chopped walnuts	250 mL
I tbsp	finely chopped dates	15 mL
I tbsp	flaxseeds	15 mL
I	piece (1 inch/2.5 cm) vanilla bean	I
2 cups	boiling water (see Tip, page 140)	500 mL

1. In a clean jar with a lid, combine walnuts, dates, flaxseeds, vanilla bean and water. Shake well and let cool in the jar.

2. In a blender or food processor, process until ingredients are liquefied.

3. Store in a clean jar with a lid in the refrigerator for up to 3 days. Shake well before using.

Coconut is naturally sweet and when blended with carob, it is even sweeter. Use coconut milk to replace dairy and sugar in shakes, puddings and other desserts.

Tip

• Use fresh coconut and shred it, freezing the remainder if necessary. If fresh coconut is unavailable, use the unsweetened dried type available at some natural food stores. Frozen shredded coconut is available at Asian and Caribbean stores.

Coconut-Carob Milk

½ cup	finely shredded fresh coconut (see Tip, left)	125 mL
3 tbsp	powdered carob	45 mL
I	piece (1 inch/2.5 cm) vanilla bean	I
½ cup	boiling water (see Tip, page 140)	125 mL

1. In a blender or food processor, combine coconut, carob, vanilla bean and water and let cool. Process until ingredients are liquefied.

2. Store in a clean jar with a lid in the refrigerator for up to 3 days. Shake well before using.

Fruit Milk

Depending on the fruit used, fruit milks tend to be sweeter-tasting. For this reason, they work well in beverages and desserts.

Makes ½ cup (125 mL)

Date sugar is commonly used in commercial products as a sweetener. Using date milk is like using sugar (although it provides some fiber and a few nutrients), so use it sparingly.

Date Milk

¼ cup	chopped dates	50 mL
1	piece (1 inch/2.5 cm) vanilla bean	1
½ cup	boiling water (see Tip, page 140)	125 mL

1. In a blender or food processor, combine dates, vanilla bean and water and let cool. Process until ingredients are liquefied.

2. Store in a clean jar with a lid in the refrigerator for up to 1 week. Shake well before using.

Makes ½ cup (125 mL)

Figs have antibacterial, cancer-fighting properties and make a sweet milk that can be used with tofu in shakes and other recipes. Use fresh figs if available.

Fig Milk

¼ cup	chopped fresh or dried figs	50 mL
1	piece (1 inch/2.5 cm) vanilla bean	1
½ cup	boiling water (see Tip, page 140)	125 mL

1. In a blender or food processor, combine figs, vanilla bean and water and let cool. Process until ingredients are liquefied.

2. Store in a clean jar with a lid in the refrigerator for up to 1 week. Shake well before using.

Makes ½ cup (125 mL)

Sweet, yet slightly tart, this fruit milk has a unique taste. Use it in baked goods and cooked cereals, fruit shakes or smoothies. Look for organic apricots with no sulfur added in the drying process.

Apricot Milk

¼ cup	chopped dried apricots	50 mL
1	piece (1 inch/2.5 cm) vanilla bean	1
½ cup	boiling water (see Tip, page 140)	125 mL

1. In a blender or food processor, combine apricots, vanilla bean and water and let cool. Process until ingredients are liquefied.

2. Store in a clean jar with a lid in the refrigerator for up to 1 week. Shake well before using.

Cream, Ice Cream and Sour Cream

Canned coconut cream (not milk) and puréed tofu may be used to replace cream in soups and some desserts. Cashew Cream (below) is another alternative for light or heavy cream in soup or casserole recipes. Only heavy (whipping) cream (30% butterfat or higher) will whip up into a cream topping, although a processed vegan aerosol whipped soy cream product is available.

Ice cream is traditionally made from custard using eggs, heavy cream and flavorings. The protein in the eggs and the butterfat in the cream freeze and solidify as the mixture is churned over ice. A vegan alternative is iced fruit sorbets or sherbets. Homemade Soy Ice Cream (page 346) is free of additives, gums and preservatives, and commercial soy ice cream-type products are also available.

Sour cream can be replaced by commercial soy sour cream products or Soy Sour Cream (page 145).

Cashew Cream

Makes 1⅓ cups (325 mL)

Use this wherever half-and-half (10%) cream is called for. You can make the sauce thicker by using another ½ cup (125 mL) of cashews. It can then substitute for heavy (whipping) cream in recipes. Only one other nut may be substituted for the cashews in this versatile cook's tool, and that is macadamia.

| ⅓ cup | cashews | 75 mL |
| 1 cup | rice milk or soy milk | 250 mL |

1. In a blender, combine cashews and milk. Blend until nuts are completely puréed and cream is smooth.

2. Store cream tightly covered in the refrigerator for up to 4 days. Shake well before using.

Soy Sour Cream

1 lb	firm tofu, drained	454 g
3 tbsp	freshly squeezed lemon juice or 2 tbsp (25 mL) cider vinegar	45 mL
2 tbsp	olive oil	25 mL
1 tbsp	brown rice syrup or agave nectar	15 mL
1 tbsp	soy milk	15 mL
Pinch	sea salt	Pinch

This is a good replacement for sour cream and a refreshing topping for both fruit and savory dishes. It thickens a bit upon refrigeration and does not separate during storage.

1. In a blender, combine tofu, lemon juice, oil, rice syrup, soy milk and salt. Process until smooth.

2. Store sour cream tightly covered in the refrigerator for up to 1 week.

Egg Replacement

Eggs thicken and bind ingredients in recipes. When whole eggs or egg whites are beaten or whipped, they hold air and cause the other ingredients to rise. Dishes such as puffy soufflés and angel food cakes rely on eggs for leavening. Vegan egg replacement powders available at natural food stores are the best bet when egg whites for meringues or whipped egg whites are required. The following substitutes may be used in place of 1 egg as a thickener or binder.

Vegan lecithin (from soybeans, peanuts and corn) can be used as an emulsifier to replace eggs in cooking.

For each egg:

- ½ mashed banana in baked goods that contain baking powder or soda
- 1 tbsp (15 mL) flaxseeds or chia seeds dissolved in 2 tbsp (25 mL) water in baked goods and where ingredients need an emulsifier
- 2 tbsp (25 mL) cornstarch + ¼ cup (50 mL) water for soups and stews
- 2 tbsp (25 mL) arrowroot flour + ¼ cup (50 mL) water or other liquid, such as vegetable stock, broth or juice, for anything that needs to be dissolved before adding to the recipe
- 1 tbsp (15 mL) chickpea flour + 2 tbsp (25 mL) water as a binder in pancakes and baked products
- 1 tbsp (15 mL) soy powder + 2 tbsp (25 mL) water for batters and doughs

Glazes

Because of their high sugar content, many of these glazes may be stored for one or two months in the refrigerator. This means they become a pantry staple, on hand for use in many recipes. Sterilizing the jar and lid before use extends the length of storage. Sterilize jars by covering them with boiling water 1 inch (2.5 cm) above their tops, and boiling strongly for 15 minutes.

Makes 2 cups (500 mL)

This slightly tart syrupy condiment is used in many Turkish and Moroccan dishes. It may be available in Middle Eastern specialty food stores but this recipe is so easy to make and store that it can become a pantry staple.

Pomegranate Molasses

• *Canning jar*

4 cups	pomegranate juice	1 L
½ cup	organic cane sugar	125 mL
¼ cup	freshly squeezed lemon juice	50 mL

1. In a heavy-bottomed saucepan, combine pomegranate juice, sugar and lemon juice. Bring to a gentle boil over medium-high heat, stirring until sugar is dissolved. Reduce heat and keep simmering gently for about 1 hour or until thick and syrupy. Liquid should be reduced by at least one half. Pour the hot liquid into canning jar before cooling. Cap and then let cool completely.

2. Store molasses in the refrigerator for up to 2 months.

Makes 2 cups (500 mL)

Use this syrup as a glaze for fresh fruit and fruit tarts.

Tip

• Make a pot of green tea using 2 teabags (or 3 tbsp/45 mL loose green tea) and 5 cups (1.25 L) boiling water. Steep for 3 minutes, strain and measure out 4 cups (1 L).

Green Tea Molasses

• *Canning jar*

4 cups	strong green tea (see Tip, left)	1 L
½ cup	organic cane sugar	125 mL
2 tbsp	freshly squeezed lemon juice	25 mL

1. In a heavy-bottomed saucepan, combine green tea, sugar and lemon juice. Bring to a gentle boil over medium-high heat, stirring until sugar is dissolved. Reduce heat and keep simmering gently for about 1 hour or until thick and syrupy. Liquid should be reduced by at least one half. Pour the hot liquid into canning jar before cooling. Cap and then let cool completely.

2. Store molasses in the refrigerator for up to 2 months.

Date Molasses

Makes 2 cups (500 mL)

This molasses has a tang and isn't as sweet or thick as brown rice syrup. It's a pantry staple that can be used as a less expensive alternative in most recipes.

4 cups	apple or orange juice	I L
I cup	chopped dates	250 mL
2 tbsp	freshly squeezed lemon juice	25 mL
2 tbsp	organic cane sugar	25 mL
2 tsp	chopped pitted tamarind	10 mL

1. In a heavy-bottomed saucepan, combine apple juice, dates, lemon juice, sugar and tamarind. Bring to a gentle boil over medium-high heat, stirring until sugar is dissolved. Reduce heat and keep simmering gently for about 1 hour or until thick and syrupy. Liquid should be reduced by at least one half. Let cool.

2. Using a blender, process the date mixture until smooth. Store molasses in a clean jar with lid in the refrigerator for up to 1 month.

Spiced Sweet Glaze

Makes 1¼ cups (300 mL)

This easy-to-make glaze transforms steamed or raw vegetables and other simple vegan dishes into gourmet fare. It enlivens them without masking their vibrant taste.

¾ cup	Pomegranate Molasses (page 146) or store-bought	175 mL
¼ cup	freshly squeezed orange juice	50 mL
I	head roasted garlic (page 132)	I
I tbsp	tamari or soy sauce	15 mL
2 tsp	finely chopped candied ginger	10 mL
I tsp	chipotle flakes or hot pepper flakes	5 mL
½ tsp	ground coriander	2 mL
¼ tsp	ground cinnamon	I mL
¼ tsp	ground cumin	I mL

1. In a blender or food processor, combine molasses, orange juice, garlic, tamari, ginger, pepper flakes, coriander, cinnamon and cumin. Blend until ingredients are liquefied.

2. Store glaze in a clean jar with a lid in the refrigerator for up to 1 month.

Maple-Roasted Garlic Glaze

2	heads roasted garlic (page 132)	2
3 tbsp	pure maple syrup	45 mL
1 tbsp	olive oil	15 mL
1 tsp	balsamic vinegar	5 mL
¼ tsp	sea salt	1 mL
¼ tsp	ground cinnamon, optional	1 mL

1. Squeeze roasted garlic cloves into a bowl and mash with a fork. Add maple syrup, oil, vinegar, salt and cinnamon, if using, and stir well to blend.

2. Store glaze tightly covered in the refrigerator for up to 1 week.

Sauces

Avocado Sauce

A versatile, creamy sauce that is used for pasta sauces, in casseroles and sometimes in desserts (see Tip, below).

Tip
• Use vanilla-flavored soy or rice milk and omit the garlic if the sauce is intended for desserts or sweet dishes.

2 tbsp	olive oil	25 mL
3 tbsp	all-purpose flour	45 mL
1 ¼ cups	rice milk or soy milk	300 mL
3 tbsp	freshly squeezed lemon juice	45 mL
1	ripe avocado, peeled	1
1	clove garlic	1
	Sea salt and freshly ground pepper	

1. In a saucepan, heat oil over medium heat. Stir in flour and cook, stirring constantly, for 1 minute. Whisk in milk. Cook, stirring, for about 4 minutes or until thickened. Let cool slightly.

2. In a blender or food processor, combine lemon juice, avocado and garlic. Process for 20 seconds. With the motor running, add rice milk mixture through the opening in the lid. Blend until sauce is liquefied and smooth. Add salt and pepper to taste.

Makes 4 cups (1 L)

A very easy sauce that is useful in main-course dishes. This basic white sauce is light and silky with a roasted, nutty taste. Use it in pasta and roasted vegetable dishes as you would a béchamel or Mornay sauce made with cream.

Creamy White Sauce

- *Preheat oven to 400°F (200°C)*
- *Rimmed baking sheet*

½	eggplant	½
½	butternut squash	½
1	apple, cut in half	1
4 tbsp	olive oil, divided	60 mL
1	whole head garlic, ¼ inch (0.5 cm) of the top removed	1
1½ cups	rice milk or soy milk	375 mL

1. Arrange eggplant, squash and apple cut side down on baking sheet and drizzle with 3 tbsp (45 mL) of the olive oil. Place garlic head cut side up on same baking sheet. Drizzle with remaining olive oil.

2. Bake in preheated oven for 30 minutes. Using a slotted spoon, remove apple halves and transfer to a bowl. Bake for another 15 minutes or until eggplant is tender. Transfer eggplant to a bowl. Continue to bake squash and garlic for another 15 minutes, for a total of 1 hour, or until tender. Let cool slightly. Scoop apple, eggplant and squash flesh out of their skins and discard skins.

3. In a blender or food processor, combine rice milk, apple, eggplant and squash. Squeeze garlic flesh out of the skin and add to the blender. Blend until sauce is liquefied and smooth. Store sauce tightly covered in the refrigerator for up to 3 days.

Garlic White Sauce

Makes 2 cups (500 mL

Many casseroles, soups and pasta dishes rely on a white sauce to bind all of the ingredients. Here is another basic vegan white sauce to have in your recipe toolbox.

Tip

• Use vanilla-flavored soy or rice milk and omit the onion and garlic if the sauce is intended for desserts or sweet dishes.

I tbsp	olive oil	15 mL
½	onion, finely chopped	½
3 tbsp	finely chopped fresh parsley	45 mL
I	clove garlic, finely chopped	I
I ½ cups	rice milk	375 mL
I	roasted eggplant, peeled (page 132)	I
I	head roasted garlic (page 132)	I

1. In a saucepan, heat oil over medium heat. Add onion and cook, stirring occasionally, for 5 minutes or until slightly softened. Add parsley and garlic and cook, stirring frequently, for 3 to 4 minutes or until onion is soft.

2. In a blender, combine onion mixture, rice milk, eggplant and garlic. Process until liquefied. Store sauce tightly covered in the refrigerator for up to 3 days.

Red Pepper Sauce

Makes 1½ cups (375 mL)

Paprika from Turkey is, in my opinion, the very best you can get. Whether you buy it smoked, sweet or hot, powdered, flaked or in a paste, it is always fresh and flavorful. Use this sauce with steamed, roasted or baked vegetables and as a pasta sauce (see Spaghetti with Red Pepper Sauce, page 300).

• *Preheat broiler*
• *Rimmed baking sheet, lightly oiled*

2	red bell peppers, halved and seeded	2
¼ cup	olive oil, divided (approx.)	50 mL
I	head garlic, ¼ inch (0.5 cm) of the top removed	I
I tbsp	sweet Turkish paprika	15 mL
I tsp	hot pepper flakes	5 mL

1. Arrange red pepper halves cut side down on prepared baking sheet. Drizzle with 1 tbsp (15 mL) of the oil. Broil on the top oven rack for 8 to 10 minutes or until skin is blackened and bubbled. Transfer peppers to a bowl and cover with a towel. Set aside and let cool.

2. Place garlic cut side up on sheet. Drizzle 1 tbsp (15 mL) of oil over. Reduce temperature to 400°F (200°C). Roast on center rack for 40 minutes or until cloves are browned and tender when pierced with a knife. Set aside and let cool.

3. When cool enough to handle, rub blackened skin off red peppers, then coarsely chop peppers and place in a blender. Squeeze roasted garlic cloves into blender. Add paprika and hot pepper flakes and blend. Slowly add remaining oil through opening in the lid and process until smooth.

Tomato Sauce

One can always find excellent canned organic tomato sauces and I recommend that they be used whenever time is short. But for a tomato sauce with bite and boldness, this is the one I make.

1 tbsp	olive oil	15 mL
2	onions, coarsely chopped	2
4	large cloves garlic, finely chopped	4
1 tbsp	finely chopped candied ginger	15 mL
1	carrot, shredded	1
1	parsnip, shredded	1
8 oz	mushrooms, chopped	250 g
1	can (28 oz/796 mL) crushed tomatoes with juice	1
¼ cup	chopped fresh parsley	50 mL
3 tbsp	chopped fresh basil	45 mL
1 tbsp	chopped fresh rosemary	15 mL
1 tbsp	Turkish red pepper paste or harissa, optional	15 mL

1. In a saucepan, heat oil over medium heat. Add onions and cook, stirring occasionally, for 5 minutes or until slightly softened. Add garlic, ginger, carrot and parsnip and cook, stirring frequently, for 5 minutes. Add mushrooms and cook, stirring frequently, for 3 minutes or until vegetables are soft.

2. Stir in tomatoes with liquid and bring to a boil. Reduce heat and simmer, stirring occasionally, for 7 minutes. Add parsley, basil, rosemary and red pepper paste, if using. Cook for 1 minute. Store sauce tightly covered in the refrigerator for up to 3 days.

Tomato Grilling Sauce

This is an all-round
great sauce for
marinating tofu and
tempeh in preparation
for the grill. It adds
a zing to grilled
vegetables as well. As
the tomatoes cook, the
skin wrinkles and pulls
away from the flesh
making them very easy
to peel.

Tip

• For a smoother sauce,
process in the blender
until smooth.

1 tbsp	olive oil	15 mL
2	onions, finely chopped	2
4	large cloves garlic, minced	4
1 tbsp	finely chopped candied ginger	15 mL
4	medium tomatoes, quartered	4
½ cup	Date Molasses (page 147)	125 mL
¼ cup	brown rice syrup or corn syrup	50 mL
1 tbsp	rice vinegar	15 mL
1 tbsp	fresh thyme leaves or chopped fresh oregano	15 mL
1 tsp	hot pepper flakes, optional	5 mL
	Sea salt and freshly ground pepper	

1. In a saucepan, heat oil over medium heat. Add onions and cook, stirring occasionally, for 5 minutes or until slightly softened. Add garlic and ginger and cook, stirring occasionally, for 5 minutes or until onions are soft. Add tomatoes and cook, stirring frequently, for 15 minutes. Using a fork, remove and discard the tomato skins.

2. Stir in molasses, rice syrup, vinegar, thyme and hot pepper flakes, if using. Simmer, stirring occasionally, for about 5 minutes or until thick and slightly reduced. Add salt and pepper to taste.

3. Store sauce in a clean jar with lid in the refrigerator for up to 2 weeks.

Fast and easy, yet very complex in flavor, this sauce serves as a dip for appetizers and as a glaze for stir-fried vegetables.

Tip

- Toasting the peanuts is optional, but it does give them a richer flavor.

Chunky Peanut Sauce

- *Preheat oven to 375°F (190°C)*
- *Rimmed baking sheet, lightly oiled*

2 cups	salted peanuts	500 mL
¾ cup	brown rice syrup	175 mL
¼ cup	rice vinegar	50 mL
3 tbsp	tamari or soy sauce	45 mL
3	cloves garlic, minced	3
3 tbsp	chopped fresh cilantro or parsley	45 mL
1 tbsp	toasted sesame oil	15 mL

1. Arrange peanuts in one layer on prepared baking sheet. Toast in preheated oven for 10 minutes. Stir and continue toasting for another 3 minutes or until light golden. Let cool and coarsely chop.

2. In a bowl, combine rice syrup, vinegar, tamari, garlic, cilantro and sesame oil. Spoon in chopped peanuts and mix well with a fork.

3. Store sauce tightly covered in the refrigerator for up to 5 days.

Use fresh, "peanuts only" peanut butter and if the taste is not sweet enough, add more brown rice syrup. For a thinner dipping sauce, add apple juice until the desired consistency is achieved.

Smooth Peanut Sauce

½ cup	freshly ground smooth peanut butter	125 mL
3 tbsp	Fruit Purée (page 139) or applesauce	45 mL
2	cloves garlic, minced	2
2 tbsp	tamari or soy sauce	25 mL
2 tbsp	freshly squeezed lemon juice	25 mL
1 tbsp	brown rice syrup, agave nectar, or Date Molasses (page 147)	15 mL
1 tbsp	freshly grated gingerroot, optional	15 mL

1. In a heavy-bottomed saucepan, combine peanut butter, fruit purée, garlic, tamari, lemon juice, rice syrup and ginger, if using. Heat over medium-low heat, stirring constantly, until combined and smooth.

2. Store sauce tightly covered in the refrigerator for up to 5 days.

Mushroom Sauce

2 tbsp	olive oil	25 mL
4 cups	sliced mushrooms	I L
I	small onion, chopped	I
I	clove garlic, finely chopped	I
I cup	vegetable stock or water	250 mL
I 1/3 cups	Cashew Cream (page 144)	325 mL

It may seem as though there are too many mushrooms, but as they cook, their volume will be reduced by about half. A deep, wide-bottomed skillet or saucepan will reduce the cooking time. The wider the pan, the faster the mushrooms will cook.

1. In a saucepan, heat oil over high heat. Add mushrooms, onion and garlic. Reduce heat to medium-low and cook, stirring frequently, for 10 to 20 minutes or until mushrooms are reduced and tender.

2. Add stock and increase heat to bring the mixture to a gentle boil. Boil gently, stirring occasionally, for 5 minutes or until the stock is reduced to about half its volume. Stir in Cashew Cream and heat through.

3. Store sauce tightly covered in the refrigerator for up to 3 days.

Teriyaki Sauce

2/3 cup	tamari or soy sauce	150 mL
1/3 cup	brown rice syrup	75 mL
2 tbsp	freshly squeezed lemon juice or rice vinegar	25 mL
2 tbsp	Cashew Butter (page 181) or store-bought cashew butter	25 mL
2	cloves garlic, minced	2

This is a versatile sauce for marinating tempeh or tofu, for dipping wraps and appetizers, for drizzling on rice cakes and for seasoning soups and casserole dishes.

1. In a bowl or jar with a tight-fitting lid, combine tamari, rice syrup, lemon juice, cashew butter and garlic. Whisk or shake to thoroughly mix together.

2. Store sauce tightly covered in the refrigerator for up to 1 week.

Put this easy-to-make sauce to work with steamed vegetables, or use it with pasta or rice as in Lentil and Rice Bowl (see recipe, page 309) or with stir-fried vegetables.

Yellow Coconut Curry Sauce

I cup	coconut milk	250 mL
¼	onion	¼
6	dried apricot halves	6
2	cloves garlic or 8 cloves roasted garlic	2
I tsp	grated lemon zest	5 mL
2 tbsp	freshly squeezed lemon juice	25 mL
I tbsp	coarsely chopped galangal	15 mL
2 tsp	miso	10 mL
I tsp	hot pepper flakes	5 mL
I tsp	coriander seeds	5 mL
½ tsp	caraway seeds	2 mL
½ tsp	fennel seeds	2 mL
½ tsp	fenugreek seeds	2 mL
I tbsp	finely chopped fresh turmeric root or I tsp (5 mL) ground turmeric	15 mL
½ cup	unsweetened shredded coconut, optional	125 mL

1. In a blender, combine coconut milk, onion, apricot halves, garlic, lemon zest and juice, galangal, miso and hot pepper flakes. Process until blended.

2. In a saucepan, combine coriander, caraway, fennel, fenugreek and turmeric root. Toast over medium-high heat until the seeds begin to pop and their fragrance is released, 2 to 3 minutes. Scrape coconut-milk mixture into saucepan and simmer, stirring occasionally, for 10 minutes. The sauce should be thick and creamy.

3. Strain into a bowl and stir in coconut, if using. Store sauce tightly covered in the refrigerator for up to 5 days.

With their delicate
taste and creamy
texture, cashews make
this sauce very different
from a peanut sauce.
Use it with pasta and
rice or with milder
tasting vegetables.

Cashew Curry Sauce

1 tbsp + 1 tsp	olive oil, divided	20 mL
1	onion, cut in half and sliced	1
1	leek, white and light green parts, sliced	1
2 tsp	cumin seeds	10 mL
2 tsp	coriander seeds	10 mL
1/3 cup	whole cashews	75 mL
1 cup	soy milk	250 mL
8	cloves roasted garlic (page 132)	8
1 tsp	chipotle flakes or hot pepper flakes	5 mL
1/2 tsp	ground cinnamon	2 mL
	Sea salt and freshly ground pepper	

1. In a skillet, heat 1 tbsp (15 mL) of the oil over high heat. Add onion and leek. Reduce heat to medium-low and cook, stirring occasionally, for 10 minutes or until soft.

2. In a small skillet over medium-high heat, toast cumin and coriander seeds until lightly colored or until the seeds begin to pop and their fragrance is released, 2 to 3 minutes. Stir into onion-leek mixture. Let cool.

3. Add remaining 1 tsp (5 mL) of oil to the skillet used for toasting seeds. Heat oil over medium-high heat. Add cashews and toast, stirring frequently, for 5 minutes or until lightly browned.

4. In a blender or food processor, combine soy milk, toasted cashews and roasted garlic. Process until smooth. Add onion-leek mixture, chipotle flakes and cinnamon and process until smooth. Season to taste with salt and pepper.

5. Store sauce tightly covered in the refrigerator for up to 3 days.

Candied Nuts

Makes 2 cups (500 mL)

Pecans are exceptionally tasty when candied, but almonds, Brazil nuts and hazelnuts also work well. Use unsalted nuts in this recipe. Save the reserved spiced syrup to make Date Molasses (page 147).

Tip

- Use a deep, heavy-bottomed saucepan and be careful to watch that the foam doesn't rise and overflow. Keep the mixture boiling but reduce the heat as much as possible so that it does not scorch on the bottom of the pan.

- *Preheat oven to 350°F (180°C)*
- *Rimmed baking sheet, lightly oiled and lined with parchment paper*

2 cups	water	500 mL
2 cups	organic cane sugar	500 mL
¼ tsp	ground cinnamon	1 mL
¼ tsp	hot pepper flakes	1 mL
Pinch	sea salt	Pinch
2 cups	nuts (see Intro, left)	500 mL

1. In a saucepan, combine water, sugar, cinnamon, hot pepper flakes and salt. Bring to a boil over medium heat, stirring until sugar is dissolved. Stir in nuts and boil gently, stirring occasionally, for 20 minutes.

2. Strain off liquid over a bowl and reserve it (see Intro, left). Arrange nuts in one layer on the prepared baking sheet. Bake in preheated oven for 15 minutes or until crisp and golden brown. Let cool completely.

3. Store nuts in an airtight tin or jar at room temperature for 3 to 4 weeks.

Crumb Nut Topping

Makes 2 cups (500 mL)

Almonds, Brazil nuts, cashews, pecans, walnuts, hazelnuts and peanuts may be used in this easy topping. Use parsley, or a mixture of basil, sage, oregano and thyme or a traditional fines herbes blend for the mixed herbs.

1 cup	chopped nuts (see Intro, left)	250 mL
1 cup	whole wheat bread crumbs	250 mL
1 tbsp	chopped fresh mixed herbs (see Intro, left)	15 mL

1. In a bowl, combine nuts, bread crumbs and herbs. Stir to combine. Store topping tightly covered in the refrigerator for up to 5 days.

Use almonds, Brazil
nuts, cashews, pecans,
walnuts, hazelnuts or
peanuts. This topping is
good on any of the
baked casseroles (see
recipes, pages 228
to 238).

Oat Nut Topping

½ cup	large-flake rolled oats, spelt or Kamut	125 mL
½ cup	cashew pieces or other nuts (see Intro, left)	125 mL
½ cup	raisins	125 mL

1. In a blender or food processor, combine oats, nuts and raisins. Blend or chop until a coarse, well-mixed crumb is achieved.

2. Store topping tightly covered in the refrigerator for up to 5 days.

Using a healthy stuffing
adds an extra serving of
whole grains, nuts and
seeds, and even fruits
and vegetables to
the diet.

Chickpea Stuffing

1 tbsp	ground flaxseeds	15 mL
2 tbsp	rice milk or soy milk	25 mL
2 cups	stale whole wheat bread crumbs	500 mL
1 cup	chopped cooked chickpeas or Mini Mushroom Burger mixture (page 168)	250 mL
1	apple, finely chopped	1

1. In a bowl, combine flaxseeds and rice milk. Let stand for 5 minutes or until thick and gel-like. Add bread crumbs, chickpeas and apple.

Use this very versatile
topping to add
piquancy to creamy
puréed soups, to
accompany creamed
vegetables, or to splash
color and tart flavor on
stir-fries and casseroles.

Caramelized Red Onions

- *Preheat oven to 400°F (200°C)*
- *9-inch (2.5 L) square baking pan*

2	red onions, cut in half and sliced	2
2 tbsp	olive oil	25 mL
1 tbsp	balsamic vinegar	15 mL
2 tbsp	Pomegranate Molasses (page 146) or store-bought	25 mL

1. Arrange onions in the pan and drizzle with oil and vinegar. Bake in preheated oven, stirring once, for 40 minutes or until crisp and brown on the edges. Toss with molasses.

Appetizers, Spreads and Dips, Pestos and Salsas

Makes 6 small or 3 large pancakes

Thanks to Priya Kothari who graciously gave me permission to use her online recipe as inspiration for this fabulously convenient recipe. It is easy, fast, great tasting and nutritious, and except for the chickpea flour, it uses ingredients that you are likely to have on hand — especially if you use frozen corn and peas. Use this as a basic recipe and then experiment by seasoning with your favorite blends and substituting your favorite vegetables.

Tips

- Chickpea flour, or *besan* (the Indian name for the flour), is produced from finely ground chickpeas. It is a silky flour that when combined with a liquid, produces a smooth and binding batter. Pan-fried vegetable cakes made with besan are called *besan ki childa*.

- Pancakes are best if cooked in a heavy well-seasoned, very hot pan.

Vegetable Pancakes

- *Preheat oven to 200°F (100°C)*
- *Baking sheet*

1	carrot, shredded	1
1	small onion, finely chopped	1
½	red or green bell pepper, diced	½
½ cup	frozen corn kernels	125 mL
½ cup	fresh or frozen green peas	125 mL
2 tbsp	chopped fresh parsley	25 mL
	Sea salt and freshly ground pepper	
1½ cups	chickpea flour (see Tips, left)	375 mL
1 cup	rice milk or soy milk (approx.)	250 mL
2 tbsp	olive oil, divided	25 mL

1. In a bowl, combine carrot, onion, bell pepper, corn, peas and parsley. Season to taste with salt and pepper.

2. In a separate bowl, combine chickpea flour and rice milk, using more or less milk to make a thick but pourable, pancake-like batter. Add vegetables to batter and stir well to combine.

3. In a cast-iron or heavy skillet, heat 1 tbsp (15 mL) of the oil over medium-high heat. Pour in about ¼ cup (50 mL) of the pancake mixture for small pancakes (or ½ cup/125 mL for larger ones) and flatten with the back of a spoon to about ½-inch (1 cm) thick. Pour another portion of batter into the skillet and flatten. Cook for 2 minutes or until the edges start to brown. Flip and cook for 2 minutes on the other side. Transfer cooked pancakes to baking sheet and keep warm in preheated oven. Repeat with remaining pancake mixture, adding more oil to the skillet as needed. Store uncooked batter tightly covered in the refrigerator for up to 2 days.

Serving Suggestion
- Serve with Apricot Tamarind Marmalade (page 183), Umeboshi Sauce (page 363), Chunky Peanut Sauce (page 153) or Smooth Peanut Sauce (page 153).

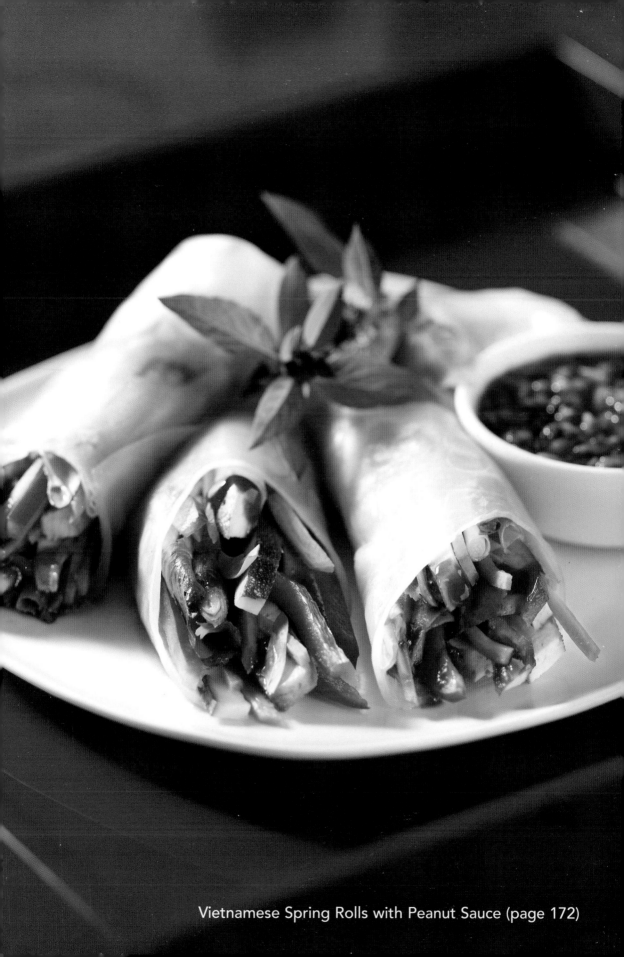

Vietnamese Spring Rolls with Peanut Sauce (page 172)

Sweet Potato Curried Cauliflower Soup (page 192)

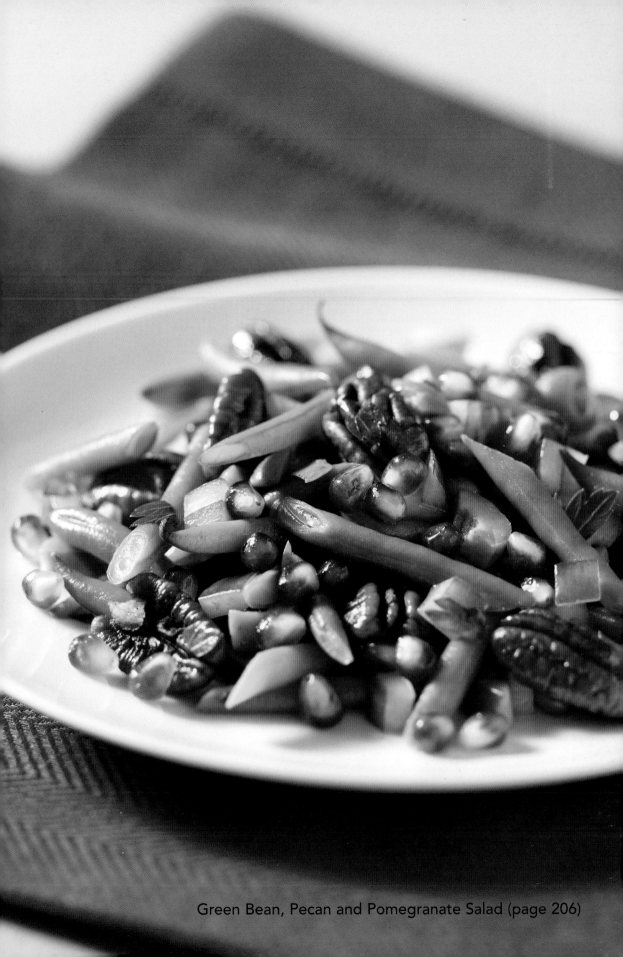

Green Bean, Pecan and Pomegranate Salad (page 206)

Okra and Broad Beans with Tomato Sauce (page 213)

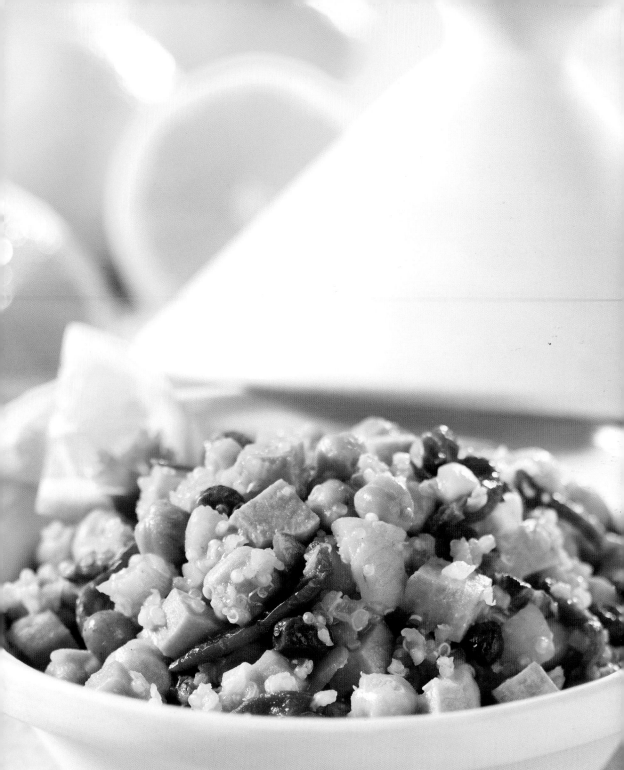

Moroccan Chickpea Tagine (page 230)

Green Pea and Asparagus Curry (page 259)

Leek, Kohlrabi, Garlic and Onion Tart (page 273)

Portobello Pot-au-feu (page 280)

Mushroom and Sweet Potato Cocktail Quesadillas

- *Preheat oven to 200°F (100°C)*
- *Baking sheet*

3 tbsp	olive oil, divided	45 mL
2 cups	sliced mushrooms	500 mL
3	green onions, thinly sliced	3
1 tbsp	fresh thyme leaves	15 mL
3 tbsp	Spiced Sweet Glaze (page 147) or Green Tea Molasses (page 146)	45 mL
	Sea salt and freshly ground pepper	
½ cup	Sweet Potato Spread (page 182)	125 mL
4	10-inch (25 cm) whole wheat flour tortillas	4
1 cup	packed fresh spinach	250 mL

1. In a skillet, heat 2 tbsp (25 mL) of the oil over medium heat. Add mushrooms and cook, stirring occasionally, for 6 to 8 minutes or until they release most of their juices and are slightly browned. Transfer to a bowl and toss with green onions, thyme and glaze. Add salt and pepper to taste.

2. Spread 2 tbsp (25 mL) of the Sweet Potato Spread over the entire surface of one tortilla, leaving a 1-inch (2.5 cm) margin around the edges. Distribute ¼ cup (50 mL) of the mushroom mixture evenly over one half only of the tortilla, leaving the margins free. Top mushrooms with ¼ cup (50 mL) of the spinach.

3. Moisten the margin edge on one half of the tortilla with tepid water. Fold it in half to enclose the filling, creating a half-moon shaped quesadilla. Using a fork, press the edges together to seal. Repeat with remaining tortillas and filling.

4. Coat a skillet with 1 tsp (5 mL) of the oil and heat over medium heat. Add 1 or 2 folded quesadillas. Cover, reduce heat and cook for about 3 minutes or until golden brown. Flip quesadillas and cook, uncovered, for about 2 minutes. The second side should be crisp and lightly browned. Transfer cooked quesadillas to baking sheet and keep warm in preheated oven. Repeat with remaining quesadillas. Cut in half and then in half again for cocktail-size wedges.

Spring Dolmades

8 oz	grape leaves in brine, drained and rinsed (see Tip, left)	250 g
3 tbsp	olive oil, divided	45 mL
3	green onions, sliced	3
¼ cup	finely chopped walnuts	50 mL
¼ tsp	ground cinnamon	1 mL
½ tsp	sea salt	2 mL
½ cup	long-grain white rice	125 mL
3 cups	vegetable stock or water, divided	750 mL
½ tsp	grated lemon zest	2 mL
2 tbsp	freshly squeezed lemon juice	25 mL
¼ cup	fresh green peas	50 mL
¼ cup	coarsely chopped fresh asparagus tips	50 mL
1 cup	Tofu Aïoli or Avocado Aïoli (page 178)	250 mL

Dolmades — from the Arabic word *dolma*, meaning "something stuffed" — are delicate parcels made by wrapping a variety of ingredients in grape leaves (also called vine leaves). Canned grape leaves packed in brine are available in specialty food stores. The North American spring vegetables bring this Mediterranean classic to the New World. Kids love making this recipe and it makes a great weekend dish.

Tip

• If you have fresh grape leaves, choose 25 to 35 small whole leaves. Reserve 5 or 6. Blanch by cooking in a large saucepan of simmering water for 1 or 2 minutes to soften them for folding. Drain and pat dry. Line the bottom of a large saucepan with reserved grape leaves. Continue with Step 2.

1. Separate and select 20 to 30 of the best grape leaves. Soak in warm water for 30 minutes. Rinse and pat dry. Trim stems if necessary. Line the bottom of a large saucepan with 5 or 6 of the remaining grape leaves.

2. Meanwhile, in a skillet, heat 1 tbsp (15 mL) of the oil over medium heat. Add onions and cook, stirring occasionally, for 4 minutes or until soft. Add walnuts and cook, stirring frequently, for 2 minutes. Stir in cinnamon, salt and rice. Cook, stirring occasionally, for 1 minute.

3. Add ¾ cup (175 mL) of the vegetable stock, lemon zest and juice and stir well. Bring to a boil over high heat. Cover, reduce heat and simmer for 10 minutes. Stir in peas and asparagus. Cover and let cool. Rice and vegetables will be only partially cooked at this point.

4. Lay out one grape leaf, vein side facing up and with stem end closest to you. Place 1 tbsp (15 mL) of the rice filling in the center of the leaf. Fold the stem end up over the filling. Neatly fold in the edges of both sides of the leaf. Roll the parcel toward the tip to finish the cigar-shaped wrap. Repeat with the remaining leaves and filling. Dolmades may be made up to this point and stored tightly wrapped in the refrigerator for up to 2 days. Bring to room temperature before steaming.

5. Arrange the rolled dolmades side by side, seam side down, in a single layer if possible in the prepared saucepan. Drizzle with remaining oil and pour over the remaining vegetable stock. Stock should cover the dolmades (add more stock if required). Bring to a boil over high heat. Cover, reduce heat and gently simmer for 1 hour or until rice is tender.

6. Using a slotted spoon, lift the dolmades out of the cooking liquid and let cool in a large colander. Serve warm or at room temperature and pass with the aïoli.

Steamed Rice and Mushroom Pockets

These morsels taste so delicious they are well worth the time it takes to make and steam them. The Chinese use bamboo leaves for this dramatic starter but they can be hard to find. Savoy cabbage leaves are not as dramatic as bamboo leaves, but they stand up to the steaming and they can be eaten if desired. (Bamboo leaves are not to be eaten.)

Tip

• If using bamboo leaves, fold one end of a bamboo leaf on the diagonal to form a cone and secure it with a toothpick. Hold in one hand and spoon in 2 tbsp (25 mL) of the rice. Add 2 tbsp (25 mL) of the mushroom mixture. Fold the other end of the bamboo leaf over to enclose the filling and secure with a toothpick. Tie securely with kitchen string. Repeat with the remaining leaves and filling and follow Step 4.

• *Steamer*

3 tbsp	olive oil, divided	45 mL
3	green onions, thinly sliced	3
1	medium zucchini, peeled and diced	1
½ cup	sliced mushrooms	125 mL
¼ cup	chopped water chestnuts	50 mL
3 tbsp	sesame seeds	45 mL
1 tbsp	Date Molasses (page 147) or blackstrap molasses	15 mL
1 tbsp	tamari or soy sauce	15 mL
1	small cayenne pepper, finely chopped, or ½ tsp (2 mL) hot pepper flakes	1
1 tbsp	chopped fresh cilantro or parsley	15 mL
2 cups	Mushroom Broth (page 138), vegetable stock or water	500 mL
1 cup	white "sticky" rice	250 mL
10	large outer leaves of Savoy cabbage or bamboo leaves (see Tip, left)	10

1. In a heavy skillet or wok, heat 2 tbsp (25 mL) of the oil over high heat. Swirl to coat the base and sides. Add onions, zucchini and mushrooms and cook, stirring constantly, for 4 minutes. Stir in water chestnuts, sesame seeds, molasses, tamari, cayenne pepper and cilantro. Transfer to a bowl and let cool.

2. In a saucepan, bring broth to a boil over high heat. Reduce heat and keep broth simmering. In the same skillet used for the vegetable mixture, heat remaining oil over medium-high heat. Add rice and stir constantly for about 2 minutes or until the rice turns translucent and glass-like. Reduce heat and stir in ½ cup (125 mL) of the hot broth. Cook and stir until all the broth has been absorbed. Keep adding broth by the ½ cup (125 mL) until all the broth is incorporated into the rice. This will take about 20 minutes or more and the rice will still be al dente.

3. *Assemble Pockets:* Fill a large saucepan to the halfway point with water. Bring to a boil over high heat. Keep the water gently boiling. Meanwhile, lay out one cabbage leaf so that it sits up like a cup. Spoon 2 tbsp (25 mL) of the rice into the center of the cup. Spoon 2 tbsp (25 mL) of the vegetables over the rice. (As the leaves get smaller, reduce the amount of rice and mushrooms accordingly.) Fold the left side of the leaf toward the right, enclosing the filling and forming a cone shape, then fold the right side over the left and secure with a toothpick. Neatly fold the top of the leaf down and secure with a toothpick. Repeat with the remaining leaves and filling.

4. Arrange the rice pockets in a steamer. Place the steamer over the boiling water, cover and steam for $1\frac{1}{2}$ hours or until the rice is tender. Keep the water in the saucepan simmering and add more boiling water as required. If you have layered the rice pockets, after 45 minutes, move the top ones to the bottom layer and the bottom pockets to the top.

Pan-Seared Artichokes with Pomegranate Molasses

If you have never
worked with fresh
artichokes, they take
just a bit of work to
prepare, and are so
much better than those
in a jar or can. Save all
the trimmings except
the hairy choke (inner
core) to use in
vegetable stock.

	Juice of 1 lemon	
4	large artichokes	4
4 tbsp	olive oil, divided	60 mL
3	cloves garlic, slivered	3
	Sea salt and freshly ground pepper	
¼ cup	Pomegranate Molasses (page 146) or store-bought	50 mL
½ cup	Romesco Tomato Tapenade (page 189), optional	125 mL

1. Pour lemon juice into a large bowl and set aside. Working with one artichoke at a time, snap off the dark-green outer leaves, leaving the pale, tender inner leaves on the stem. Trim off all but 1 inch (2.5 cm) of the stem. Trim away the top third of the artichoke leaves. Use a paring knife to peel away the tough outer layer of the stem and to remove the base of the leaves. Cut the artichoke in half and then half again. Trim away and discard the hairy choke and any thorny inner leaves from each quarter. As the artichokes are cut and trimmed, toss the quarters into the bowl with the lemon juice.

2. Add 2 tbsp (25 mL) of the oil to the bowl and toss to coat the artichoke quarters. In a heavy skillet, heat remaining oil over medium-high heat. Using tongs, add artichokes to the skillet and arrange them with one cut side down. Reserve the lemon juice and oil. Cook for 2 to 3 minutes or until browned on the one edge.

3. Add garlic to pan. Turn and cook artichoke wedges on the other edge for 2 or 3 minutes or until browned. Turn artichokes onto their curved side. Season to taste with salt and pepper. Drizzle molasses and reserved lemon juice and oil over all. Cover, reduce heat and simmer for about 7 minutes or until the artichokes are tender when pierced with the tip of a knife.

4. *To serve:* Place 4 artichoke wedges on each serving plate. Drizzle with pan juices and spoon 2 tbsp (25 mL) of the tapenade onto the plate, if using.

Portobello Mushrooms with Olive Tapenade

This easy starter is delicious with any favorite filling recipe. Try Basil Pesto (page 188) or Roasted Corn Salsa (page 190) in place of the Olive Tapenade. You can increase the amounts to serve any number. Use whole mushrooms as a starter or side dish, or cut in half or quarters and serve as canapés.

- *Preheat oven to 375°F (190°C)*
- *Rimmed baking sheet, lightly oiled*

4	portobello mushrooms	4
2 tbsp	olive oil	25 mL
	Sea salt and freshly ground pepper	
¼ cup	Olive Tapenade (page 188)	50 mL

1. Arrange mushrooms on prepared baking sheet, gill side down. Brush or drizzle with olive oil. Season to taste with salt and pepper. Bake in preheated oven for 15 minutes.

2. Turn mushrooms over and spoon 1 tbsp (15 mL) of the Olive Tapenade into the centers. Bake for another 5 to 10 minutes or until mushrooms are tender when pierced with a sharp knife and filling is bubbly.

Mini Mushroom Burgers with Apricot Tamarind Marmalade

Make this mixture often — and in great quantities because it is so versatile. Use it as a meat substitute in pasta sauces, to stuff vegetables, as a seasoning for rice and potato pancakes (see Potato Rösti, page 224), and in vegetable salads. Shaped into a roll before freezing, it can be easily measured out and added frozen to baked and roasted dishes.

- *2 pieces waxed or parchment paper, cut into 18-inch (45 cm) lengths*
- *Rimmed baking sheet*

3 tbsp	whole chia seeds	45 mL
2 tbsp	ground flaxseeds	25 mL
½ cup	tomato juice	125 mL
2 tbsp	olive oil	25 mL
1 cup	chopped mushrooms	250 mL
1 cup	chopped onion	250 mL
1	clove garlic, finely chopped	1
1	carrot, shredded	1
½ cup	hulled pumpkin seeds, chopped	125 mL
½ cup	macadamia or Brazil nuts, chopped	125 mL
¼ cup	chopped fresh parsley	50 mL
1 tbsp	tamari or soy sauce	15 mL
1 tbsp	fresh thyme leaves	15 mL
	Sea salt and freshly ground pepper	
2 cups	finely chopped walnuts, divided	500 mL
1 cup	Apricot Tamarind Marmalade (page 183) or store-bought tandoori chutney	250 mL

1. In a bowl, combine chia seeds, flaxseeds and tomato juice. Let stand for at least 20 minutes or until thickly gelled.

2. Meanwhile, in a skillet, heat oil over medium heat. Add mushrooms and onion and cook, stirring occasionally, for 10 minutes or until soft. Add garlic and cook for 2 minutes. Remove from heat and let cool.

3. In a bowl, combine carrot, pumpkin seeds, macadamia nuts, parsley, tamari and thyme leaves. Stir in mushroom mixture and seed mixture. Season to taste with salt and pepper.

4. Scatter 1 cup (250 mL) of the walnuts evenly over one piece of waxed paper. Scrape the mushroom mixture into the center of the walnuts. Roll into a 2-inch (5 cm) diameter log. Wrap in waxed paper and refrigerate for at least 30 minutes. Logs may be made to this point and stored in the refrigerator for up to 3 days.

5. Preheat oven to 325°F (160°C). Spread the remaining walnuts on the second sheet of waxed paper. Slice chilled mushroom log into 1-inch (2.5 cm) disks. Coat the cut sides of the disks with the walnuts. Arrange patties on baking sheet and bake for 15 minutes until lightly browned. Top each patty with marmalade.

Serving Suggestion

- Place a patty on the broad end of an endive leaf and top with 1 tbsp (15 mL) of the marmalade.

This easy chunky mix
is a quick and
great-tasting dip for raw
veggies or as a spread
on crackers, or it can be
served with radicchio
leaves as a first course.
It may be made one day
in advance but tends to
darken during storage.

Tip

• For a smoother dip,
blend in a food
processor or blender.

Country-Style Eggplant

4 tbsp	olive oil, divided	60 mL
1½ cups	finely chopped onions	375 mL
4 cups	diced eggplant, about 1 medium	1 L
3 tbsp	freshly squeezed lemon juice	45 mL
2	cloves garlic, minced	2
½ tsp	sea salt	2 mL
2 tbsp	Spiced Sweet Glaze (page 147) or pure maple syrup	25 mL
1	jar (6 oz/175 g) marinated artichokes, drained and coarsely chopped	1
1 cup	green olives, pitted and chopped, optional	250 mL
	Toast points or radicchio leaves, optional	

1. In a saucepan, heat 2 tbsp (25 mL) of the oil over medium heat. Add onions and cook, stirring occasionally, for 6 to 8 minutes or until soft. Add 1 to 2 tbsp (15 to 25 mL) of the remaining oil and heat. Stir in eggplant, lemon juice, garlic and salt. Cover, reduce heat to low and cook, stirring occasionally, for 15 minutes. Check periodically and add small amounts of water by the tablespoon (15 mL) if eggplant appears to be sticking. Eggplant should be very soft. Add glaze, artichokes and olives, if using, and cook, stirring occasionally, for 5 minutes. Serve with toast points, if using.

When spring brings wild leeks (ramps) and fresh asparagus, this is one way to combine their fresh tastes. Serve this easy dish as a starter for a light lunch.

Cream of Leek and Asparagus on Toast Points

3 tbsp	olive oil, divided	45 mL
1	bunch wild leeks (about 20), white part and green leaves, sliced, or 1 cup (250 mL) sliced leeks, white and tender green parts	1
2 tbsp	all-purpose flour	25 mL
2 cups	rice milk or soy milk	500 mL
1 lb	fresh asparagus, trimmed and cut into 1-inch (2.5 cm) pieces	500 g
4	slices whole wheat bread, toasted	4
4	wild leek leaves, optional	4

1. In a saucepan, heat 2 tbsp (25 mL) of the oil over medium heat. Add leeks and cook, stirring occasionally, for 6 to 8 minutes or until soft. Using a slotted spoon, lift out leeks and set aside. Add remaining oil to saucepan and stir in flour. Cook, stirring constantly, for 1 minute. Whisk in rice milk and cook, stirring constantly, for 4 minutes or until sauce thickens. Add leeks and asparagus and cook, stirring frequently, for 5 minutes or until asparagus is tender-crisp.

2. Cut each slice of toast into 4 wedges and arrange on plates. Spoon creamed vegetables over toast points and garnish with leek leaves, if using.

Serves 4 to 6

Rice paper rounds or squares are available in most Asian supermarkets. There is a definite knack to softening and rolling them, but after one or two tries, they are very easy to assemble — something kids love to do.

Vietnamese Spring Rolls with Peanut Sauce

- *4 lint-free cloth kitchen towels, soaked and wrung out*

14 oz	firm tofu, cut into ½-inch (1 cm) slices	410 g
5 tbsp	tamari or soy sauce, divided (approx.)	75 mL
½ cup	olive oil, divided (approx.)	125 mL
	Sea salt and freshly ground pepper	
½ tsp	hot pepper flakes	2 mL
10 to 12	8-inch (20 cm) rice paper rounds	10 to 12
4	green onions, trimmed and thinly sliced lengthwise	4
1	carrot, cut into 2-inch (5 cm) long matchsticks	1
1	zucchini, cut into 2-inch (5 cm) long matchsticks	1
1	red bell pepper, cut into 2-inch (5 cm) long matchsticks	1
1 cup	coarsely shredded fresh spinach	250 mL
10 to 12	fresh cilantro sprigs	10 to 12
6 to 8	large fresh basil leaves, cut into chiffonade	6 to 8
¼ cup	Umeboshi Sauce (page 363) or Green Tea Molasses (page 146)	50 mL
½ cup	Chunky Peanut Sauce (page 153), Smooth Peanut Sauce (page 153) or store-bought	125 mL

1. Arrange tofu slices in a shallow dish and brush or drizzle with 3 tbsp (45 mL) of the tamari. Flip and brush the other sides. In a skillet, pour enough oil to reach about ½ inch (1 cm) up the sides. Heat over medium-high heat to just below the point of smoking. Add tofu slices and fry, in batches, turning once, for about 3 minutes per side or until crisp on the outside. Using a slotted spoon, transfer tofu to paper towels to drain and season to taste with salt and pepper and hot pepper flakes. Reheat oil as necessary between batches. Cut tofu into thin strips and set aside. Tofu may be prepared up to this point several hours ahead of time.

2. Fill a bowl two-thirds full with tepid water. Lay a damp kitchen towel on a work surface. Grasping a rice paper round between the thumb and index fingers of both hands, quickly immerse it in the water and place on the damp towel. Do not let the rice paper sit in the water or it will get too soft. Repeat with a second rice paper round and place it next to the first one on the towel. Cover the two rice paper rounds with a second damp towel. Repeat until you have 6 rice paper rounds softening between damp towels. Gently turn the pile of towels and wrappers over so the first ones are now on top.

3. Place one rice paper round on a work surface. Place 3 or 4 tofu slices horizontally centered in the lower third of the round (closest to you). Place one slice of green onion and a few sticks of carrot, zucchini and red pepper sticks over the tofu, all lining up horizontally with the tofu slices. Add a few spinach leaves, a sprig of cilantro and a couple of basil strands. Drizzle 1 tsp (5 mL) of the Umeboshi Sauce over all.

4. Roll the rice paper away from you, snugly but gently over the filling, tucking in the ends as you roll. It may take one or two attempts before you achieve the right amount of tension in the rolling — too tight and the paper will tear, too loose and the rolls fall apart when cut. Place the roll seam side down on a serving platter. Stuff and roll the remaining rice paper rounds in the same way. When you have the first 6 rounds completed, cover tightly with plastic wrap and refrigerate. Repeat Steps 2 and 3 with the remaining rice paper rounds and filling. The spring rolls can be prepared up to this point and refrigerated for up to 4 hours.

5. *To serve:* Cut the rolls in half on the diagonal. In a bowl, stir 1 or 2 tbsp (15 or 25 mL) of the tamari into the peanut sauce until it reaches the desired dipping consistency.

Any sweet bell pepper or fiery hot cayenne peppers may be roasted in this manner.

Tip

• Peppers can be stuffed ahead of time and refrigerated overnight.

Spinach-Stuffed Red Pepper Rolls

• *Preheat broiler, with oven rack in top position, directly under heat*
• *Baking sheet*

4	red bell peppers	4

Spinach Stuffing

2 tbsp	olive oil	25 mL
½ cup	chopped onion	125 mL
2	cloves garlic, minced	2
⅓ cup	rice milk or soy milk	75 mL
2 tbsp	Cashew Butter (page 181) or store-bought nut butter	25 mL
2 cups	chopped fresh spinach	500 mL
1 tbsp	pure maple syrup, optional	15 mL
	Olive oil for brushing	

1. *Peppers:* Place peppers on a baking sheet. Broil in preheated oven, turning often, for 5 to 8 minutes or until the skin is evenly charred and blistered.

2. Place baking sheet on a cooling rack and cover peppers with a clean towel. Let cool. Remove the charred skin from peppers. It should slip off easily when rubbed. Carefully slit peppers open from stem to base on one side only. Remove stem, ribs and seeds.

3. *Spinach Stuffing:* Meanwhile, in a skillet, heat oil over medium heat. Add onion and cook, stirring occasionally, for 5 minutes or until slightly softened. Add garlic and cook, stirring frequently, for 3 minutes or until onion is soft. Add rice milk and cashew butter and stir until butter is blended into the sauce. Add spinach and maple syrup, if using, and cook, stirring for 1 minute or until spinach is wilted.

4. *To assemble rolls:* Divide the stuffing into 4 portions and spoon along the inside edge of a roasted pepper. Roll pepper tightly around stuffing and secure with a toothpick. Repeat with remaining peppers and stuffing. Arrange on baking sheet and brush with olive oil. Broil in preheated oven on top rack (or grill on the barbecue) for 1 or 2 minutes or until rolls are partly browned and stuffing is bubbly.

Brazil Nut Rissoles

Although these little rice packets are delicate, they hold together for finger-food platters. I like them best as an appetizer served with a punchy condiment such as Olive Tapenade (page 188) or Kiwi and Avocado Salsa with Pomegranate and Red Onion (page 189).

- *Preheat oven to 375°F (190°C)*
- *Baking sheet*

I tbsp	ground flaxseeds	15 mL
3 tbsp	water or tomato juice	45 mL
I cup	cooked brown rice	250 mL
½ cup	finely chopped Brazil nuts	125 mL
2 tbsp	chopped fresh tarragon	25 mL
	Sea salt and freshly ground pepper	
I cup	fresh bread crumbs	250 mL

1. In a bowl, combine flaxseeds and water. Let stand for 10 minutes or until gelatinous.

2. Meanwhile, in a separate bowl, combine brown rice, Brazil nuts and tarragon. Season to taste with salt and pepper. Stir in flaxseeds. Using two spoons, press the mixture into small "eggs." Roll the rissoles in bread crumbs to coat and arrange on a baking sheet. Rissoles can be assembled to this point. Cover tightly and refrigerate overnight.

3. Bring to room temperature and bake in preheated oven for 15 minutes or until lightly browned. Serve hot or at room temperature.

Baked Cauliflower

This cauliflower isn't really coated because the breading doesn't stick, but the taste of the tender cauliflower and toasted crumbs is very much like a breaded and deep-fried dish — with far fewer calories.

- *Preheat oven to 375°F (190°C)*
- *Rimmed baking sheet, lightly oiled*

½	large cauliflower	½
2 tbsp	rice milk or soy milk	25 mL
½ cup	fresh whole wheat bread crumbs	125 mL
½ cup	chopped almonds, Brazil nuts or pistachio nuts	125 mL
1 tbsp	chopped fresh rosemary	15 mL
1 tbsp	chopped fresh parsley	15 mL
	Sea salt and freshly ground pepper	

1. In a bowl, toss cauliflower with rice milk. Add bread crumbs, almonds, rosemary and parsley and mix well. Season to taste with salt and pepper.

2. Spread cauliflower mixture on prepared baking sheet. Bake in preheated oven for 25 minutes or until cauliflower is lightly browned and pierces easily with a sharp knife.

Serving Suggestions

- Divide the cauliflower and bread crumbs evenly into 4 portions. Spoon each into a lettuce-leaf cup.
- Garnish with any pesto or salsa (pages 187 to 190).
- Serve over Sweet Potato Crackers (page 177).

Sweet Potato Crackers

Serves 4

This is so easy and such a tasty way to enjoy the nutrients in sweet potatoes. Serve them as is or with a spread or dip; top with tomato sauce for an easy first course; or spread with a tablespoon of pesto or tapenade.

Tip

- For the herbs, use parsley, thyme, oregano, chives, rosemary, tarragon, dill or chervil.

- *Preheat oven to 375°F (190°C)*
- *Rimmed baking sheet, lightly oiled*

1	sweet potato	1
1 tbsp	olive oil	15 mL
1 tbsp	chopped fresh herbs (see Tip, left)	15 mL
	Sea salt and freshly ground pepper	

1. Peel sweet potato and slice lengthwise into ¼-inch (0.5 cm) thick slices. Arrange slices on prepared baking sheet. Brush one side with oil and sprinkle with herbs, salt and pepper. Bake in preheated oven, turning once, for 25 minutes or until lightly browned on both sides.

Herbed Carrot and Turnip Fritters

Makes 8 to 10 fritters

Make these fritters small for passing as hors d'oeuvres or a bit larger for a first course. Dress them with any of the sauces (pages 148 to 156) or spreads (pages 178 to 187).

Tip

- For the herbs, use parsley, thyme, oregano, chives, rosemary, tarragon, dill or chervil.

- *Preheat oven to 375°F (190°C)*
- *Baking sheet, lightly oiled*

1 tbsp	ground flaxseeds	15 mL
3 tbsp	water or tomato juice	45 mL
2	medium carrots, shredded	2
½	small onion, shredded	½
¼	medium turnip, shredded	¼
1 cup	cooked brown rice	250 mL
1 tbsp	chopped fresh herbs (see Tip, left)	15 mL
	Sea salt and freshly ground pepper	
½ cup	Kiwi and Avocado Salsa with Pomegranate and Red Onion (page 189) or Roasted Corn Salsa (page 190)	125 mL

1. In a bowl, combine flaxseeds and water. Let stand for 10 minutes or until gelatinous.

2. Meanwhile, in a separate bowl, combine carrots, onion, turnip, brown rice and herbs. Season to taste with salt and pepper. Stir in flaxseeds. Scoop ¼ cup (50 mL) at a time and press into small fritters on prepared baking sheet. Bake in preheated oven for 25 minutes or until lightly browned. Serve hot topped with salsa.

Tofu Mayonnaise

I	clove garlic	I
8 oz	medium-soft or regular tofu, drained	250 g
2 tbsp	freshly squeezed lemon juice	25 mL
I tbsp	olive oil	I5 mL
I tsp	Dijon mustard	5 mL
	Sea salt	

1. In a blender or food processor, chop garlic. Add tofu, lemon juice, oil and mustard and process for 20 seconds or until smooth. Add salt to taste and process for 5 seconds to blend.

2. Transfer mixture to a clean container with lid. Store mayonnaise tightly covered in the refrigerator for up to 3 days.

Tofu Aïoli

I cup	Soy Sour Cream (page 145) or non-dairy sour cream	250 mL
4	cloves garlic, minced	4
Pinch	sea salt	Pinch

1. In a bowl, combine sour cream, garlic and salt.

2. Store aïoli tightly covered in the refrigerator for up to 5 days.

Avocado Aïoli

2	ripe avocados, peeled	2
I tbsp	freshly squeezed lemon juice	I5 mL
I cup	Soy Sour Cream (page 145) or non-dairy sour cream	250 mL
2	cloves garlic, minced	2
¼ tsp	sea salt	I mL

1. In a bowl, using a fork, mash avocado with lemon juice. Whisk in sour cream, garlic and sea salt.

2. Store aïoli tightly covered in the refrigerator for up to 5 days.

Almond Garlic Spread

The advantage of this spread is that it can be made thick or thin, for use as a salad dressing, a sandwich spread or with cooked vegetables in place of butter.

8	large cloves garlic	8
1 tbsp	coarse sea salt	15 mL
1 ½ cups	whole or chopped almonds (unblanched)	375 mL
1	small potato, cooked and peeled	1
	Juice of 1 lemon	
½ cup	olive oil	125 mL
½ to 1 cup	hot water	125 to 250 mL

1. Using a mortar and pestle or a food processor, mash or blend garlic and sea salt together. Add almonds and smash or process until finely chopped. Add potato and mash or process until combined with garlic and almonds. Whisk or blend in lemon juice. Slowly whisk in oil by hand or through the feed tube of food processor until all the oil is combined into the sauce. Whisk in a little hot water at a time until mixture reaches desired consistency.

2. Transfer mixture to a clean container with lid. Store spread tightly covered in the refrigerator for up to 1 week.

Roasted Garlic and Artichoke Spread

With its taste of the Mediterranean, this spread may be used as an impromptu sauce for steamed vegetables, as a substitute for mayonnaise, a dip for raw vegetables or a spread for crackers and breads. It is easy and may be made up to 3 days in advance.

- *Preheat oven to 400°F (200°C)*
- *Small heatproof baking dish with lid or foil*

3	whole heads garlic	3
5 tbsp	olive oil, divided	75 mL
1	can (14 oz/398 mL) artichokes, drained	1
1 tbsp	chopped fresh rosemary	15 mL
	Sea salt and freshly ground pepper	

1. Remove loose, papery skin from garlic heads. Slice off and discard ¼ inch (0.5 cm) from tops of the cloves in entire heads. Place the garlic heads cut side up in baking dish and drizzle with oil. Cover with a lid or foil. Bake in preheated oven for about 40 minutes or until garlic is quite soft. Transfer to a wire rack and let cool. If using a clay garlic roaster with a lid, roast at 375°F (190°C) for 35 to 40 minutes or until garlic is quite soft.

2. When garlic is cool enough to handle, squeeze cloves from their skins into a blender or food processor. Add artichokes and rosemary. Purée, adding remaining oil through opening in the lid, until soft and creamy. Season to taste with salt and pepper.

3. Transfer to a clean container with lid. Store spread tightly covered in the refrigerator for up to 3 days.

Cashew Butter

½ cup	unsweetened apple juice	125 mL
2 cups	lightly salted roasted cashews	500 mL
2 tbsp	brown rice syrup or Date Molasses (page 147)	25 mL
2 tbsp	freshly squeezed lemon juice (see Tip, left)	25 mL

Easy and delicious, this nut butter is great for breakfast on toasted whole wheat bread. It is a very good substitute for tahini, a sesame paste, because it is milder than peanut butter, which is often used to replace tahini.

Tip

• Omit lemon juice if using the Date Molasses.

1. In a blender or food processor, combine apple juice, cashews, rice syrup and lemon juice. Blend until smooth.

2. Transfer to a clean container with lid. Store spread tightly covered in the refrigerator for up to 1 week.

Fig Spread

12	dried or fresh figs, chopped	12
¾ cup	unsweetened apple juice	175 mL
½ cup	Pomegranate Molasses, Green Tea Molasses, Date Molasses (pages 146 and 147) or store-bought	125 mL
¼ cup	white wine or additional apple juice	50 mL

The reason some people do not like figs is because of the seeds and unfortunately, they are unavoidable in this spread. If you don't mind them, this spread is heavenly.

1. In a saucepan, combine figs, apple juice, molasses and wine. Bring to a boil over medium heat. Reduce heat and simmer, swirling pan occasionally, for 35 minutes or until very thick. Let cool. In a blender or food processor, blend until smooth.

2. Transfer mixture to a clean container with lid. Store spread tightly covered in the refrigerator for up to 1 month.

This spread makes a
sweet-tasting butter
replacement. Use it
for sandwiches and on
pancakes or toast just
as you would butter.
It is easy to make, but
the almonds must be
soaked ahead of time,
so it is not a spur-of-
the-moment
preparation.

Tip

• To cook sweet
potatoes you can
either prick them
and roast at
400°F (200°C) for
40 minutes, or
simmer in water for
20 to 30 minutes,
until soft.

Variation

• For a fruity-tasting
spread at breakfast
or for desserts, use
apple juice in place
of the vegetable
stock. For a savory
spread, add 1 clove
of garlic in Step 3.

Sweet Potato Spread

1 cup	whole almonds (unblanched)	250 mL
1 cup	water	250 mL
2	cooked small sweet potatoes (about 14 oz/420 g) (see Tip, left)	2
1/3 cup	vegetable stock or water	75 mL
2 tbsp	freshly squeezed lemon juice	25 mL
1 tbsp	olive oil	15 mL
1/4 tsp	ground nutmeg	1 mL
Pinch	sea salt	Pinch

1. In a small bowl, combine almonds and water. Cover and let stand in the refrigerator for at least 6 hours or overnight.

2. Peel and cut sweet potatoes into large chunks and wrap. Refrigerate until ready to make the spread.

3. Drain and rinse almonds. In a blender, combine almonds, sweet potatoes, vegetable stock, lemon juice, oil and nutmeg. Process for 30 seconds or until mixture is smooth and creamy. Add salt to taste.

4. Transfer mixture to a clean container with lid. Store spread tightly covered in the refrigerator for up to 5 days.

Apricot Tamarind Marmalade

Fruity and tart-sweet, this spread makes a healthy accompaniment to savory baked and roasted dishes.

Tips

- Be sure to check the tamarind for seeds. They are very smooth and hard and easy to miss but a hazard for teeth in a finished dish.

- Jaggery or "gur" is a coarse, unrefined sugar found throughout South and Southeast Asia. It is sometimes available at Indian markets or natural food stores and comes in solid cakes or blocks that range from rock-hard to crumbly. Made from the sap of date palm trees or from sugar cane juice, it contains more mineral salts and is included in Ayurvedic medicine for some throat and lung ailments. Use jaggery as you would brown sugar in recipes.

¾ cup	freshly squeezed orange juice	175 mL
2 tbsp	freshly squeezed lemon juice	25 mL
1 tbsp	rice vinegar	15 mL
¾ cup	chopped dried apricots	175 mL
¼ cup	chopped pitted tamarind (see Tips, left)	50 mL
¼ cup	chopped dates	50 mL
2 tbsp	jaggery or brown sugar (see Tips, left)	25 mL
½ tsp	ground cinnamon	2 mL
½ tsp	ground turmeric	2 mL
¼ tsp	ground mace	1 mL
	Sea salt and freshly ground pepper	

1. In a heavy-bottomed saucepan, combine orange juice, lemon juice and vinegar. Bring to a boil over high heat. Add apricots, tamarind, dates, jaggery, cinnamon, turmeric and mace. Stir well to combine and bring to a boil, stirring constantly. Reduce heat to medium-low and simmer, stirring occasionally, for 40 minutes or until mixture is soft and thick. Season to taste with salt and pepper.

2. Cool and transfer mixture to a clean container with lid. Store marmalade in the refrigerator for up to 3 weeks.

Red Hot Hummus

Go easy on the chili
paste until you get the
heat just the way you
like it. Substitute 1 to
2 tsp (5 to 10 mL)
powdered chili pepper
or hot pepper flakes for
the paste.

Tip

• You can use 2 cups
  (500 mL) cooked
  chickpeas, drained
  and rinsed, instead
  of canned.

	Juice of 1 lime or lemon	
2 tbsp	whole chia seeds	25 mL
½ cup	coarsely chopped sun-dried tomatoes	125 mL
1 cup	hot water	250 mL
1	can (14 to 19 oz/398 to 540 mL) chickpeas, drained and rinsed (see Tip, left)	1
2	cloves garlic	2
1 tbsp	toasted sesame oil	15 mL
¼ cup	olive oil	50 mL
1 to 2 tbsp	chili paste	15 to 25 mL
	Sea salt and freshly ground pepper	

1. In a bowl, combine lemon juice and chia seeds. In a separate bowl, combine sun-dried tomatoes and hot water. Set both aside for at least 20 minutes or until gelatinous.

2. In a food processor, combine chickpeas, garlic and sesame oil. Process for 20 seconds. With the motor running, add lemon juice and chia seed mixture and sun-dried tomato mixture through the feed tube. Keep the motor running and slowly add olive oil through the opening. Process until well blended, about 20 seconds. Add chili paste, salt and pepper to taste and process for 5 seconds to blend into the hummus.

3. Transfer mixture to a clean container with lid. Store hummus in the refrigerator for up to 3 days.

Roasted Vegetable Hummus

Cinnamon gives a spicy nudge to this Middle Eastern staple. This is a fairly thick dip that is best made in a food processor (see Tips, below).

Tips
- To use a blender, add ¼ cup (50 mL) apple juice before processing in Step 2.
- You can use 2 cups (500 mL) cooked chickpeas, drained and rinsed, instead of canned.

- *Preheat oven to 400°F (200°C)*
- *Rimmed baking sheet*

6	cloves garlic	6
2	onions, quartered	2
2	carrots, cut into 1-inch (2.5 cm) pieces	2
I	red bell pepper, quartered	I
5 tbsp	olive oil, divided	75 mL
I	can (14 to 19 oz/398 to 540 mL) chickpeas, drained and rinsed (see Tips, left)	I
2 tbsp	freshly squeezed lemon juice	25 mL
2 tbsp	Smooth Peanut Sauce (page 153) or tahini	25 mL
½ tsp	ground cinnamon	2 mL
½ tsp	sea salt	2 mL

1. On baking sheet, combine garlic, onions, carrots and red pepper. Drizzle 2 tbsp (25 mL) of the oil over and toss well to coat. Roast in preheated oven for 40 minutes or until soft and browned. Edges of vegetables may be slightly burnt and crisp. Let cool.

2. In a food processor, combine roasted vegetables, remaining olive oil, chickpeas, lemon juice, peanut sauce, cinnamon and salt. Blend until smooth.

3. Transfer mixture to a clean container with lid. Store hummus tightly covered in the refrigerator for up to 3 days.

Roasted Eggplant and Artichoke Dip

Without the cream cheese and fat-laden sauces typically used in dips, this vegan version is tasty and much healthier.

Tip

• You can use 2 cups (500 mL) cooked black beans, drained and rinsed, instead of canned.

• *Preheat oven to 400°F (200°C)*
• *Rimmed baking sheet*

6	cloves garlic	6
2	onions, quartered	2
I	eggplant, peeled and cut into eighths	I
4 tbsp	olive oil, divided	60 mL
2 tbsp	freshly squeezed lemon juice	25 mL
I	can (14 oz/398 mL) artichokes, drained	I
I	can (14 to 19 oz/398 to 540 mL) black beans, drained and rinsed (see Tip, left)	I
½ tsp	ground cumin	2 mL
½ tsp	sea salt	2 mL
¼ cup	unsweetened apple juice (approx.)	50 mL

1. On baking sheet, combine garlic, onions and eggplant. Drizzle 2 tbsp (25 mL) of the oil over and toss well to coat. Roast in preheated oven for 40 minutes or until soft and browned. Let cool.

2. In a food processor, combine roasted vegetables, remaining olive oil, lemon juice, artichokes, black beans, cumin and salt. Blend until smooth. With the motor running, add apple juice though the feed tube until desired consistency is reached.

3. Transfer mixture to a clean container with lid. Store dip tightly covered in the refrigerator for up to 3 days.

Vegetable Raita

This is such a favorite vegan standby, it had to be included. I added the carrot and green onion for a slight twist.

Tip

- To drain cucumber, set the cucumber in a sieve over a bowl and allow the water to drain out. This will take about 30 minutes. (Alternatively, cover and let stand overnight in the refrigerator.) Draining the cucumber keeps the dip from separating.

1	cucumber, shredded and drained (see Tip, left)	1
1	carrot, shredded	1
2	green onions, thinly sliced	2
2 cups	Soy Sour Cream (page 145) or non-dairy sour cream	500 mL

1. In a bowl, combine drained cucumber, carrot, green onions and sour cream. Stir well to mix.

2. Transfer mixture to a clean container with lid. Store dip tightly covered in the refrigerator for up to 3 days.

Pestos and Salsas

Pumpkin Seed Pesto

This is a great spread to use on toast in the morning. Pumpkin seeds are rich in healthy amino acids.

1 cup	hulled pumpkin seeds	250 mL
½ cup	sesame seeds	125 mL
¼ cup	whole almonds (unblanched)	50 mL
3 tbsp	brown rice syrup	45 mL
1 tbsp	ground flaxseeds	15 mL
3 tbsp	hemp oil or walnut oil (approx.)	45 mL

1. In a blender or food processor, combine pumpkin seeds, sesame seeds, almonds, rice syrup and flaxseeds. Process for 30 seconds or until blended. With the motor running, add oil through the opening in the lid just until a smooth spread is achieved.

2. Transfer mixture to a clean container with lid. Store pesto tightly covered in the refrigerator for up to 5 days.

Basil Pesto

2	large cloves garlic	2
½ cup	pine nuts or toasted sunflower seeds	125 mL
3 cups	lightly packed fresh basil leaves	750 mL
¾ cup	freshly grated Parmesan soy cheese	175 mL
¾ cup	olive oil (approx.)	175 mL
½ tsp	sea salt	2 mL

1. In a food processor, combine garlic and pine nuts. Process for 10 seconds or until chopped. Add basil and soy cheese and pulse 3 to 5 times. With the motor running, slowly add oil in a steady stream through the feed tube. Keep adding oil and blending until pesto has reached the desired consistency. Add salt and process for 3 seconds to blend.

2. Transfer mixture to a clean container with lid. Store pesto tightly covered in the refrigerator for up to 1 week or in freezer bags in the freezer for up to 3 months.

Olive Tapenade

1	large clove garlic	1
2 tbsp	pine nuts or sunflower seeds	25 mL
2 cups	drained pitted black or green olives (see Tip, left)	500 mL
1 tbsp	fresh thyme leaves	15 mL
1 tbsp	chopped fresh oregano or parsley	15 mL
1 tsp	drained capers	5 mL
¼ cup	olive oil	50 mL

Like pesto, olive tapenade has a strong taste on its own. But when used as a spread or mixed with other ingredients in canapés, tortillas or pita pockets, as a base for sandwich spreads and as a flavor booster for sauces and stir-fries, it is pleasant and very versatile.

Tip
• You can use a 14-oz (398 mL) can of olives for this recipe.

1. In a food processor or blender, process garlic and pine nuts for about 30 seconds or until finely chopped. Add olives, thyme, oregano and capers and pulse 2 to 3 times to chop. With the motor running, slowly add oil in a steady stream through the feed tube. Process just until oil is mixed in well.

2. Transfer mixture to a clean container with lid. Store tapenade tightly covered in the refrigerator for up to 1 week.

Romesco Tomato Tapenade

Romesco is a traditional
Spanish sauce often
served with fish and
seafood dishes. Use this
vegan version to dress
up spring vegetables
such as peas, turnips or
asparagus. Sun-dried
tomatoes packed in oil
tend to be softer and
easier to work with than
dry-packed in this dish.

2	large cloves garlic	2
½ cup	whole almonds (unblanched)	125 mL
2 cups	oil-packed sun-dried tomatoes, drained	500 mL
½	red bell pepper, cut in chunks	½
¼ cup	fresh basil or oregano leaves	50 mL
2 tbsp	red wine vinegar	25 mL
¼ to ½ cup	olive oil	50 to 125 mL
¼ tsp	sea salt	1 mL

1. In a food processor or blender, combine garlic and almonds. Process for 10 seconds or until chopped. Add sun-dried tomatoes, red pepper and basil. Process for 1 minute or until tomatoes are coarsely chopped. With the motor running, add vinegar and then oil in a steady stream through the feed tube. Keep adding and blending the oil until tapenade has reached the desired consistency — it should be finely chopped and easy to spread but not excessively oily. Add salt.

2. Transfer mixture to a clean container with lid. Store tapenade tightly covered in the refrigerator for up to 1 week.

Kiwi and Avocado Salsa with Pomegranate and Red Onion

Use this salsa as a
garnish for baked and
roasted dishes. If the
ingredients are cut into
a fairly small dice (close
to ¼ inch/0.5 cm),
the salsa will be easier
to use as you might
a sauce.

4	kiwifruits, peeled and chopped	4
1	avocado, peeled and diced	1
½	red onion, diced	½
½ cup	fresh pomegranate seeds, optional	125 mL
3 tbsp	freshly squeezed lemon juice	45 mL
¼ cup	grapeseed oil or hemp oil	50 mL
1 tbsp	Pomegranate Molasses (page 146) or store-bought	15 mL
	Sea salt and freshly ground pepper	

1. In a bowl, combine kiwifruits, avocado, onion and pomegranate seeds, if using. Toss with lemon juice. Drizzle oil and molasses over the salsa and toss well to combine. Season to taste with salt and pepper.

2. Store salsa tightly covered in the refrigerator for up to 2 days.

Roasted Corn Salsa

• *Preheat oven to 400°F (200°C)*
• *9-inch (2.5 L) baking pan*

In the summer, try grilling the corn, carrots and red pepper whole on the barbecue. Then strip the kernels from the cob and chop the vegetables. If you really like cilantro and wish to add more, this corn salsa is accommodating.

Tip

• To remove kernels from an ear of corn, stand the corn, broad end down in a pie plate. Run a French knife down the cob removing the kernels and letting them fall into the plate. Keep turning the cob and slicing the kernels until all have been removed. Refrigerate or freeze the cob for use in vegetable stock.

2	ears corn, kernels removed, or 1 can (12 oz/341 mL) corn kernels, drained (see Tip, left)	2
2	carrots, diced	2
½	red bell pepper, diced	½
2 tbsp	olive oil	25 mL
1	avocado	1
3 tbsp	freshly squeezed lime or lemon juice	45 mL
2	green onions, thinly sliced	2
¼ cup	chopped fresh cilantro or Italian parsley	50 mL
1 tbsp	fresh thyme leaves	15 mL
½ tsp	sea salt	2 mL
2 tbsp	Pomegranate Molasses (page 146) or store-bought	25 mL

1. In baking pan, combine corn, carrots and red pepper. Drizzle with oil and bake in preheated oven for 35 minutes or until carrots are tender when pierced with a knife. The corn and red pepper may be a bit charred around the edges. Let cool.

2. Peel and dice avocado. In a bowl, toss avocado with lemon juice. Add corn, carrots, red pepper, green onions, cilantro and thyme. Season with salt and drizzle molasses over. Toss well to combine.

Soups, Salads and Sides

This is a delightfully sweet and tasty soup with just a hint of complex spices. Omit or reduce the dates for a more savory dish. For a creamy soup, purée the mixture using an immersion blender or in batches using either a blender or a food processor.

Sweet Potato Curried Cauliflower Soup

I tsp	whole cumin seeds	5 mL
½ tsp	whole fennel seeds	2 mL
½ tsp	whole coriander seeds	2 mL
5 tbsp	olive oil, divided	75 mL
¼	head cauliflower, chopped into coarse pieces	¼
I	onion, finely chopped	I
2	cloves garlic, finely chopped	2
I	piece (I inch/2.5 cm) candied ginger, finely chopped	I
I	large sweet potato, peeled and cut into I-inch (2.5 cm) cubes	I
4 cups	vegetable stock or water	I L
2 tbsp	tamari or soy sauce	25 mL
6	dates, coarsely chopped	6
I tbsp	Yellow Curry Spice (page 253) or curry powder	15 mL

1. In a large, heavy skillet, toast cumin, fennel and coriander seeds over medium-high heat until the seeds begin to pop and their fragrance is released, about 2 minutes. Do not allow to smoke or burn. Add 2 tbsp (25 mL) of the oil to pan and heat. Stir in cauliflower. Reduce heat to medium-low and cook, stirring frequently, for 8 minutes or until cauliflower is caramelized and tender when pierced with the tip of a knife. Set the pan aside.

2. In a soup pot, heat 2 tbsp (25 mL) of the oil over medium heat. Stir in onion and cook, stirring occasionally, for 5 minutes or until slightly softened. Add remaining oil, garlic, ginger and sweet potato and cook, stirring frequently, for 2 minutes. Stir in stock, tamari and dates. Increase heat and bring to a light boil. Reduce heat and simmer for 20 minutes or until sweet potato is soft.

3. Using a potato masher or fork, mash sweet potato in pot to thicken soup. Add curry and cauliflower. Simmer for 3 minutes or until cauliflower is heated through.

Moroccan Pumpkin Soup

Like most Moroccan dishes, this is not overly spicy — it has just the right amount of complex tastes to make it interesting. Any small, thick-skinned cooking pumpkin or butternut squash will work in this recipe.

Tip

• Pressed curry powder is available in cubes and can usually be found in gourmet food or natural food stores.

I tsp	whole cumin seeds	5 mL
I tsp	whole coriander seeds	5 mL
½ tsp	whole fennel seeds	2 mL
3 tbsp	olive oil, divided	45 mL
2	red onions, chopped	2
I tbsp	Pomegranate Molasses (page 146) or blackstrap molasses	15 mL
I	onion, sliced	I
I	leek, white and green parts, sliced	I
I tbsp	organic cane sugar	15 mL
I	sweet or pie pumpkin (2 lbs/1 kg), peeled and cut into 1-inch (2.5 cm) cubes	I
2	apples, chopped	2
I tbsp	curry powder or cube (see Tip, left)	15 mL
I tsp	ground turmeric	5 mL
½ tsp	ground cinnamon	2 mL
4 cups	vegetable stock or water	I L
I cup	rice milk	250 mL
½ cup	cashews	125 mL

1. In a large saucepan, toast cumin, coriander and fennel seeds over high heat until the seeds begin to pop and their fragrance is released, about 2 minutes. Do not allow to smoke or burn. Add 2 tbsp (25 mL) of the oil to pan and heat. Stir in red onions. Reduce heat to medium and cook, stirring frequently, for 10 minutes or until onions are soft and caramelized. Transfer ¾ cup (175 mL) to a bowl and add molasses. Stir and set aside.

2. Add remaining oil to onions in pan and heat over high heat. Stir in leek. Reduce heat to medium and cook, stirring frequently, for 6 minutes or until soft. One at a time, add sugar, pumpkin, apples, curry powder, turmeric and cinnamon, stirring after each addition. Cook, stirring, for 1 minute. Add vegetable stock and bring to a gentle boil over high heat. Cover, reduce heat to medium-low and gently boil for 40 minutes or until vegetables are tender when pierced with the tip of a knife.

3. In a blender, combine rice milk and cashews. Blend until smooth. Ladle 2 cups (500 mL) of the soup mixture into blender. Blend with nut mixture until smooth. Stir into soup and heat through. Ladle soup into bowls and float 2 tbsp (25 mL) of the reserved red onion on top of each.

Hearty Potato and Leek Soup

Tomato is an unusual ingredient in potato and leek soup but in the fall when tomatoes are abundant, they add a cheery note to this winter favorite. Omit them in the winter when fresh ripe organic tomatoes are not available.

Tip

• You can use 2 cups (500 mL) cooked chickpeas, drained and rinsed, instead of canned.

2 tbsp	olive oil	25 mL
3	onions, chopped	3
2	leeks, white and green parts, sliced	2
3	cloves garlic, finely chopped	3
2	tomatoes, seeded and chopped, optional	2
4 cups	vegetable stock or water (approx.)	I L
4 to 5	potatoes, cut into 1-inch (2.5 cm) cubes (about 4 cups/1 L)	4 to 5
I tsp	crushed dried rosemary	5 mL
	Sea salt and freshly ground pepper	
I	can (14 to 19 oz/398 to 540 mL) chickpeas with liquid, optional (see Tip, left)	I
2 cups	fresh spinach, optional	500 mL

1. In a large saucepan, heat oil over medium heat. Add onions and cook, stirring occasionally, for 3 minutes or until slightly soft. Stir in leeks and cook, stirring occasionally, for 6 minutes or until soft. Add garlic and cook, stirring occasionally, for 3 minutes. Add tomatoes, if using.

2. Add vegetable stock, potatoes and rosemary. Stir and bring to a boil over medium-high heat. Cover, reduce heat to low and cook for 20 minutes or until potatoes are tender when pierced with the tip of a knife.

3. Using a ladle, transfer 3 cups (750 mL) of the soup mixture to a blender. Blend until mixture is smooth. Return to saucepan and season to taste with salt and pepper. Stir in chickpeas with liquid and spinach, if using. Cook over low heat for about 2 minutes, until chickpeas are heated and spinach is wilted. Add more vegetable stock or water if a thinner soup is desired.

Creamy Asparagus Soup

Fresh spring asparagus is best in this soup but frozen may be used.

3 tbsp	olive oil	45 mL
1 cup	chopped onion	250 mL
8 oz	mushrooms, chopped	250 g
3	cloves garlic, finely chopped	3
4 cups	vegetable stock or water	1 L
1 lb	asparagus, trimmed and broken into 1-inch (2.5 cm) pieces	500 g
2 tbsp	pure maple syrup	25 mL
½ tsp	sea salt	2 mL
2 cups	Soy Sour Cream (page 145), Cashew Cream (page 144) or non-dairy sour cream	500 mL

1. In a large saucepan, heat oil over medium heat. Stir in onion and mushrooms. Cook, stirring frequently, for about 10 minutes or until soft. Add garlic and cook, stirring, for 1 minute.

2. Stir in vegetable stock, asparagus, maple syrup and sea salt. Increase heat and bring to a boil. Reduce heat and simmer for about 20 minutes or until asparagus is tender when pierced with the tip of a knife. Whisk in sour cream and heat through.

Use shiitake, portobello, cremini, white button or smoky nutty-flavored black morel mushrooms for this earthy soup. If you use all portobello mushrooms or some in combination, the soup will be beautifully black.

Variation

• Add 1 can (19 oz/ 540 mL) drained and rinsed black beans at the end of Step 3. Cook over medium heat until heated through.

Roasted Mushroom and Wild Rice Soup

- *Preheat oven to 375°F (190°C)*
- *Rimmed baking sheet, lightly oiled*

10 oz	mushrooms (see Intro, left) cut into ½-inch (1 cm) pieces	300 g
1 cup	cubed (½ inch/1 cm) sweet potato or squash	250 mL
4	cloves garlic	4
4 tbsp	olive oil, divided	60 mL
2 tbsp	tamari or soy sauce	25 mL
1 tbsp	rice vinegar	15 mL
1	onion, diced	1
1	carrot, diced	1
¼ cup	red wine or grape juice	50 mL
½ cup	wild rice	125 mL
½ tsp	ground cinnamon	2 mL
¼ tsp	ground nutmeg	1 mL
	Sea salt and freshly ground pepper	
6 cups	Mushroom Broth (page 138), vegetable stock or water	1.5 L

1. On prepared baking sheet, spread mushrooms, sweet potato and garlic in one layer. Drizzle 2 tbsp (25 mL) of the oil, tamari and rice vinegar over vegetables. Bake in preheated oven for 30 minutes.

2. Meanwhile, in a large saucepan, heat remaining oil over medium heat. Add onion and cook, stirring occasionally, for 3 minutes or until slightly softened. Add carrots and cook for 5 minutes or until vegetables are softened.

3. Stir in roasted mushrooms, sweet potatoes, garlic and any pan juices. Add red wine and cook, stirring often, for 3 to 5 minutes, until wine is evaporated. Stir in wild rice, cinnamon, nutmeg, salt and pepper. Cook, stirring for 30 seconds to mix well. Add broth and bring to a boil over high heat. Cover, reduce heat to medium-low and simmer for 45 minutes or until rice is tender.

Roasted Garlic and Lentil Soup

Use fresh tomatoes in season and substitute 1 cup (250 mL) of crushed canned tomatoes in winter. Best if served immediately. When stored, even in the refrigerator, this soup thickens, absorbing the liquid.

Tips

- Designer rice (mahogany, black, red; short- and long-grain varieties) is becoming very popular and widely available. Look for red rice in gourmet food or natural food stores.

- You can use 2 cups (500 mL) cooked lentils plus ½ cup (125 mL) vegetable stock, instead of canned.

- *Preheat oven to 375°F (190°C)*
- *10-inch (25 cm) pie plate or baking dish*

10	small (2 inch/5 cm diameter) tomatoes	10
12	cloves garlic	12
4 tbsp	olive oil, divided	60 mL
1 tbsp	chopped fresh rosemary	15 mL
1 cup	chopped onion	250 mL
1 tsp	ground cumin	5 mL
½ tsp	crushed fennel seeds	2 mL
½ tsp	sea salt	2 mL
Pinch	ground ginger	Pinch
Pinch	ground nutmeg	Pinch
1 cup	red or brown rice (see Tips, left)	250 mL
3 cups	vegetable stock or water, divided (approx.)	750 mL
1	can (19 oz/540 mL) lentils with liquid (see Tips, left)	1

1. In pie plate, combine tomatoes and garlic and toss with 2 tbsp (25 mL) of the oil and rosemary. Bake in preheated oven for 40 minutes or until garlic is soft. Let cool.

2. Meanwhile, in a large saucepan, heat remaining oil over medium heat. Add onion and cook, stirring occasionally, for 6 to 8 minutes or until soft. Add cumin, fennel, salt, ginger, nutmeg and rice. Cook, stirring constantly, for 1 minute. Add 2 cups (500 mL) of the vegetable stock. Increase heat to high and bring to a boil. Cover, reduce heat to low and simmer for 40 minutes or until rice is tender.

3. When tomatoes and garlic are cool enough to handle, transfer to a blender and add remaining vegetable stock. Blend until smooth. Add tomato purée and lentils with liquid to rice in saucepan. Bring to a simmer and cook for 1 to 2 minutes or until heated through. Add more vegetable stock or water if a thinner soup is desired.

Using the flavorful tomatoes of summer and fresh red peppers, this robust soup is perfect for the beginning of a light lunch or dinner.

Roasted Tomato and Red Pepper Soup

- *Preheat oven to 375°F (190°C)*
- *Rimmed baking sheet, lightly oiled*

5	small tomatoes	5
2	red bell peppers, cut in half	2
I	onion, quartered	I
12	cloves garlic	12
2 tbsp	olive oil	25 mL
I tbsp	chopped fresh rosemary or basil	15 mL
3 cups	vegetable stock or water, divided	750 mL
I tbsp	pure maple syrup, optional	15 mL
	Sea salt and freshly ground pepper	

1. On prepared baking sheet, combine tomatoes, red peppers, onion and garlic in one layer. Drizzle with oil and bake in preheated oven for 40 minutes. Remove onion and garlic, if tender, and continue roasting tomatoes and peppers for another 10 minutes or until skin on peppers is bubbly and black in places and tomatoes are soft and runny. Let cool.

2. In a blender or food processor, combine half of the roasted tomatoes, red peppers, onion and garlic with 1½ cups (375 mL) of the vegetable stock. Blend until smooth. Pour into a saucepan. Repeat with remaining vegetables and vegetable stock.

3. Add maple syrup, if using, and salt and pepper to taste. Soup may be transferred to a jar or bowl tightly covered and refrigerated for up to 2 days before using. To serve, in a saucepan, bring to a boil over high heat. Reduce heat and simmer, stirring constantly, for 1 minute.

Avocado Vichyssoise

Serves 4

Avocados are actually a semitropical fruit native to Mexico and Central America. Now grown in California for export, the Hass variety accounts for up to 85% of the more than 80 varieties known. Rich in dietary fiber, vitamins K, A, B6, C and folate, avocados also provide unsaturated fats containing oleic acid. It is the fats in avocados that lend their creamy texture to this soup and to other dishes such as sauces and dips.

Tip

• Avocado Vichyssoise may be made up to 2 days in advance and stored tightly covered in the refrigerator.

2	large ripe avocados	2
	Juice of 1 lemon	
4 cups	Mushroom Broth (page 138), vegetable stock or water	1 L
1	potato, peeled and cut into ½-inch (1 cm) cubes	1
	Sea salt and freshly ground pepper	
¼ tsp	hot pepper flakes	1 mL
½ cup	rice milk or soy milk	125 mL
4 tbsp	chopped fresh chives or Basil Pesto (page 188), optional	60 mL

1. Peel, pit and slice avocados in half and place in a bowl with lemon juice.

2. In a saucepan, bring broth to a gentle boil over high heat. Add avocados with lemon juice and potato. Season to taste with salt, pepper and hot pepper flakes. Cover, reduce heat and simmer for 15 minutes or until potato is soft. Let cool.

3. In a blender, combine rice milk and avocado mixture and blend until smooth. Transfer to a bowl, cover and refrigerate for 1 hour or until well chilled. Ladle into soup bowls and garnish with chopped chives, if using.

Spinach Cream Gazpacho

Simple and yet sophisticated, this soup is great for summer entertaining because it may be made up to 1 day in advance. Spice it up by adding half a seeded jalapeño pepper.

1 cup	chopped tomatoes with juice	250 mL
2 tbsp	freshly squeezed lemon juice	25 mL
6	pitted dates	6
3 cups	chopped spinach leaves	750 mL
1 cup	rice milk or soy milk	250 mL
½ cup	unsalted cashews	125 mL
1	cucumber, peeled and cut into cubes	1
2	green onions, white and light green parts, sliced	2
	Sea salt and freshly ground pepper	

1. In a saucepan, combine tomatoes with juice, lemon juice and dates. Bring to a boil over high heat. Reduce heat and simmer, stirring often, for 5 minutes or until dates are well blended into tomatoes. Add spinach and stir until wilted. Let cool.

2. In a blender, combine rice milk, cashews, cucumber and green onions. Blend until smooth. Add half of the spinach mixture to blender and blend until smooth. Add to remaining spinach mixture in saucepan and season to taste with salt and pepper. Chill for at least 30 minutes or overnight. Serve cold or at room temperature.

French Canadian Onion Soup

With its slightly sweet maple syrup-spiked flavor, this soup is a North American version of a classic European peasant soup.

Tip

- Use milder, sweeter onions such as Vidalia, Walla Walla or Honey Sweet for this soup. Cut onions in half and slice thinly crosswise.

2 tbsp	olive oil	25 mL
2	large sweet onions, thinly sliced (about 3 cups/750 mL) (see Tip, left)	2
2	leeks, white part only, thinly sliced	2
4 cups	Mushroom Broth (page 138), vegetable stock or water	1 L
2 tbsp	pure maple syrup	25 mL
1 tbsp	tamari or soy sauce	15 mL
1 tsp	finely chopped fresh tarragon	5 mL
	Sea salt and freshly ground pepper	
4	slices of baguette bread	4
1	clove garlic	1

1. In a saucepan, heat oil over medium-high heat. Add onions and leeks. Cover, reduce heat to low and sweat, stirring once or twice, for 15 minutes or until onions are soft and translucent. Keep temperature high enough to gently steam-cook but not so high that they brown or burn on the bottom of the pan.

2. Add broth, maple syrup, tamari and tarragon. Increase heat and bring to a boil. Reduce heat and simmer for 20 minutes. Taste and add salt and pepper if required.

3. Just before serving, toast bread slices and rub both sides with clove of garlic. Float one slice of toast on each bowl of soup.

Borscht

Roasting the vegetables gives a slightly smoky flavor to this soup. Serve it piping hot in the winter and chilled in the summer.

- *Preheat oven to 400°F (200°C)*
- *11- by 7-inch (2 L) baking pan, lightly oiled*

4	medium beets, peeled and quartered (about 2 lbs/1 kg)	4
2	medium carrots, halved lengthwise	2
1	onion, halved	1
3 tbsp	olive oil	45 mL
4 cups	vegetable stock or water, divided	1 L
	Juice of 1 lemon	
1	piece (1 inch/2.5 cm) fresh gingerroot, grated	1
	Salt and freshly ground pepper	
¼ cup	Soy Sour Cream (page 145) or non-dairy sour cream, optional	50 mL

1. In prepared baking pan, arrange beets, carrots and onion in one layer. Drizzle with oil. Roast in preheated oven for 1 hour or until tender when pierced with the tip of a knife. Let cool and chop into small pieces. Divide roasted vegetables into 2 batches for blending.

2. In a blender, combine half of the vegetable stock, lemon juice and ginger. Add half of the roasted vegetables and blend until smooth. Transfer to a saucepan. Blend the second batch of stock and vegetables and transfer to the pan. Heat over medium heat and season to taste with salt and pepper. Serve hot or chilled. Garnish each bowl of soup with 1 tbsp (15 mL) sour cream, if using.

Makes ¾ cup (175 mL)

Use this classic, garlicky sauce to dress raw and cooked greens and vegetables.

Caesar Salad Dressing

2 tbsp	ground flaxseeds	25 mL
¼ cup	soy milk or rice milk	50 mL
3	large cloves garlic	3
2 tbsp	freshly squeezed lemon juice	25 mL
1 tsp	balsamic vinegar	5 mL
½ tsp	dry mustard	2 mL
½ cup	olive oil	125 mL

1. In a blender, combine flaxseeds and soy milk. Let stand for at least 10 minutes or until gelatinous.

2. Add garlic, lemon juice, vinegar and mustard. Blend until smooth. With the motor running, slowly pour oil through the opening in the lid. Blend until oil is incorporated into the dressing.

3. Transfer dressing to a clean jar with lid. Store tightly covered in the refrigerator for up to 5 days.

Makes 1 cup (250 mL)

Tahini is a paste made from sesame seeds and is available at Middle Eastern grocery stores and some supermarkets. A very good substitute for tahini is Cashew Butter (page 181).

Tropical Tahini Dressing

1 cup	pineapple juice	250 mL
3 tbsp	tahini or Cashew Butter (page 181)	45 mL
2 tbsp	freshly squeezed lemon juice	25 mL
2 tbsp	olive oil	25 mL
1 tbsp	brown rice syrup or Date Molasses (page 147)	15 mL
	Sea salt	

1. In a blender or food processor, combine pineapple juice, tahini, lemon juice, oil and rice syrup. Blend until smooth. Season to taste with salt. Serve in a sauce bowl with a fork to whisk because it tends to separate upon sitting.

2. Transfer dressing to a clean jar with lid. Store tightly covered in the refrigerator for up to 5 days.

Kiwi Dressing

3	well-ripened kiwifruits, cut into quarters	3
⅓ cup	grapeseed oil	75 mL
2 tbsp	rice vinegar	25 mL

Some things happen as a result of accidents or necessity. When a few kiwifruits reached the critical point of becoming overripe, I decided to use them to make a salad and vegetable dressing. The result is a creamy, tart-sweet and fresh-tasting dressing that is good with both fruit and vegetables.

1. In a blender or bowl, blend or mash kiwifruits. In a jar with a tight-fitting lid, combine mashed kiwifruit, oil and vinegar. Place lid on jar and shake well.

2. Store dressing tightly covered in the refrigerator for up to 5 days.

Fennel and Cucumber Salad with Ginger Dressing

1	English cucumber	1
½	fennel or kohlrabi bulb	½
½	red onion	½

Allowing the natural water in the cucumber to drain away before tossing it with the dressing keeps it from being diluted (see Tip, below). This is one of those salads that marinates in the dressing and improves with time, so it can be made up to 2 days before serving.

Ginger Dressing

2 tbsp	grapeseed oil	25 mL
2 tbsp	rice vinegar	25 mL
1 tbsp	tamari or soy sauce	15 mL
2 tsp	grated fresh gingerroot	10 mL
1 tsp	organic cane sugar	5 mL
¼ tsp	hot pepper flakes	1 mL

Tip

• Try sprinkling a bit of salt on the vegetables and allowing them to drain. The salt draws out the water more quickly than just letting them stand in a colander. Rinse the salt off before adding the vegetables to the dressing.

1. Using a mandoline or food processor, slice cucumber and fennel very thin. Let stand in a colander to drain for at least 30 minutes or for up to 1 hour (see Tip, left). Thinly slice red onion by hand.

2. *Ginger Dressing:* In a salad bowl, whisk together oil, vinegar, tamari, ginger, sugar and hot pepper flakes. Add cucumber, fennel and onion and toss well to coat.

Serves 4

In winter, the warmed pears make a cozy starter but this salad is just as nice without warming the pears — simply slice and pile on top of the other salad ingredients.

Warm Pear and Snow Pea Salad with Miso Dressing

- *Preheat oven to 400°F (200°C)*
- *Rimmed baking sheet, lightly oiled*

2	ripe pears, halved lengthwise and cored, stem intact	2
¼ cup	agave nectar or Pomegranate Molasses (page 146)	50 mL
1 tbsp	freshly squeezed lemon juice	15 mL
1 tbsp	fresh thyme leaves	15 mL
1½ cups	bean sprouts	375 mL
2 oz	snow peas, cut lengthwise into matchsticks	60 g
2	green onions, halved lengthwise and sliced crosswise on the diagonal	2
1	carrot, shredded	1
3 tbsp	sesame seeds	45 mL

Miso Dressing

2 tbsp	tamari or soy sauce	25 mL
2 tbsp	agave nectar or Pomegranate Molasses	25 mL
2 tbsp	grapeseed oil	25 mL
1 tbsp	rice vinegar	15 mL
2 tsp	toasted sesame oil	10 mL
2 tsp	miso	10 mL

1. Place a pear half on working surface, cut side down. Starting ½ inch (1 cm) down from stem, cut lengthwise to bottom of pear into scant ½-inch (1 cm) slices, keeping pear intact at stem. Arrange on prepared baking sheet and press to fan slices.

2. In a bowl, combine agave nectar, lemon juice and thyme. Drizzle over pears. Bake in preheated oven for 10 to 15 minutes or until tender. Let cool slightly.

3. In a salad bowl, combine bean sprouts, snow peas, green onions and carrot.

4. *Miso Dressing:* In a jar with a tight-fitting lid, combine tamari, agave nectar, grapeseed oil, vinegar, sesame oil and miso. Place lid on jar and shake well.

5. Arrange bean sprout mixture on a salad plate. Lift pear halves onto salad, drizzle with dressing and sprinkle sesame seeds over salad.

Fast, easy and great tasting, this salad can step in as an appetizer or side dish. Serve it with whole grains for a light lunch. Do not be tempted to cook the beans for more than 3 minutes or their texture will soften too much.

Green Bean, Pecan and Pomegranate Salad

1 lb	green beans, cut into 2-inch (5 cm) pieces	500 g
½ cup	diced red onion	125 mL
1 cup	whole pecans	250 mL
1 cup	pomegranate seeds	250 mL
¼ cup	chopped green olives, optional	50 mL

Pomegranate Dressing

⅓ cup	olive oil	75 mL
3 tbsp	Pomegranate Molasses (page 146) or store-bought	45 mL
1 tbsp	chopped fresh parsley	15 mL

1. In a pot of boiling salted water, cook green beans for 3 minutes. Drain and rinse with cold water. Let cool to room temperature. In a bowl, combine green beans, red onion, pecans, pomegranate seeds and olives, if using.

2. *Pomegranate Dressing:* Meanwhile, in a jar with a tight-fitting lid, combine oil, molasses and parsley. Shake well to combine and drizzle over salad.

Spinach and Whole-Grain Salad with Kiwi Dressing

Whole grains, such as Kamut or spelt add a chewy texture to this salad combination.

Variation

• Use 1 cup (250 mL) halved green grapes if kiwifruit is not in season.

2 tbsp	olive oil	25 mL
1 cup	chopped red onion	250 mL
1 cup	cooked Kamut or spelt kernels (see Instructions, page 331)	250 mL
2 cups	packed fresh spinach or seasonal greens	500 mL
½ cup	chopped fresh parsley	125 mL
⅓ cup	sunflower seeds	75 mL
⅓ cup	chopped walnuts	75 mL
1	kiwifruit, sliced	1
⅓ cup	Kiwi Dressing (page 204)	75 mL

1. In a skillet, heat oil over medium heat. Add onion and cook, stirring occasionally, for 6 minutes or until soft. Stir in Kamut and heat through.

2. Meanwhile, in a bowl, combine spinach and parsley. Drizzle with hot onion mixture along with any pan juices. Add sunflower seeds, walnuts, kiwi slices and dressing. Toss to combine.

Roasted Vegetable Salad

In summer the grill is easy and fast for grilling vegetables. Use an oiled basket or skewer the veggies whole to grill, then cut into serving-size bites. When combined with balsamic vinegar, the plums morph into a tart-sweet self-basting dressing.

Tip

• You can use 2 cups (500 mL) cooked chickpeas, drained and rinsed, instead of canned.

• *Preheat oven to 375°F (190°C)*
• *Rimmed baking sheet, lightly oiled*

2	black plums, cut into eighths	2
I	red bell pepper, cut into eighths	I
I	carrot, cut in half lengthwise and then crosswise into eighths	I
I	onion, cut into eighths	I
2	cauliflower florets, thinly sliced	2
	Sea salt and freshly ground pepper	
4 tbsp	olive oil, divided	60 mL
2 cups	packed seasonal greens	500 mL
2 tbsp	balsamic vinegar	25 mL
I	can (14 to 19 oz/398 to 540 mL) chickpeas, drained and rinsed (see Tip, left)	I

1. On prepared baking sheet, combine plums, red pepper, carrot, onion and cauliflower. Season to taste with salt and pepper. Toss with 2 tbsp (25 mL) of the oil and arrange in a single layer. Bake in preheated oven for 30 to 40 minutes or until tender when pierced with the tip of a knife.

2. In a salad bowl, toss greens with roasted vegetables and pan juices. Add remaining oil, vinegar and chickpeas. Taste and add more salt and pepper, if required.

Chickpeas with Kiwi and Avocado Salsa

Make this in summer or winter and serve chilled or at room temperature. It is easy and fresh tasting as a starter or as a side dish for baked or roasted casseroles.

I	can (14 to 19 oz/398 to 540 mL) chickpeas, drained and rinsed (see Tip, above)	I
3 cups	Kiwi and Avocado Salsa with Pomegranate and Red Onion (page 189)	750 mL

1. In a bowl, combine chickpeas and salsa. Recipe may be made ahead and stored tightly covered in the refrigerator for up to 2 days.

Citrus Greens with Fig Dressing

Light and refreshing, this salad may be served at the end of the meal in place of dessert. It is an easy dish for entertaining because the ingredients may be made the day before and tossed together just before serving.

Variations

- Use pure maple syrup or brown rice syrup in place of the molasses, if necessary.

- You may substitute fig or apricot jam for the Fig Spread.

6	oranges, peeled and sectioned	6
I tbsp	chopped fresh tarragon	I5 mL
I tbsp	freshly squeezed lemon juice	I5 mL
I tbsp	Date Molasses (page I47), Pomegranate Molasses (page I46) or store-bought	I5 mL
3 cups	mesclun greens	750 mL
8	dates, thinly sliced	8

Fig Dressing

¼ cup	olive oil	50 mL
3 tbsp	Fig Spread (page I8I)	45 mL
I tbsp	freshly squeezed lemon juice	I5 mL
¼ tsp	ground cinnamon	I mL

1. In a bowl, combine oranges, tarragon, lemon juice and molasses. Cover tightly and refrigerate for at least 30 minutes or overnight.

2. *Fig Dressing:* In a clean jar with a tight-fitting lid, combine oil, Fig Spread, lemon juice and cinnamon. Shake well to combine. Set aside. Prepare salad ingredients and dressing to this point, cover and refrigerate for up to 24 hours, if desired.

3. *Assemble salad:* In a salad bowl, combine chilled orange mixture and its juices with the mesclun greens. Drizzle with Fig Dressing and toss well to combine. Arrange date slices over top.

Grilled Mediterranean Vegetable and Lentil Salad

Using the grill keeps the kitchen cool in the summertime, but the vegetables may be roasted in the oven (see Tip, below).

Tip

- To roast vegetables in the oven, place on a lightly oiled rimmed baking sheet and roast in a 400°F (200°C) oven for 30 minutes or until soft.

- *Preheat barbecue grill to high*
- *2 grilling baskets, lightly oiled*

I	red bell pepper, cut in half	I
2	small zucchini	2
2 tbsp	olive oil, divided	25 mL
I	eggplant, cut into ½-inch (I cm) rounds	I

Dressing

¼ cup	olive oil	50 mL
I tbsp	freshly squeezed lemon juice	15 mL
I tbsp	balsamic vinegar	15 mL
I tbsp	tamari or soy sauce	15 mL
I	clove garlic, minced	I
I tbsp	chopped fresh oregano	15 mL
I tbsp	chopped fresh mint or tarragon	15 mL

Salad

½	red onion, thinly sliced	½
½	cucumber, diced	½
I cup	cooked lentils or black-eyed peas, drained and rinsed	250 mL
	Sea salt and freshly ground pepper	

1. Arrange red pepper halves and zucchini in a prepared grilling basket. Brush with 1 tbsp (15 mL) of the oil and grill for 8 to 10 minutes or until tender when pierced with the tip of a knife. Arrange eggplant in remaining basket and brush with remaining oil. Grill for 3 to 4 minutes or until tender. Let vegetables cool enough to handle. Peel and slice red pepper and cut zucchini and eggplant into chunks.

2. *Dressing:* Meanwhile, in a large bowl, whisk together oil, lemon juice, vinegar, tamari, garlic, oregano and mint.

3. *Assemble Salad:* Add red onion, cucumber and lentils to dressing. Add grilled vegetables and stir to combine well. Taste and season with salt and pepper, if required.

Mango and Red Onion with Chili Sauce Salsa

Tropical mango and herbed chili sauce make an unusual combination in this flavorful summer starter.

4	large ripe mangoes, sliced	4
½	red onion, thinly sliced	½
2 tbsp	Date Molasses (page 147), Pomegranate Molasses (page 146) or store-bought	25 mL

Chili Sauce Salsa

¼ cup	chili sauce, store-bought or homemade	50 mL
2 tbsp	olive oil	25 mL
1 tbsp	balsamic vinegar	15 mL
1 tbsp	chopped fresh cilantro	15 mL
1 tbsp	shredded fresh basil	15 mL

1. In a salad bowl, combine mangoes, onion and molasses. Cover tightly and refrigerate for 30 minutes or overnight.

2. *Chili Sauce Salsa:* In a clean jar with a tight-fitting lid, combine chili sauce, oil, vinegar, cilantro and basil. Shake well to combine. Toss with chilled mango mixture.

Bulgur Asparagus Salad

In this salad, the bulgur and asparagus are made piquant with lemon juice and almonds.

Tip

• When whole wheat berries are steamed, hulled, dried and cracked, the resulting product is called bulgur. It is often confused with couscous, a totally different wheat product.

• *Preheat oven to 400°F (200°C)*
• *Rimmed baking sheet, lightly oiled*

1 lb	asparagus, trimmed	500 g
5 tbsp	olive oil, divided	75 mL
3 tbsp	freshly squeezed lemon juice	45 mL
½ cup	finely chopped onion	125 mL
1	clove garlic, minced	1
2 tbsp	finely chopped fresh parsley	25 mL
1 cup	fine or coarse bulgur (see Tip, left)	250 mL
1¼ cups	boiling water or vegetable stock	300 mL
½ cup	finely chopped almonds	125 mL

1. Arrange asparagus on prepared baking sheet in a single layer. Drizzle or brush 2 tbsp (25 mL) of the oil and the lemon juice over. Bake in preheated oven for 20 minutes or until tender when pierced with the tip of a knife.

2. Meanwhile, in a skillet, heat 2 tbsp (25 mL) of the oil over medium heat. Add onion and garlic and cook, stirring occasionally, for 6 to 8 minutes or until soft. Add parsley, bulgur and water. Cover, reduce heat to medium-low and simmer for 15 to 20 minutes or until the liquid has been absorbed. Fluff with a fork and transfer to a bowl.

3. Add remaining oil to skillet and return to medium heat. Stir in almonds and toast, stirring frequently, for 2 minutes or until lightly browned.

4. Divide bulgur evenly among 4 salad plates. Top each plate with 4 or 5 asparagus spears and sprinkle with toasted almonds. Serve warm or at room temperature.

Serves 4 to 6

Okra is not native to North America, having originated, it is thought, in Ethiopia. The tall plant produces seed pods that have an unusually mucilaginous juice and a sweet flavor. Okra was grown and added to stews in the Deep South. The stews were called gumbo, a word derived from the Bantu dialects from southern and central Africa.

Tip

• Fresh okra is not always available. Use frozen, thawed, or drained canned okra and add in the last few minutes of cooking.

Okra and Broad Beans with Tomato Sauce

3 tbsp	olive oil	45 mL
1	onion, chopped	1
1	leek, white and light green parts, sliced	1
2	cloves garlic, finely chopped	2
10 oz	okra (see Tip, left)	300 g
10 oz	shelled fresh broad beans or green beans, cut into 1-inch (2.5 cm) pieces	300 g
1	can (28 oz/796 mL) diced tomatoes with juice	1
2 tbsp	freshly squeezed lemon juice	25 mL
1 tbsp	Date Molasses (page 147) or blackstrap molasses	15 mL
2 tbsp	finely shredded fresh basil	25 mL
1/4 tsp	ground nutmeg	1 mL

1. In a skillet, heat oil over medium heat. Add onion and leek and cook, stirring frequently, for 8 to 10 minutes or until soft. Add garlic, okra, broad beans, tomatoes with juice, lemon juice and molasses. Simmer over medium-low heat for 7 to 10 minutes or until beans are tender when pierced with the tip of a knife. Stir in basil and nutmeg.

Maple and Orange–Glazed Eggplant

This dish makes a light start to dinner, and may be turned into a light lunch by serving over Braised Greens with Cherries and Pine Nuts (page 223), rice or seasonal greens.

- *Preheat oven to 375°F (190°C)*
- *13- by 9-inch (3 L) baking pan, lightly oiled*

2	eggplants	2
2 tbsp	olive oil	25 mL
1 cup	finely chopped onion	250 mL
2	cloves garlic, finely chopped	2
1 cup	freshly squeezed orange juice	250 mL
1	piece (1 inch/2.5 cm) candied ginger, finely chopped	1
3 tbsp	tamari or soy sauce	45 mL
3 tbsp	pure maple syrup	45 mL
1 tbsp	rice vinegar	15 mL

1. Trim ends from eggplants and pare the skin lengthwise in strips, leaving some skin running lengthwise in $\frac{1}{2}$-inch (1 cm) strips. Cut eggplants in half lengthwise and cut each half into 3 wedges. Arrange wedges, skin side down, in a single layer in prepared baking pan. Set aside.

2. Meanwhile, in a saucepan, heat oil over medium heat. Add onion and garlic and cook, stirring occasionally, for 6 to 8 minutes or until soft. Add orange juice and bring to a boil, stirring occasionally. Stir in ginger, tamari, maple syrup and rice vinegar and simmer for 1 to 2 minutes or until slightly thick.

3. Pour glaze over eggplant wedges. Cover with foil and bake in preheated oven for 40 minutes. Remove foil, turn wedges over and bake, uncovered, for another 20 minutes or until eggplant is soft and glaze is bubbly.

Roasted Spice-Glazed Root Vegetables

Adding garlic to the roasted vegetables gives them extra sweetness. This side dish is very easy to prepare.

- *Preheat oven to 400°F (200°C)*
- *Rimmed baking sheet, lightly oiled*

6	cloves garlic	6
2	onions, quartered	2
2	carrots, quartered lengthwise and cut in half	2
2	parsnips, quartered lengthwise and cut in half	2
1	medium sweet potato, cut lengthwise into wedges	1
½	rutabaga, cut in half lengthwise, then cut into wedges	½
3 tbsp	olive oil	45 mL
	Sea salt and freshly ground pepper	
3 tbsp	Spiced Sweet Glaze (page 147) or pure maple syrup	45 mL

1. On prepared baking sheet, arrange garlic, onions, carrots, parsnips, sweet potato and rutabaga in one layer. Drizzle with oil and season to taste with salt and pepper.

2. Bake in preheated oven for 45 minutes or until tender when pierced with the tip of a knife. Transfer to a bowl and toss with glaze.

Look for small yellow lentils in Middle Eastern supermarkets or use the widely available red lentils in this dish. Save leftover Yellow Curry Dal for use in soups and Lentil and Broccoli Casserole (page 231).

Yellow Curry Dal

2 tbsp	olive oil	25 mL
1 cup	chopped onion	250 mL
2	cloves garlic, finely chopped	2
1 tbsp	Yellow Curry Spice (page 253) or curry powder	15 mL
1 tsp	grated fresh gingerroot	5 mL
1 ¼ cups	dried yellow lentils (see Intro, left), rinsed	300 mL
2 cups	vegetable stock or water	500 mL
	Sea salt and freshly ground pepper	

1. In a saucepan, heat oil over medium heat. Add onion and garlic and cook, stirring occasionally, for 6 to 8 minutes or until soft. Stir in curry and ginger. Cook, stirring frequently, for 1 minute.

2. In a strainer, pick over and remove any small stones or grit from lentils. Add lentils and vegetable stock to saucepan. Stir well and bring to a boil. Reduce heat and simmer for 15 minutes, stirring occasionally for the first 10 minutes and frequently during the last 5 minutes of cooking. Cook only until water is absorbed and lentils are soft. Season to taste with salt and pepper. Serve warm or at room temperature.

This is a very easy yet sophisticated side dish. Use it as a base for main-dish entrées.

Tip

• You may use a blender or food processor to purée the rutabaga.

Fruited Rutabaga Purée

| 1 | rutabaga (about 2 ½ lbs/ 1.25 kg), cut into 1-inch (2.5 cm) cubes | 1 |
| 1 cup | Fruit Purée (page 139) or applesauce | 250 mL |

1. In a saucepan of boiling salted water, cook rutabaga for 25 minutes or until soft. Drain and return to pot. Using an immersion blender or potato masher, mash rutabaga. Add Fruit Purée and stir well to combine.

Roasting beets is an easy and delicious way to cook them. Their sugars caramelize and their sweet and slightly nutty flavor is brought out with this method.

Variation

• In the spring use 1 to 2 pounds (500 g to 1 kg) of asparagus, trimmed in place of the beets. Reduce roasting time to 35 to 40 minutes or until asparagus is tender when pierced with the tip of a knife.

Roasted Beets with Pomegranate Molasses

• *Preheat oven to 375°F (190°C)*
• *Pie plate or baking dish, lightly oiled*

6	medium beets, trimmed and quartered	6
2	onions, quartered	2
3 tbsp	olive oil	45 mL
1 tbsp	chopped fresh rosemary	15 mL
1 tbsp	Pomegranate Molasses (page 146) or store-bought	15 mL

1. In prepared pie plate, combine beets, onions, oil and rosemary. Bake in preheated oven for 50 minutes or until beets are tender when pierced with the tip of a knife. Drizzle with molasses.

With this recipe, you can afford to spend the time it takes to slice the green vegetables because the cooking time is so short. The added bonus is that a shorter cooking time avoids bringing out the sulfur in cruciferous vegetables, which is responsible for their unpleasant smell. This recipe keeps the time to a minimum and the taste is sweeter — even without the maple syrup. Use a deep, heavy-bottomed pan and cook the greens just before sitting down to the meal.

Maple-Glazed Cabbage Greens with Pecans

12	Brussels sprouts, halved lengthwise and cored	12
4	kale leaves, thick rib removed	4
1/4	green cabbage, cored	1/4
2 tbsp	olive oil	25 mL
4 tbsp	freshly squeezed lemon juice, divided	60 mL
3 tbsp	pure maple syrup	45 mL
	Sea salt and freshly ground pepper	
1/2 cup	toasted pecans or Candied Nuts (page 157)	125 mL

1. Thinly slice Brussels sprouts and kale leaves. Shred cabbage.

2. In a large skillet, heat oil over high heat. Add Brussels sprouts, kale and cabbage. Sprinkle 2 tbsp (25 mL) of the lemon juice over the greens and cook, stirring constantly, for 2 minutes. Remove from heat and add maple syrup and remaining lemon juice. Season to taste with salt and pepper. Serve garnished with pecans.

Gingered Carrot-Turnip Purée

Warm the plates and
serve immediately
because if the purée
hits a cold plate or sits
too long before being
served, some of the
liquid may separate out.

3	large carrots, cut into chunks	3
½	rutabaga, cut into chunks	½
1 tsp	finely grated orange zest, optional	5 mL
	Juice of 1 orange	
1 tbsp	agave nectar or brown rice syrup	15 mL
1 tsp	finely grated fresh gingerroot	5 mL
1 tsp	toasted sesame oil	5 mL
	Sea salt	

1. In a large saucepan or deep skillet, combine carrots and rutabaga. Fill with just enough water to cover the vegetables. Bring to a boil over high heat. Cover, reduce heat to medium-low and simmer for 30 minutes or until the vegetables are tender when pierced with the tip of a knife. Drain and let cool slightly.

2. In a blender or food processor, combine vegetables, orange zest, if using, orange juice, agave nectar, ginger, sesame oil and salt to taste. Blend or process until puréed or smooth. Serve immediately.

This makes an excellent main dish, or serve smaller portions as a warm salad course or vegetable side dish. The best thing about it is that it takes less than half an hour from start to finish.

Tip

• If cumin seeds are not available, use 2 tsp (10 mL) ground cumin and skip the toasting and grinding in Step 1.

Garlic Greens with Chickpeas and Cumin

1 tbsp	cumin seeds (see Tip, left)	15 mL
1 tsp	hot pepper flakes	5 mL
½ tsp	ground cinnamon	2 mL

Garlic Greens

3 tbsp	olive oil	45 mL
2	onions, coarsely chopped	2
4	cloves garlic, chopped	4
8	dried apricot halves, thinly sliced	8
1	can (14 to 19 oz/398 to 540 mL) chickpeas with liquid (see Tip, page 222)	1
	Juice of 1 lemon	
4 cups	packed fresh spinach, trimmed (about 10 oz/300 g)	1 L
	Sea salt and freshly ground pepper	

1. In a small skillet, toast cumin seeds over medium heat until aromatic, 1 to 2 minutes. Remove from heat and let cool. Using a mortar and pestle or spice grinder, pulverize or grind the toasted seeds. In a bowl, combine with hot pepper flakes and cinnamon. Set aside.

2. *Garlic Greens:* In a deep skillet or saucepan, heat oil over medium heat. Add onions and cook, stirring frequently, for 6 to 8 minutes or until soft.

3. Stir in cumin mixture, garlic and apricots and cook, stirring occasionally, for 2 minutes. Add chickpeas with liquid and lemon juice. Bring to a boil and add spinach. Cover, reduce heat and simmer, stirring once, for 5 minutes. Season to taste with salt and pepper.

Roasted Red Peppers with Moroccan Couscous

Served with rice or a green salad, this makes a colorful side dish.

- *Preheat oven to 375°F (190°C)*
- *Baking sheet, lightly oiled*

3	red bell peppers, halved crosswise	3
2 tbsp	olive oil	25 mL

Moroccan Couscous

1 tbsp	olive oil	15 mL
½ cup	chopped onion	125 mL
1	clove garlic, minced	1
1½ cups	couscous	375 mL
1 cup	vegetable stock or water	250 mL
¼ cup	raisins	50 mL
¼ cup	Apricot Tamarind Marmalade (page 183) or orange marmalade	50 mL
¼ tsp	ground cinnamon	1 mL
¼ tsp	ground cumin	1 mL
	Sea salt and freshly ground pepper	

1. Arrange pepper halves, cut side down, on prepared baking sheet. Brush or drizzle with oil. Bake in preheated oven for 40 minutes or until the skin bubbles and blackens in places. Transfer to a bowl and let cool. Slip the skins off and arrange, cut sides up, on a serving platter.

2. *Moroccan Couscous:* Meanwhile, in a skillet, heat oil over medium heat. Add onion and cook, stirring occasionally, for 6 to 8 minutes or until onion is soft. Add garlic and cook, stirring, for 1 minute.

3. Add couscous and cook, stirring constantly, for 1 minute to lightly toast the grains. Add vegetable stock, raisins, marmalade, cinnamon and cumin. Increase heat to high and bring to a boil. Turn off heat, leaving the pan on the burner or element, and cover pan. Let stand for 10 minutes or until liquid is absorbed. Fluff with a fork and season to taste with salt and pepper. Divide couscous into 6 portions and stuff each portion into a pepper half. Serve warm or cold.

Roasted Fingerling Potatoes with Shallots and Rosemary

Fingerling potatoes are just that — long, thin or stubby potatoes that resemble fingers. Fingerling potatoes such as Russian Banana are creamy, with a butter-colored flesh that roasts well. If fingerlings are not available, any waxy variety of potato (such as Charlotte, Maris Peer or any of the red potatoes) works well in this recipe.

Variations

- You can use regular-size potatoes here instead of fingerlings. Just cut them into wedges.
- If long "banana" shallots are available, use them here in place of regular shallots.

- *Preheat oven to 375°F (190°C)*
- *13- by 9-inch (3 L) baking pan, oiled*

2 lbs	yellow fingerling potatoes	I kg
6	shallots	6
6	cloves garlic	6
I	sprig fresh rosemary, chopped	I
I tbsp	chopped fresh anise, optional	15 mL
2 tbsp	olive oil	25 mL

I. In prepared dish, combine potatoes, shallots, garlic, rosemary and anise, if using. Drizzle with oil and bake in preheated oven for 45 minutes or until potatoes are lightly browned and tender when pierced with the tip of a knife.

Citrus Beets

Chill and serve as a condiment or spoon directly from the pan for a colorful side dish or salad. Leftovers may be frozen and added to soups and vegetable stews.

4 cups	shredded beets (about I ½ lbs/750 g)	I L
I cup	freshly squeezed orange juice	250 mL
¼ cup	freshly squeezed lemon juice	50 mL
2 tbsp	agave nectar or I tbsp (15 mL) brown rice syrup	25 mL
I tbsp	rice vinegar	15 mL
I tbsp	finely chopped candied ginger, optional	15 mL
	Sea salt and freshly ground pepper	

I. In a saucepan or skillet, combine beets, orange juice and lemon juice. Bring to a boil over medium heat. Stir in agave nectar, vinegar and ginger. Reduce heat to medium-low and simmer, stirring occasionally, until liquid is nearly evaporated, sauce is syrupy and beets are tender, about 1 hour. Season to taste with salt and pepper.

Shredded Vegetable Bake

Kids love vegetables cooked this way because the sugars are caramelized and the potatoes resemble french fries. Use any variety of potato — Russet, Yukon Gold and Kennebec are good varieties for this method.

Tip

- You can use 2 cups (500 mL) cooked chickpeas, drained and rinsed, instead of canned.

- *Preheat oven to 400°F (200°C)*
- *Two 13- by 9-inch (3 L) baking pans, lightly oiled*

3	potatoes, shredded	3
I	onion, shredded	I
I	carrot, shredded	I
¼	rutabaga, shredded	¼
I cup	whole wheat bread crumbs	250 mL
2 tbsp	trail mix or nuts, finely chopped	25 mL
2	cloves garlic, minced	2
3 tbsp	olive oil	45 mL
	Sea salt and freshly ground pepper	
I	can (14 to 19 oz/398 to 540 mL) chickpeas, drained and rinsed (see Tip, left)	I

1. In a large bowl, toss together potatoes, onion, carrot, rutabaga, bread crumbs, trail mix, garlic and oil. Divide in two and spread in a thin layer on prepared pans. Sprinkle liberally with salt and pepper. Bake in preheated oven for 20 minutes.

2. Stir and spread in a thin layer again and grind more salt and pepper over vegetables and bake for another 20 minutes.

3. Divide chickpeas in half and stir into vegetables in pans, spreading out. Bake for 10 to 15 minutes or until vegetables are crisp and lightly browned.

Serves 4

Use spinach, kale, Swiss chard, bok choy (see Tip, below) or any other leafy green in this recipe.

Tip

• If using bok choy in this recipe, use 1 bunch (approximately 1½ lbs/750 g). Thinly slice the white stalks and add to the wok with the sesame oil in Step 1. Stir-fry for 3 minutes. Add sliced leafy tops and stir-fry for 1 minute or until wilted. Continue with Step 2.

Variation

• Use dried cranberries, dried apricots or raisins in place of the cherries.

Braised Greens with Cherries and Pine Nuts

1 tbsp	olive oil	15 mL
1	sweet onion (such as Vidalia), sliced	1
1	clove garlic, finely chopped	1
1 tsp	toasted sesame oil	5 mL
1 lb	leafy greens (see Intro, left), sliced	500 g
¼ cup	dried cherries	50 mL
2 tbsp	pine nuts	25 mL
Pinch	ground nutmeg	Pinch
2 tbsp	Pomegranate Molasses (page 146) or store-bought, optional	25 mL

1. In a wok or skillet, heat olive oil over medium-high heat. Add onion and stir-fry for 3 minutes. Add garlic and stir-fry for 1 minute. Add sesame oil and greens and stir-fry for 1 minute or until wilted.

2. Stir in cherries, pine nuts and nutmeg and stir until heated through. Drizzle some molasses on each plate, if using, and pile braised greens beside it.

Potato Rösti

- *Preheat oven broiler, position rack on top shelf*
- *10-inch (25 cm) cast-iron skillet*

1 tbsp	ground flaxseeds	15 mL
2 tbsp	rice milk or soy milk	25 mL
2	medium potatoes, shredded	2
½	small onion, shredded	½
1 cup	Mini Mushroom Burger mixture (page 168) or chopped cooked chickpeas	250 mL
	Sea salt and freshly ground pepper	
3 tbsp	olive oil	45 mL

1. In a bowl, combine flaxseeds and rice milk. Let stand for 5 minutes or until gelatinous.

2. Add potatoes, onion and Mini Mushroom Burger mixture. Season to taste with salt and pepper.

3. In skillet, heat oil over high heat. Scrape potato mixture into skillet and press down with the back of a spoon. Reduce heat to medium and cook for 7 minutes or until potatoes start to brown around edge of pan. Place skillet on top rack of oven and broil for 5 minutes or until top is crisp and golden. Cut into wedges to serve.

Garlic Mashed Potatoes

6	medium potatoes, quartered	6
1	head roasted garlic (page 132)	1
¼ cup	Soy Sour Cream (page 145) or rice milk	50 mL
2 tbsp	safflower oil	25 mL
1 tsp	sesame oil	5 mL
	Sea salt and freshly ground pepper	

1. In a saucepan, cover potatoes with water and bring to a boil. Cover, reduce heat to medium and simmer for 15 minutes or until potatoes are soft. Drain. Let cool enough to handle. Slip skins off and return to saucepan.

2. Squeeze roasted cloves of garlic into saucepan with potatoes. Using a potato masher, mash potatoes and garlic. Add Soy Sour Cream, safflower oil, sesame oil and salt and pepper to taste. Beat until smooth.

Serve this spicy vegetable hot or cold, with other vegetables, as a starter, or with a rice dish.

Madras Cauliflower

3 cups	sliced cauliflower florets	750 mL
2 tbsp	olive oil	25 mL
1 cup	chopped onion	250 mL
2	green onions, chopped	2
2 tbsp	Madras Curry Paste (page 255) or curry powder, or to taste	25 mL
½ cup	whole wheat bread crumbs	125 mL

1. In a saucepan, cover cauliflower with water. Bring to a boil over high heat. Reduce heat and simmer for 3 minutes. Drain and let cool slightly.

2. In a wok, heat oil over medium-high heat. Add onion and green onions and stir-fry for 2 minutes. Add curry paste and bread crumbs and stir-fry for 1 minute. Add blanched cauliflower and stir-fry for 3 to 5 minutes or until cauliflower is browned and tender-crisp.

Use a smaller amount of the Madras Curry Paste if you are unsure about the heat.

Madras Frites

- *Preheat oven to 425°F (220°C)*
- *Rimmed baking sheet, lightly oiled*

2	large potatoes, cut into wedges	2
2 tbsp	Madras Curry Paste (page 255) or curry powder	25 mL
2 tbsp	olive oil	25 mL

1. In a bowl, toss potato wedges with curry paste and oil. On prepared baking sheet, arrange wedges in a single layer. Bake in preheated oven for 20 minutes. Turn and bake for another 15 minutes or until wedges are crisp and browned.

Curried Green Sauté

Serve this dish as you would mashed potatoes. It adds both color and extra hot spicy flavor to main-course dishes.

1 cup	water	250 mL
1 tbsp	freshly squeezed lemon juice	15 mL
2 tsp	grated fresh gingerroot	10 mL
¼	head cabbage, shredded	¼
1 lb	fresh spinach, trimmed and coarsely chopped	500 g
2 tbsp	olive oil	25 mL
1 cup	finely chopped onion	250 mL
1 to 2 tbsp	Green Curry Paste (page 256) or curry powder	15 to 25 mL

1. In a saucepan over medium-high heat, bring water, lemon juice and ginger to a gentle boil. Add cabbage. Cover and reduce heat to low. Simmer for 5 minutes or until tender when pierced with the tip of a knife. Add spinach. Increase heat to medium and cook, uncovered, stirring frequently, for 3 minutes or until spinach is soft and most of the water is evaporated. Drain and set aside.

2. Meanwhile, in a skillet, heat oil over medium heat. Add onion and cook, stirring occasionally, for 6 to 8 minutes or until soft. Add curry paste to taste and cook, stirring constantly, for 1 minute. Add curried onions to greens and mix well.

Casseroles, Stews and Curries

Serves 4

Mushroom-Stuffed Fennel and Red Peppers

The combination of red peppers and anise-flavored fennel is intensified by the use of fresh tarragon. For a more subtle herb combination, substitute parsley or oregano for the tarragon.

- *Preheat oven to 375°F (190°C)*
- *13- by 9-inch (3 L) baking pan, lightly oiled*

1	fennel bulb, trimmed and halved lengthwise	1
2	red bell peppers	2

Mushroom Filling

4 tbsp	olive oil, divided	60 mL
1 cup	chopped onion	250 mL
2 cups	sliced mushrooms	500 mL
½ cup	whole wheat bread crumbs	125 mL
3 tbsp	chopped fresh parsley	45 mL
2 tbsp	chopped fresh tarragon or chervil (see Intro, left)	25 mL
	Sea salt and freshly ground pepper	

1. In a saucepan, cover fennel halves with water. Bring to a boil over high heat. Reduce heat and simmer for 10 minutes or until almost tender (the tip of a knife should meet with some resistance when the fennel is pierced). Drain, reserving cooking liquid for vegetable stock or another use. Slice red peppers in half lengthwise.

2. *Mushroom Filling:* Meanwhile, in a skillet, heat 2 tbsp (25 mL) of the oil over medium heat. Add onion and mushrooms and cook, stirring frequently, for 8 to 10 minutes or until soft. Remove from heat and stir in bread crumbs, parsley and tarragon. Season to taste with salt and pepper.

3. Split fennel halves in half again and arrange, cut sides up, in prepared baking pan. Add red pepper halves, cut sides up. Divide stuffing into 8 portions. Stuff into the peppers and press between the layers of fennel. Drizzle with remaining oil and bake in preheated oven for 15 minutes or until filling is browned and crispy and vegetables are tender when pierced with the tip of a knife.

Lentil Tagine

If using a tagine, be sure that the base is flameproof so it can sit directly on an electric or gas stovetop. If the tagine is clay and not flameproof, use a Dutch oven or enamel pan with a lid; or use a saucepan for Steps 1 and 2 and transfer to the tagine to bake. Save leftover Lentil Tagine for use in soups and Lentil and Broccoli Casserole (page 231).

- *Preheat oven to 375°F (190°C)*
- *Flameproof tagine or Dutch oven*

1 cup	dried red lentils	250 mL
1 tbsp	olive oil	15 mL
1	onion, chopped	1
1	carrot, finely chopped	1
2	cloves garlic, minced	2
1	slice or cube (1 inch/2.5 cm) candied ginger, finely chopped	1
1 tbsp	Garam Masala Spice Blend (page 254) or store-bought	15 mL
1 tsp	Red Curry Spice (page 252), Yellow Curry Spice (page 253) or curry powder	5 mL
½ cup	brown rice (see Tip, page 316)	125 mL
1	can (19 oz/540 mL) sliced peaches with juice	1
3 cups	Mushroom Broth (page 138), vegetable stock or water	750 mL
¼ cup	red or white wine, optional	50 mL
	Sea salt and freshly ground pepper	

1. In a strainer, pick over and remove any small stones or grit from lentils. Rinse under cool water. Drain and set aside.

2. In base of tagine, heat oil over medium heat. Add onion and carrot. Cook, stirring frequently, for 5 minutes or until slightly softened. Add garlic and cook, stirring frequently, for 2 minutes or until onion and garlic are soft. Stir in garam masala and curry. Cook, stirring constantly, for 30 seconds.

3. Add lentils, rice, peaches with juice, broth and red wine, if using, to tagine. Bring to a boil. Cover and bake in preheated oven for 1 hour, stirring once halfway through cooking, until lentils and rice are soft. Season to taste with salt and pepper.

Moroccan Chickpea Tagine

This is a very nice slow-cooked stew but to save time, it may be cooked on the stovetop (see Tips, below).

Tips

• *To cook Moroccan Chickpea Tagine on the stovetop:* In a Dutch oven or large saucepan, heat 1 tbsp (15 mL) olive oil over high heat. Reduce heat to medium. Add onion and cook, stirring frequently, for 6 to 8 minutes or until soft. Add all other ingredients. Reduce heat to low, cover and cook, stirring once or twice, for 45 minutes or until sweet potato is tender.

• Use 1¼ cups (300 mL) vegetable stock if using canned chickpeas and their liquid.

• *Preheat oven to 350°F (180°C)*
• *Tagine or Dutch oven*

4 cups	cooked chickpeas, rinsed and drained, or 2 cans (14 to 19 oz/398 to 540 mL) chickpeas with liquid (see Tips, left)	1 L
2 cups	vegetable stock or water	500 mL
	Juice of 1 lemon	
2 cups	diced sweet potato, sweet or pie pumpkin or butternut squash	500 mL
½ cup	quinoa, rinsed	125 mL
1	onion, chopped	1
¼ cup	chopped dried apricots	50 mL
¼ cup	chopped raisins	50 mL
4	sun-dried tomato halves, thinly sliced	4
2	slices (⅛ inch/0.25 cm) fresh gingerroot, finely chopped	2
½ tsp	ground cumin	2 mL
½ tsp	ground coriander	2 mL
¼ tsp	ground cinnamon	1 mL
¼ tsp	hot pepper flakes	1 mL
	Sea salt and freshly ground pepper	

1. In the base of tagine, combine chickpeas, stock, lemon juice, sweet potato, quinoa, onion, apricots, raisins, sun-dried tomatoes, ginger, cumin, coriander, cinnamon and hot pepper flakes.

2. Bake in preheated oven for 1½ hours or until sweet potato is tender when pierced with the tip of a knife. Season to taste with salt and pepper.

This is a very easy casserole to make with leftover cooked Yellow Curry Dal (page 216) or Lentil Tagine (page 229). Omit the onion if using leftover lentils.

Lentil and Broccoli Casserole

- *Preheat oven to 375°F (190°C)*
- *8-inch (2 L) baking pan or casserole dish*

3 cups	broccoli florets	750 mL
½ cup	rice milk or soy milk	125 mL
1 cup	chickpea flour	250 mL
2 cups	cooked lentils or leftover cooked lentil mixture (see Intro, left), well drained	500 mL
½ cup	finely chopped onion	125 mL
	Vegetable oil	
2 cups	tomato sauce	500 mL

1. In a saucepan, cover broccoli with water. Bring to a boil over high heat. Reduce heat and simmer for 6 minutes or until almost tender (the tip of a knife should meet with some resistance when stems are pierced). Drain, reserving cooking liquid for another use.

2. Meanwhile, in a bowl, whisk rice milk into chickpea flour. Add lentils and onion. Form into balls 1½ inches (4 cm) in diameter. Pour oil into a large skillet until it reaches about ¼ inch (0.5 cm) up sides of pan. Heat over medium-high heat. Add lentil balls, in one layer with room to turn and cook, turning often, for 1 or 2 minutes per side or until lightly browned all over. Adjust heat to keep balls gently sizzling without splattering. Using a slotted spoon, transfer to a paper towel-lined plate to drain. Repeat with remaining balls.

3. In a mixing bowl, combine broccoli, lentil balls and tomato sauce. Scrape into baking pan and bake in preheated oven for 15 minutes or until bubbly.

You can choose seasonal greens for this year-round dish — spinach and dandelion greens in spring, or cabbage, Swiss chard and kale in winter.

Roasted Vegetable Lasagna

- *Preheat oven to 375°F (190°C)*
- *2 rimmed baking sheets, lightly oiled*
- *11- by 7-inch (2 L) baking pan, lightly oiled*

l	large eggplant, trimmed and cut lengthwise into ¼-inch (0.5 cm) slices	l
2	red bell peppers, halved lengthwise	2
5 tbsp	olive oil, divided	75 mL
l tbsp	balsamic vinegar	15 mL
l	large onion, chopped	l
2 cups	sliced mushrooms	500 mL
2	cloves garlic, minced	2
2 tbsp	chopped fresh mixed herbs, such as oregano, thyme and basil	25 mL
l	can (19 oz/540 mL) crushed tomatoes	l
l	can (14 to 19 oz/398 to 540 mL) lima beans, drained and rinsed	l
3 cups	shredded greens (see Intro, left)	750 mL

1. Arrange eggplant slices on one baking sheet and brush with 1 tbsp (15 mL) of the oil. Arrange red pepper halves, cut side down, on the other baking sheet and brush with 1 tbsp (15 mL) of the oil. Bake in preheated oven for 15 minutes or until the tip of a knife easily pierces the eggplant and the skin of the red peppers is dark and blistered. Do not overcook the eggplant. Let cool completely. Slip skin off red peppers and slice into wide strips. In a bowl, toss pepper strips with 1 tbsp (15 mL) of the oil and the vinegar and set aside.

2. In a skillet, heat remaining oil over medium heat. Add onion and mushrooms and cook, stirring frequently, for 6 to 8 minutes or until slightly softened. Add garlic and cook, stirring frequently, for 2 minutes or until onion and garlic are soft. Add herbs and tomatoes. Reduce heat to medium-low and simmer, stirring occasionally, for 10 minutes. Add lima beans and greens and cook for 1 to 5 minutes or until greens are wilted or, in the case of winter greens, tender when pierced with the tip of a knife.

3. Line prepared baking pan with one-third of the eggplant slices. Lay half the red pepper over the eggplant. Spread with one-third of the tomato sauce. Layer another one-third of the eggplant slices and the remaining red pepper slices and spread another one-third of the sauce over. Top with remaining eggplant slices and spread with remaining tomato sauce. Lasagna may be covered and stored in the refrigerator overnight. Bring back to room temperature before baking. Bake in preheated oven for 40 minutes or until sauce is bubbly.

Serves 4 to 6

This is an easy dish to prepare after a long day at work, and almost any vegetables will work in it (see Variations, below).

Variations

- Use ½ cup (125 mL) sliced celery or shredded cabbage instead of the fennel.

- For a crunchy topping, after the scallop is baked, spread 1 cup (250 mL) Crumb Nut Topping (page 157) or Oat Nut Topping (page 158) over the scallop and bake for 10 to 15 minutes or until browned.

Potato and Vegetable Scallop

- *Preheat oven to 350°F (180°C)*
- *8-cup (2 L) casserole dish, lightly oiled*

1	potato, thinly sliced	1
1	can (14 to 19 oz/398 to 540 mL) lentils, drained and rinsed	1
1	onion, thinly sliced	1
1	leek, white and light green parts, thinly sliced	1
2	carrots, thinly sliced	2
¼	fennel bulb, thinly sliced	¼
¼ cup	spelt flour	50 mL
1 cup	rice milk	250 mL

1. Arrange one-third of the potato slices on bottom of prepared dish. Layer one-third each of the lentils, onion, leek, carrots and fennel over potatoes. Sprinkle with about 2 tbsp (25 mL) of the flour. Drizzle with about ⅓ cup (75 mL) of the rice milk. Arrange another layer of one-third each of the potatoes, lentils, onion, leek, carrots, fennel, the remaining flour and ⅓ cup (75 mL) rice milk. Layer remaining lentils, onion, leek, carrots and fennel, ending with potatoes. Drizzle remaining rice milk over casserole.

2. Cover and bake in preheated oven for 40 to 45 minutes or until vegetables are tender when pierced with the tip of a knife and mixture is bubbly.

Cranberry Baked Beans

The cranberries add a
citrus-tart twist to an
old favorite.

Tip

* You can use 2 cups
(500 mL) cooked
kidney beans, drained
and rinsed, instead
of canned.

* *Preheat oven to 350°F (180°C)*
* *8-cup (2 L) casserole dish, lightly oiled*

1	can (14 to 19 oz/398 to 540 mL) red kidney beans, drained and rinsed (see Tip, left)	1
1 cup	chopped onion	250 mL
½ cup	dried cranberries	125 mL
½ cup	cranberry juice	125 mL
2 tbsp	Date Molasses (page 147) or blackstrap molasses	25 mL
1 tbsp	brown rice syrup	15 mL
1 tsp	dried mustard	5 mL
¼ tsp	ground ginger	1 mL

1. In prepared casserole dish, combine kidney beans, onion,
cranberries, cranberry juice, molasses, rice syrup, mustard
and ginger. Bake in preheated oven for 40 minutes or until
thick and bubbly.

Vegetable and Tempeh Pie

A hearty and delicious one-dish meal for a dinner party or weekend family meal. For easier preparation, make the Avocado Sauce and Garlic Mashed Potatoes as well as the tempeh a day in advance. Cover tightly and refrigerate until ready to roast vegetables, then remove from the refrigerator and let return to room temperature before proceeding with the recipe.

- *Preheat oven to 350°F (180°C)*
- *Rimmed baking sheet, lightly oiled*
- *9-inch (2.5 L) baking pan or casserole dish, lightly oiled*

2	small zucchini, cut into 1-inch (2.5 cm) chunks	2
2	small carrots, cut into 1-inch (2.5 cm) chunks	2
2	small parsnips, cut into 1-inch (2.5 cm) chunks	2
2 tbsp	olive oil	25 mL
1 tbsp	chopped fresh rosemary or thyme	15 mL

Tempeh

2 tbsp	olive oil	25 mL
1	onion, chopped	1
2	cloves garlic, chopped	2
1 tbsp	fresh chopped herbs, such as oregano, sage and thyme	15 mL
2 tbsp	tamari or soy sauce	25 mL
2 cups	cubed (½ inch/1 cm) tempeh	500 mL
½ cup	Mushroom Broth (page 138), vegetable stock or water, divided	125 mL
3 cups	spinach leaves	750 mL
2 cups	Avocado Sauce (page 148)	500 mL
1½ cups	Garlic Mashed Potatoes (page 224) (half the recipe)	375 mL

1. On prepared baking sheet, combine zucchini, carrots and parsnips. Toss with oil and rosemary. Bake in preheated oven for 30 minutes or until almost tender (the tip of a knife should meet with some resistance when vegetables are pierced).

2. *Tempeh:* Meanwhile, in a skillet, heat oil over medium heat. Add onion and cook, stirring occasionally, for 5 minutes or until slightly softened. Add garlic and herbs and cook, stirring frequently, for 3 minutes or until soft. Add tamari and tempeh and cook, stirring constantly, for 1 minute. Add ¼ cup (50 mL) of the broth and bring to a boil. Reduce heat and simmer, stirring constantly, for about 10 minutes, until broth has been absorbed. Add remaining broth and cook, stirring constantly, for 10 minutes. Add spinach and cook, stirring, for about 3 minutes or until wilted.

3. *Assemble pie:* In prepared baking pan, toss together roasted vegetables, tempeh mixture and Avocado Sauce. Spread Garlic Mashed Potatoes evenly over top of vegetables. Bake in preheated oven for 45 minutes or until top is lightly browned and sauce is bubbly. Let stand for 5 minutes before serving.

Succotash and Corn Dumplings

It is thought that the word *succotash* is a Native American word from the Narragansett language. Succotash has come to mean a baked dish whose main ingredients are lima beans and corn, although other vegetables and some meat and fish are often added. This recipe combines another North American classic: cornbread in the form of soft dumplings. It looks more complicated than it really is — the dumplings are easy and are added halfway through the cooking time.

Succotash Casserole

2 tbsp	olive oil	25 mL
1 cup	chopped onion	250 mL
½ cup	chopped green bell pepper	125 mL
3 cups	acorn or other squash, cut into 1-inch (2.5 cm) cubes	750 mL
2 tbsp	finely chopped jalapeño pepper, or to taste	25 mL
2	cloves garlic, finely chopped	2
1½ cups	Mushroom Broth (page 138), vegetable stock or water	375 mL

Corn Dumplings

⅓ cup	whole wheat flour	75 mL
⅓ cup	unbleached all-purpose flour	75 mL
1 tsp	baking powder	5 mL
1 cup	rice milk or water	250 mL
⅓ cup	yellow cornmeal	75 mL
½ tsp	sea salt	2 mL
1 tbsp	grapeseed oil	15 mL
1 tbsp	Fruit Purée (page 139) or applesauce	15 mL
1	can (12 oz/341 mL) whole kernel corn, drained	1
1	can (14 to 19 oz/398 to 540 mL) lima beans, drained and rinsed	1
1	can (14 oz/398 mL) creamed corn	1

1. *Succotash Casserole:* In a saucepan, heat oil over medium heat. Add onion and green pepper and cook, stirring occasionally, for 6 to 8 minutes or until soft. Add squash, jalapeño and garlic and cook, stirring frequently, for 3 minutes or until vegetables start to soften. Stir in broth and bring to a boil. Cover, reduce heat and simmer, stirring occasionally, for 15 minutes.

2. *Corn Dumplings:* Meanwhile, in a bowl, whisk together whole wheat flour, all-purpose flour and baking powder. Set aside. In a saucepan over medium heat, combine rice milk, cornmeal and salt. Cook, stirring constantly, for 3 minutes or until mixture is thickened and bubbly but not dry. Remove from heat and beat in oil, fruit purée and corn kernels. Add flour mixture to cornmeal mixture and beat well to incorporate.

3. When dumpling batter is ready and casserole has been simmering for at least 15 minutes, stir in lima beans and creamed corn. Bring back to a boil. Using a $\frac{1}{4}$-cup (50 mL) measure, drop dumplings into simmering casserole. Cover and simmer over low heat for 12 minutes or until dumplings are soft and slightly sticky from steaming but still cooked (do not lift lid to check dumplings until after 12 minutes).

Cashew Cream adds a rich taste and texture to the baked vegetables in this versatile dish.

Tip

- You can use 2 cups (500 mL) cooked chickpeas, drained and rinsed, instead of canned.

Variation

- For a crunchy topping, after the casserole is baked, spread 1 cup (250 mL) Crumb Nut Topping (page 157) or Oat Nut Topping (page 158) over vegetables and bake for 10 to 15 minutes or until browned.

Chickpeas and Potatoes in Cashew Cream

- *Preheat oven to 350°F (180°C)*
- *8-cup (2 L) casserole dish, lightly oiled*

3	medium potatoes, quartered	3
1 cup	cauliflower or broccoli florets	250 mL
1	onion, quartered	1
1	can (14 to 19 oz/398 to 540 mL) chickpeas, drained and rinsed (see Tip, left)	1
1⅓ cups	Cashew Cream (page 144)	325 mL
1 tsp	hot pepper flakes, or to taste	5 mL
	Sea salt and freshly ground pepper	

1. In a saucepan, combine potatoes, cauliflower and onion and cover with water. Bring to a boil over medium-high heat. Reduce heat and simmer for 8 minutes or until vegetables are almost tender (the tip of a knife should meet with some resistance when vegetables are pierced). Drain, reserving cooking liquid.

2. In prepared casserole dish, combine blanched vegetables, chickpeas, Cashew Cream and hot pepper flakes. If mixture seems too thick, add up to ¼ cup (50 mL) of the reserved cooking liquid. Bake in preheated oven for 35 minutes or until bubbly and lightly browned on top. Season to taste with salt and pepper.

The Pomegranate Molasses adds a sweet citrus dimension without overpowering the overall flavor. This is a traditional Turkish method of preparing vegetables. A heavy-bottomed casserole or Dutch oven provides a steady heat without burning the bottom of the stew.

Eggplant and Lentil Stew

- *3-quart (3 L) flameproof enameled cast-iron casserole dish or Dutch oven, lightly oiled*

½ cup	dried lentils or 1 cup (250 mL) cooked lentils, rinsed and drained	125 mL
1	onion, chopped	1
4	cloves garlic, minced	4
2 cups	chopped tomatoes or 1 can (19 oz/540 mL) diced tomatoes, drained	500 mL
2 cups	chopped carrots	500 mL
1 tbsp	chopped fresh oregano	15 mL
¼ tsp	hot pepper flakes	1 mL
	Sea salt and freshly ground pepper	
2	small eggplants (about 1½ lbs/750 g)	2
½ cup	olive oil	125 mL
¼ cup	Pomegranate Molasses (page 146) or store-bought	50 mL

1. If using dried lentils, in a strainer, pick over and remove any small stones or grit. Rinse under cool water and drain. In a saucepan, cover lentils with water, allowing a good 1 inch (2.5 cm) over top of them. Bring to a boil over high heat. Cover and reduce heat to medium-low. Simmer for 15 minutes or until tender. Skip step if using cooked lentils.

2. In a bowl, toss together onion, garlic, tomatoes, carrots, oregano and hot pepper flakes. Season to taste with salt and pepper. Spread half of the tomato mixture over bottom of prepared casserole dish.

3. Trim ends from eggplants and pare the skin lengthwise in strips, leaving some skin running lengthwise in ½-inch (1 cm) strips. Slice into ½-inch (1 cm) rounds. Layer half of the eggplant rounds over top of onion mixture in casserole dish. Spread half of the cooked lentils over eggplant.

4. Repeat layering onion mixture, eggplant rounds and lentils in casserole dish. Pour oil around edge and over top and then drizzle with molasses. Bring to a gentle boil over medium heat. Cover, reduce heat to low and simmer gently for 1 hour or until vegetables in stew are very soft.

The different peppers used in this Portuguese favorite — the unofficial national dish of Brazil — give it a rich and complex taste reminiscent of the original meat-filled dish.

Tip

• You can use 2 cups (500 mL) cooked black beans, drained and rinsed, instead of canned.

Black Bean and Four-Pepper Stew

1 tsp	whole cumin seeds	5 mL
½ tsp	whole coriander seeds	2 mL
1 tsp	sea salt	5 mL
½ tsp	ground cinnamon	2 mL
¼ tsp	ground nutmeg	1 mL
2 tbsp	olive oil	25 mL
1	small red onion, diced	1
1 cup	diced green bell pepper	250 mL
3	cloves garlic, finely chopped	3
	Zest and juice of 1 lime	
2 cups	chunks (1 inch/2.5 cm) acorn or butternut squash	500 mL
2 cups	Mushroom Broth (page 138), vegetable stock or water (approx.)	500 mL
2	roasted red bell peppers, cut into ½-inch (1 cm) pieces	2
1	roasted poblano chile, cut into ½-inch (1 cm) pieces	1
1	can (5 oz/127 mL) chipotle chiles in adobo sauce, drained and diced, sauce reserved	1
1	can (14 to 19 oz/398 to 540 mL) black beans, drained and rinsed (see Tip, left)	1
¼ cup	chopped fresh cilantro, optional	50 mL

1. In a small skillet over medium-high heat, toast cumin and coriander seeds until the seeds begin to pop and their fragrance is released, about 2 minutes. Do not let seeds smoke or burn. Remove from heat and add salt, cinnamon and nutmeg. Set aside.

2. In a saucepan, heat oil over medium heat. Add onion and green pepper. Cook, stirring occasionally, for 5 minutes or until slightly softened. Add garlic and cook, stirring frequently, for 2 to 3 minutes or until onion and garlic are soft. Add toasted spices and lime zest and juice. Cook, stirring constantly, for 1 minute.

3. Add squash and pour broth over, adding just enough to cover squash. Bring to a boil over high heat. Cover, reduce heat to medium-low and simmer for 25 minutes or until squash is tender when pierced with the tip of a knife. Add roasted red peppers, poblano chile, chipotle chiles and adobo sauce and black beans. Cook for 2 or 3 minutes or until peppers and beans are heated through. Add cilantro, if using, or pass separately.

Roasted Squash and Parsnip Stew

Roasting the vegetables mellows their flavor and brings out their natural sugars. This is a satisfying winter stew that is even better the day after it is made.

Tip

• *To prepare stew ahead:* Complete through to the point of adding squash, onions, parsnips, garlic and pan juices to the saucepan in Step 3 but do not simmer. Cool, cover and refrigerate for up to 24 hours. Bring to room temperature and simmer on medium-low heat for 12 minutes.

• *Preheat oven to 375°F (190°C)*
• *2 rimmed baking sheets, lightly oiled*

1	butternut squash, cut in half lengthwise, seeds removed	1
3	large onions, quartered	3
2	parsnips, cut into chunks	2
10	cloves garlic	10
3 tbsp	olive oil, divided	45 mL
2 tbsp	balsamic vinegar	25 mL
2	leeks, white and light green parts, sliced	2
3 cups	tomato sauce	750 mL
	Sea salt and freshly ground pepper	

1. Arrange squash, cut side down, on prepared baking sheet. Bake in preheated oven for 40 minutes or until tender when pierced with the tip of a knife. Let cool completely. Peel off skin and cut into 1-inch (2.5 cm) pieces. Set aside.

2. Meanwhile, on second prepared baking sheet, combine onions, parsnips and garlic. Drizzle with 2 tbsp (25 mL) of the oil and vinegar. Bake alongside squash for 30 minutes or until caramelized and tender when pierced with the tip of a knife.

3. In a large saucepan, heat remaining oil over high heat. Add leeks and reduce heat to medium. Cook, stirring occasionally, for 6 to 8 minutes or until soft. Add tomato sauce, squash, onions, parsnips, garlic and pan juices and simmer over low heat for 12 minutes to blend flavors and heat through. Season to taste with salt and pepper.

Ready in under an hour, this hearty stew makes great leftovers for lunch the next day — truly a time-saving recipe.

Tips

- Scotch barley is coarsely ground hulled barley and has as many of the nutrients as pot barley.

- You can use 2 cups (500 mL) cooked chickpeas, drained and rinsed, instead of canned.

- I prefer Lundberg short-grain brown rice, which is soft and chewy when cooked, but long-grain brown rice, red rice or a blend of your favorites will also work.

Chickpea and Swiss Chard Ragoût

2 tbsp	olive oil	25 mL
I	onion, chopped	I
I	leek, white part only, sliced	I
2	cloves garlic, minced	2
½ tsp	ground cumin	2 mL
¼ tsp	ground nutmeg	I mL
I	can (28 oz/796 mL) stewed tomatoes with juice	I
¼ cup	dry red wine	50 mL
I cup	cauliflower florets	250 mL
I cup	sliced carrots	250 mL
½ cup	Scotch barley or brown rice (see Tips, left)	125 mL
I lb	Swiss chard, ribs removed and leaves chopped (about 3 cups/750 mL)	500 g
I	can (14 to 19 oz/398 to 540 mL) chickpeas, drained and rinsed (see Tips, left)	I
I tbsp	freshly squeezed lemon juice	15 mL
¼ cup	chopped fresh flat-leaf parsley	50 mL

1. In a saucepan, heat oil over medium heat. Add onion and leek and cook, stirring occasionally, for 6 to 8 minutes or until soft. Add garlic, cumin and nutmeg and cook, stirring frequently, for 1 minute. Add tomatoes with juice, red wine, cauliflower, carrots and barley. Bring to a boil. Reduce heat and simmer, stirring once or twice, for 30 to 40 minutes or until vegetables and barley are tender.

2. Add Swiss chard, chickpeas and lemon juice. Simmer for 3 minutes or until Swiss chard is tender. Ladle into shallow bowls and garnish with parsley.

Sweet Potato Ragoût

3 tbsp	olive oil, divided	45 mL
1	onion, coarsely chopped	1
2 cups	sliced mushrooms	500 mL
2 cups	vegetable stock or water	500 mL
12	cloves roasted garlic (page 132)	12
2	small sweet potatoes, cut into 1-inch (2.5 cm) pieces (about 4 cups/1 L)	2
2 cups	shredded cabbage	500 mL
1/2 cup	red or white wine	125 mL
1	bay leaf	1
1 cup	cooked lentils (see Instructions, page 309)	250 mL
	Sea salt and freshly ground pepper	

1. In a large saucepan, heat 2 tbsp (25 mL) of the oil over medium heat. Add onion and cook, stirring occasionally, for 5 minutes or until slightly softened. Add remaining oil and stir in mushrooms. Cook, stirring frequently, for 5 minutes or until vegetables are soft.

2. Add stock and bring to a gentle boil. Add roasted garlic, sweet potatoes, cabbage, wine and bay leaf. Reduce heat and simmer, stirring once or twice, for 30 minutes or until sweet potatoes are cooked. Remove bay leaf. Stir in lentils and heat through. Season to taste with salt and pepper.

Serving Suggestion
* Serve with Braised Greens with Cherries and Pine Nuts (page 223) or Spiced Lemon Rice (page 315).

Lima Bean and Wheat Berry Stew

Whole grains such as wheat berries, Kamut and spelt add a chewy texture to stews and casserole dishes.

Tips

- To soak the wheat berries, cover with water and let stand for an hour or overnight. The longer they soak, the shorter the cooking time. Drain and rinse before adding to the stew.

- You can use 2 cups (500 mL) cooked lima or fava beans, drained and rinsed, instead of canned.

2 tbsp	olive oil	25 mL
I	red onion, halved and thinly sliced	I
I	carrot, chopped	I
I	clove garlic, finely chopped	I
½ cup	whole wheat berries or spelt kernels, soaked (see Tip, left)	125 mL
I	can (19 oz/540 mL) crushed tomatoes with juice	I
I cup	Mushroom Broth (page 138), vegetable stock or water	250 mL
I	can (14 to 19 oz/398 to 540 mL) lima or fava beans, drained and rinsed (see Tips, left)	I

1. In a saucepan, heat oil over medium heat. Add onion and carrot and cook, stirring occasionally, for 6 to 8 minutes or until slightly softened. Add garlic and cook, stirring frequently, for 3 minutes or until onion and garlic are soft. Stir in wheat berries and cook, stirring constantly, for 1 minute.

2. Add tomatoes with juice and broth and bring to a boil. Cover, reduce heat and simmer, stirring once or twice, for 1 to 1½ hours or until wheat berries are tender but chewy. Add lima beans and heat through.

Summer Vegetable Ragoût

Summer vegetables, especially fresh peas, zucchini and tomatoes combine to lend a distinctly summertime taste to this stew.

3 tbsp	olive oil, divided	45 mL
I	onion, chopped	I
I	leek, white and green parts, sliced	I
I cup	sliced stemmed shiitake mushrooms	250 mL
2	small zucchini, sliced	2
2	carrots, sliced	2
2	tomatoes, chopped	2
3 cups	Mushroom Broth (page 138), vegetable stock or water	750 mL
I tbsp	tamari or soy sauce	15 mL
I cup	fresh or frozen green peas	250 mL
2 tbsp	shredded fresh basil	25 mL
	Sea salt and freshly ground pepper	

1. In a saucepan, heat 2 tbsp (25 mL) of the oil over medium heat. Add onion and leek. Cover, reduce heat to low and sweat, stirring once or twice, for 10 minutes or until soft. Add remaining oil and increase heat to medium-high. Add mushrooms and cook, stirring frequently, for 6 to 8 minutes or until mushrooms are reduced by about half.

2. Add zucchini, carrots, tomatoes, broth and tamari. Simmer for 10 minutes or until vegetables are almost tender. Add peas and basil and cook for 3 to 5 minutes or until peas are tender. Season to taste with salt and pepper.

Here is another great stuffing for wraps and vegetables. Once baked and cooked in the stew, the plantains or bananas lose their characteristic "banana" taste. They are an excellent stew ingredient because they thicken the mixture.

Tips

• Plantains usually arrive at supermarkets green and hard. Store in a paper bag for 1 or 2 days to ripen quickly. Plantains turn yellow with solid black splotches when ripe.

• I prefer Lundberg short-grain brown rice, which is soft and chewy when cooked, but long-grain brown rice, red rice or a blend of your favorites will also work.

Baked Plantain and Peanut Stew

• *Preheat oven to 375°F (190°C)*
• *Baking sheet*

2	large ripe plantains (see Tips, left) or 3 large ripe bananas	2
2 tbsp	olive oil	25 mL
I	onion, chopped	I
2	cloves garlic, minced	2
I	jalapeño pepper, finely chopped	I
½ cup	brown rice (see Tips, left)	125 mL
I tbsp	grated fresh gingerroot	15 mL
I tsp	ground cumin	5 mL
I to 2 tsp	Garam Masala Spice Blend (page 254) or store-bought	5 to 10 mL
I tsp	sea salt	5 mL
¼ tsp	ground nutmeg	I mL
2 cups	Mushroom Broth (page 138), vegetable stock or water	500 mL
I	can (28 oz/796 mL) stewed or crushed tomatoes with juice	I
½ cup	Cashew Butter (page 181) or chunky peanut butter	125 mL
½ cup	coarsely chopped peanuts	125 mL

1. Trim tops off plantains and place on baking sheet. Bake in preheated oven for 15 minutes or until peel is charred and puffy. Let cool. Slice in half lengthwise and peel off skin. Coarsely chop flesh and set aside.

2. In a saucepan, heat oil over medium heat. Add onion and cook, stirring occasionally, for 5 minutes or until slightly softened. Add garlic and jalapeño pepper and cook, stirring frequently, for 3 minutes or until vegetables are tender. Add rice, ginger, cumin, garam masala to taste, salt and nutmeg and cook, stirring constantly, for 1 minute.

3. Stir in broth and tomatoes with juice and bring to a boil. Add baked plantains and cashew butter and stir well. Cover, reduce heat to low and simmer for 45 minutes or until rice is tender. Ladle into bowls and garnish with peanuts.

West African Mafé

Popular in West Africa from Senegal to the Congo, *mafé,* or groundnut stew is, of course, based on groundnuts — the African word for peanuts. For an authentic groundnut stew, grind whole raw peanuts to a paste using a blender or food processor and use in place of the Cashew Butter.

Tip

• Cassava root looks like a long, narrow sweet potato and is starchy, being the root of a tropical plant. It is found in Latin American and African food stores and some urban supermarkets. If cassava root is unavailable, use 2 sweet potatoes instead of the 1 called for.

3 tbsp	olive oil	45 mL
2	onions, chopped	2
1	green bell pepper, chopped	1
2	tomatoes, chopped	2
1	canned chipotle pepper in adobo sauce or jalapeño pepper, finely chopped	1
1	sweet potato, cut into $\frac{1}{2}$-inch (1 cm) cubes	1
1	small acorn squash, cut into $\frac{1}{2}$-inch (1 cm) cubes	1
1	medium cassava root, cut into $\frac{1}{2}$-inch (1 cm) cubes (see Tip, left)	1
$\frac{1}{4}$	rutabaga, cut into $\frac{1}{2}$-inch (1 cm) cubes	$\frac{1}{4}$
1 cup	coarsely chopped cabbage	250 mL
3 cups	Mushroom Broth (page 138), vegetable stock or water	750 mL
$\frac{1}{2}$ cup	Cashew Butter (page 181) or chunky peanut butter	125 mL
	Sea salt and freshly ground pepper	

1. In a saucepan, heat oil over medium heat. Add onions and green pepper and cook, stirring occasionally, for 6 to 8 minutes or until soft. Add tomatoes, chipotle pepper, sweet potato, squash, cassava, rutabaga, cabbage and broth. Bring to a boil. Reduce heat and simmer, stirring once or twice, for 40 minutes.

2. In a small bowl, blend $\frac{1}{2}$ cup (125 mL) of the hot cooking liquid with cashew butter. Add to pot. Cover and simmer for 30 more minutes. Season to taste with salt and pepper.

Jerusalem Artichoke Stew

While most stews are robust and full of texture and flavor, this one is delicate with a subtle yet no less complex taste. It takes advantage of the autumn harvest of Jerusalem artichokes but when these are not available, use potatoes instead.

Tip

• You can use 2 cups (500 mL) cooked white beans, drained and rinsed, instead of canned.

I tbsp	olive oil	15 mL
I	onion, chopped	I
2	stalks celery, chopped	2
2	cloves garlic, finely chopped	2
4 cups	vegetable stock or water	I L
2 cups	diced Jerusalem artichokes or potatoes	500 mL
I	medium carrot, diced	I
½ cup	shredded rutabaga or green cabbage	125 mL
¼ cup	dry white wine	50 mL
I	can (14 to 19 oz/398 to 540 mL) cannellini beans or flageolets, drained and rinsed (see Tip, left)	I
3 tbsp	chopped fresh parsley	45 mL
2 tbsp	freshly squeezed lemon juice	25 mL
	Sea salt and freshly ground pepper	

1. In a large saucepan, heat oil over medium heat. Add onion and celery and cook, stirring occasionally, for 6 to 8 minutes or until soft. Add garlic and cook, stirring frequently, for 2 minutes. Add stock. Increase heat to high and bring to a boil. Add Jerusalem artichokes, carrot, rutabaga and white wine. Cover, reduce heat to medium-low and simmer, stirring once or twice, for 15 minutes or until vegetables are tender when pierced with the tip of a knife.

2. Add beans, parsley and lemon juice and heat through. Season to taste with salt and pepper. Using a potato masher, mash some of the vegetables to thicken the stew.

Basic Curry Blends

Curries, like fine wines, have a distinctive bouquet and flavor that can be subtle or strong, hot or diversely savory, and there are as many different curry combinations as there are wines. Most important, curry flavoring offers welcome variety to vegan fare. A good curry is balanced, with each of the spices, herbs and other ingredients supporting the others. Chile peppers increase the heat, but they should not overpower the spices in the overall flavor combination.

Makes ½ cup (125 mL)

This curry spice is rich and complex, with an overall red color. Use it when a slightly hotter boost is called for.

Red Curry Spice

I	dried cayenne chile pepper	I
I tbsp	whole yellow or brown mustard seeds	I5 mL
I tbsp	whole red peppercorns	I5 mL
I tbsp	whole allspice berries	I5 mL
I tbsp	whole fennel seeds	I5 mL
2 tbsp	ground paprika	25 mL
I tbsp	ground turmeric	I5 mL

I. Using scissors, cut cayenne pepper pod into small pieces. In a small spice wok or dry cast-iron skillet, combine pepper pieces with mustard seeds, peppercorns, allspice and fennel seeds. Toast over medium-high heat until the seeds begin to pop and their fragrance is released, 2 to 3 minutes. Let cool.

2. Using a mortar and pestle or a small electric grinder, pound or grind toasted spices until coarse or finely ground, as desired. Add paprika and turmeric to ground spices and mix well.

3. Transfer mixture to a small clean jar with lid. Label and store in the refrigerator or a cool, dark place for up to 2 months.

Yellow Curry Spice

Pungent and gingery, with citrus notes, turmeric is one of two key curry spices. Fenugreek seeds create the overriding aroma of most curry powders. Both lend their distinctive flavors and color to this somewhat milder curry blend.

1	dried cayenne chile pepper	1
1 tbsp	whole yellow mustard seeds	15 mL
1 tbsp	whole coriander seeds	15 mL
1 tbsp	whole cumin seeds	15 mL
1 tsp	whole allspice berries	5 mL
1 tsp	fenugreek seeds	5 mL
1 tbsp	ground turmeric	15 mL
½ tsp	ground ginger	2 mL

1. Using scissors, cut cayenne pepper pod into small pieces. In a small spice wok or dry cast-iron skillet, combine pepper pieces with mustard, coriander, cumin, allspice and fenugreek seeds. Toast over medium-high heat until the seeds begin to pop and their fragrance is released, 2 to 3 minutes. Let cool.

2. Using a mortar and pestle or a small electric grinder, pound or grind toasted spices until coarse or finely ground, as desired. Add turmeric and ginger to ground spices and mix well.

3. Transfer mixture to a small clean jar with lid. Label and store in the refrigerator or a cool, dark place for up to 2 months.

Garam Masala Spice Blend

1	piece (2 inches/5 cm) cinnamon stick	1
2 tbsp	whole coriander seeds	25 mL
1 tbsp	whole cumin seeds	15 mL
2 tsp	whole cardamom seeds (see Tip, left)	10 mL
2 tsp	black peppercorns	10 mL
3	whole cloves	3
1	whole star anise	1
¼ tsp	ground nutmeg	1 mL

Masala is the Indian word for a blend of spices. A masala may be hot or sweetly fragrant, ground fine or crushed. It is added at different stages of the cooking process. Garam masala is the most common ground spice blend and is usually added towards the end of the cooking time. This masala is aromatic and not very hot; it can be used in small amounts in sweet dishes and beverages.

Tip

• When purchasing cardamom (*Elettaria cardamomum*), look for brown (called "black") or green pods that are bulging with seeds. White pods are either green or "black" pods that have been bleached. Seeds in the pods keep their unique spice essence longer. The small brown seeds are arranged in three double rows inside each pod. The whole pod and its seeds may be used in spice mixtures, but it is more common in North America to split the papery pod and remove and use only the seeds.

1. Break cinnamon into small pieces. In a small spice wok or dry cast-iron skillet, combine cinnamon, coriander, cumin and cardamom seeds, peppercorns, cloves and star anise. Toast over medium-high heat until the seeds begin to pop and their fragrance is released, 4 to 5 minutes. Let cool.

2. Using a mortar and pestle or a small electric grinder, pound or grind toasted spices until coarse or finely ground, as desired. Add nutmeg to ground spices and mix well.

3. Transfer mixture to a small clean jar with lid. Label and store in the refrigerator or a cool, dark place for up to 2 months.

Curry Pastes

For their curry powders and pastes, Indian, Thai and other Southeast Asian cooks toast whole spices one by one and then grind them, adding other ground spices, fresh herbs and piquant fresh ingredients. I have shortened the preparation time by toasting all of the seeds together. This means that extra-careful watching is required so that the smaller, lighter seeds do not smoke and burn. The pan may have to be removed before all the seeds have reached their maximum aroma, but that is the trade-off for shortening the time. Ghee (clarified butter) is the carrier widely used for the ground spice essences in spice pastes, but I have substituted grapeseed oil in the following curry paste recipes. Any lighter oil such as organic canola oil (not olive oil) will work. I prefer to add salt to the pastes because it is more convenient, but the salt may be removed from these recipes if desired. Each of the paste recipes makes about ½ cup (125 mL), enough for 4 to 8 dishes. While the curry paste recipes may be doubled, it is best to make small fresh batches rather than store them for more than a few weeks.

In my opinion, the curry pastes here are not intensely hot, but to judge for yourself, use 1 tbsp (15 mL) in recipes and add more after you have experienced the heat.

Madras Curry Paste

Makes ½ cup (125 mL)

Even with the peppercorns and chile peppers, this curry is not over-the-top hot. The mixture is more crumbly than the other pastes but adding more oil would only dilute the blend. Use this curry paste in combination with Garam Masala Spice Blend (left) for an even richer effect in hearty rice, legume and root vegetable dishes.

2 tbsp	whole coriander seeds	25 mL
1 tbsp	whole yellow or brown mustard seeds	15 mL
1 tbsp	whole cumin seeds	15 mL
1 tbsp	black peppercorns	15 mL
2	dried cayenne chile peppers	2
1	clove garlic	1
1 tbsp	sea salt	15 mL
1 tbsp	grated fresh gingerroot	15 mL
2 tbsp	grapeseed oil	25 mL
1 to 2 tsp	cider vinegar	5 to 10 mL

1. In a small spice wok or dry cast-iron skillet, combine coriander, mustard and cumin seeds, peppercorns and chile peppers. Toast over medium-high heat until seeds begin to pop and their fragrance is released, 2 to 3 minutes. Let cool.

2. Using a mortar and pestle or small electric grinder, pound or grind toasted spices until finely ground. Add garlic, salt and ginger and grind into spices. Add grapeseed oil, a few drops at a time, and grind together with spices. Add cider vinegar in drops until a thick, paste-like consistency is achieved.

3. Label and store paste in a small clean jar with a lid in the refrigerator for up to 1 month. If the paste becomes too dry, add a few more drops of oil and/or cider vinegar.

Green Curry Paste

Offering a hot and fresh curry taste with citrus overtones, this blend is very good with lentils and in vegetable curry dishes.

Tips

• Use any fresh culinary herb, alone or in combination, in place of the cilantro.

• Galangal is a root similar in appearance to ginger. The white flesh is sharp and pungent with a perfume-like, slightly sweet taste. Used in Southeast Asian dishes, galangal is available in most natural food stores.

1 tbsp	whole coriander seeds	15 mL
1 tbsp	whole fennel seeds	15 mL
2 tsp	whole cumin seeds	10 mL
2 tsp	whole fenugreek seeds	10 mL
2 tsp	sea salt	10 mL
1 or 2	fresh jalapeño or serrano chile peppers, chopped	1 or 2
¼ cup	chopped fresh cilantro or flat-leaf Italian parsley (see Tips, left)	50 mL
2	green onions, chopped	2
2	cloves garlic	2
2 tbsp	chopped fresh lemongrass	25 mL
1 tbsp	chopped galangal or grated fresh gingerroot (see Tips, left)	15 mL
1 tsp	grated lime zest	5 mL
1 tsp	freshly squeezed lime juice, optional	5 mL

1. In a small spice wok or dry cast-iron skillet, combine coriander, fennel, cumin and fenugreek seeds. Toast over medium-high heat until the seeds begin to pop and their fragrance is released, 2 to 3 minutes. Let cool.

2. Using a mortar and pestle or small electric grinder, pound or grind toasted spices until finely ground. Add salt, chile pepper and cilantro and grind into spices. Add green onions and garlic and grind into spices. Add lemongrass, galangal and lime zest and grind into spices. The mixture should have a paste-like consistency at this point, but a few drops of lime juice may be added, if desired.

3. Label and store paste in a small clean jar with a lid in the refrigerator for up to 1 month.

Roasted Zucchini Shells with Almond Filling
and Red Pepper Sauce (page 281)

Bok Choy, Mushroom and Black Bean Stir-Fry (page 288)

Udon Noodles with Tofu and
Gingered Peanut Sauce (page 304)

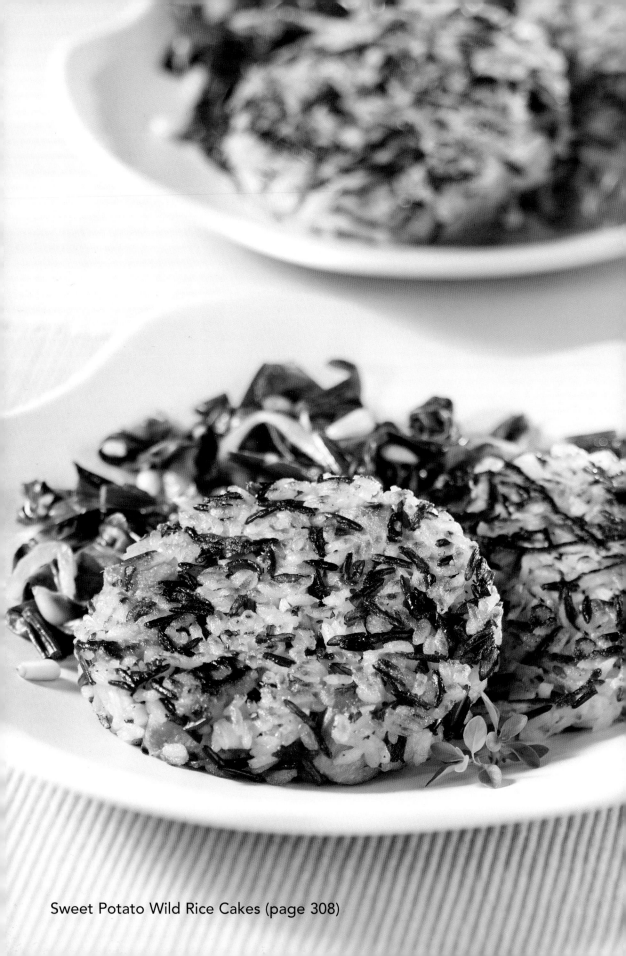

Sweet Potato Wild Rice Cakes (page 308)

Citrus Wheat Berries and Greens (page 323)

Pomegranate Smoothie (page 337)
and Mango Pineapple Mocktail (page 335)

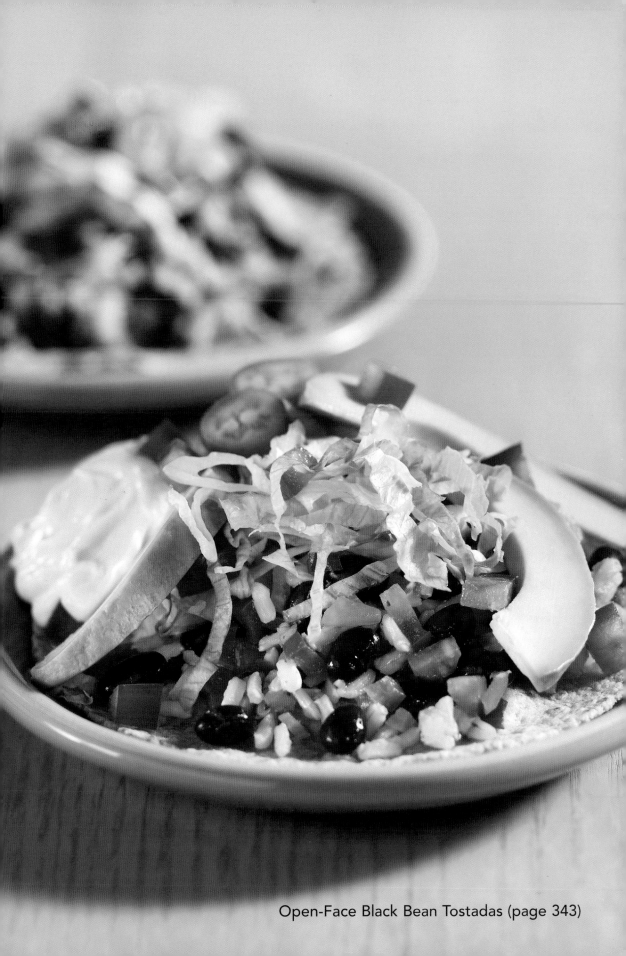

Open-Face Black Bean Tostadas (page 343)

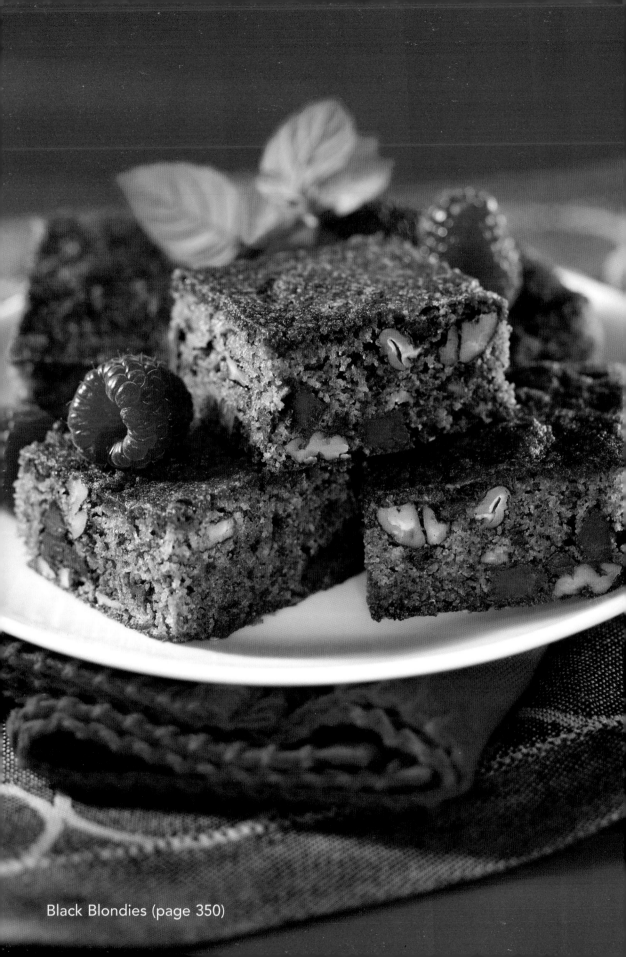

Black Blondies (page 350)

This is subtle and rich without the hot, spicy bite of many curries. I use 2 tbsp (25 mL) in stews, and less in soups that serve only 4 people.

Yellow Curry Paste

2 tbsp	whole coriander seeds	25 mL
2 tbsp	whole fenugreek seeds	25 mL
2 tsp	whole cumin seeds	10 mL
1 tbsp	ground turmeric	15 mL
½ tsp	sea salt	2 mL
3	cloves garlic	3
2 tbsp	chopped fresh lemongrass	25 mL
1	piece (1 inch/2.5 cm) fresh gingerroot	1
1 tsp	grated lemon zest	5 mL
1 tbsp	grapeseed oil	15 mL
1 to 2 tsp	freshly squeezed lemon juice	5 to 10 mL

1. In a small spice wok or dry cast-iron skillet, combine coriander, fenugreek and cumin seeds. Toast over medium-high heat until the seeds begin to pop and their fragrance is released, 2 to 3 minutes. Let cool.

2. Using a mortar and pestle or small electric grinder, pound or grind toasted spices until finely ground. Add turmeric, salt, garlic and lemongrass and grind into spices. Add ginger and lemon zest and grind into spices. Add grapeseed oil, a few drops at a time, and grind together with spices. Add lemon juice in drops until a thick paste-like consistency is achieved.

3. Label and store paste in a small clean jar with a lid in the refrigerator for up to 1 month. If the paste becomes too dry, add a few more drops of oil and/or lemon juice.

Red Curry Cauliflower

Serves 4 to 6

The coconut milk lends a tropical flavor to this faintly sweet-spicy dish. It is a fast and easy main dish that goes well with other vegetables, rice or rice noodles.

1	small head cauliflower	1
3 tbsp	olive oil	45 mL
2	onions, quartered	2
½	red bell pepper, thinly sliced	½
¼	fennel bulb, thinly sliced	¼
1 cup	shredded squash or sweet or pie pumpkin	250 mL
2	cloves garlic, minced	2
1	can (14 oz/400 mL) coconut milk	1
2 tbsp	Red Curry Spice (page 252)	25 mL
½ tsp	hot pepper flakes	2 mL
	Sea salt and freshly ground pepper	

1. Trim cauliflower and cut florets in half. Set aside.

2. In a wok, heat oil over medium-high heat. Add onions and stir-fry for 3 or 4 minutes or until golden. Stir in cauliflower and stir-fry for 4 minutes. Stir in red pepper, fennel, squash and garlic and stir-fry for 4 minutes.

3. Add coconut milk. Increase heat to high and bring to a boil. Stir in Red Curry Spice and hot pepper flakes and cook another 2 minutes. Season to taste with salt and pepper.

The onions melt into a sweet, spicy sauce for the fresh peas and asparagus.

Tip

- To chop the onions for this sauce, use a food processor, not a blender, which will liquefy them. The onions should be chopped into a fine mash, but not liquefied because the water will separate out at that point. Yellow cooking onions are best for this purpose (sweet varieties have a higher water content).

Variations

- Substitute shelled fresh or frozen edamame (green soy beans) for the peas.

- Substitute green beans or fresh garlic scapes for the asparagus.

Green Pea and Asparagus Curry

4	medium onions, cut in half, divided	4
2 tbsp	vegetable oil	25 mL
1 to 2 tbsp	Green Curry Paste (page 256) or curry powder	15 to 25 mL
2 tsp	organic cane sugar, optional	10 mL
2	medium tomatoes, chopped	2
2 cups	fresh or frozen green peas	500 mL
2 cups	fresh or frozen asparagus pieces	500 mL
1 tbsp	freshly squeezed lemon juice	15 mL
¼ cup	chopped fresh cilantro or flat-leaf Italian parsley	50 mL

1. Thinly slice 1½ onions and set aside. Using a food processor, chop remaining onions into a coarse pulp (see Tip, left).

2. In a saucepan or skillet, heat oil over medium-high heat. Add sliced onions. Cover, reduce heat to low and sweat onions for 8 to 10 minutes or until very soft. Add onion pulp and curry paste. Cook over medium-high heat, stirring frequently, for 5 minutes or until any liquid has disappeared. Add sugar, if using, and stir until dissolved. Add tomatoes, green peas, asparagus and lemon juice. Reduce heat and simmer, stirring once or twice, for 8 to 10 minutes or until vegetables are tender when pierced with the tip of a knife. Garnish with cilantro.

Eggplant Curry

The creamy eggplant texture is brought out by cooking slowly with the lid on. Serve with rice or noodles. If there are any leftovers, use them for wraps and burritos.

¼ cup	finely chopped peanuts	50 mL
¼ cup	flaked coconut	50 mL
3 tbsp	olive oil	45 mL
2 tbsp	Madras Curry Paste (page 255) or curry powder, or to taste	25 mL
3	tomatoes, chopped	3
I	large eggplant, trimmed and cut lengthwise into ½-inch (1 cm) slices (about 1½ lbs/750 g)	I
⅓ cup	coconut milk	75 mL
¼ cup	chopped fresh cilantro or flat-leaf Italian parsley, optional	50 mL

1. In a wok, lightly toast peanuts and coconut over medium-high heat for 30 seconds or until lightly browned. Add oil and curry paste and stir-fry for 1 minute. Add tomatoes and stir-fry for 2 minutes.

2. Add eggplant. Cover, reduce heat to low and simmer for 30 minutes. At the end of the 30 minutes, lift lid and stir, breaking up eggplant with a spoon. Stir in coconut milk. Simmer, stirring occasionally, for 20 minutes, until eggplant is very soft. Garnish with cilantro, if using.

The stuffing transforms a lowly potherb into an upscale dish. Use the highly flavored Chestnut Filling to top or stuff other vegetables and baked dishes.

Tips

- *To roast chestnuts:* Preheat oven to 425°F (220°C). Cut an "x" in the bottom of each chestnut shell. Arrange in one layer on a rimmed baking sheet with the cut sides up. Roast in preheated oven for 20 minutes. Let cool and peel.

- *To roast Brazil nuts:* Preheat oven to 375°F (190°C). Arrange shelled nuts in one layer on a rimmed baking sheet and roast in preheated oven for 10 to 15 minutes or until lightly browned.

- Use a combination of two or three of the following fresh herbs: sage, thyme, oregano, marjoram, basil, rosemary or tarragon.

Curried Chestnut–Stuffed Cabbage

- *Preheat oven to 375°F (190°C)*
- *9-inch (2.5 L) baking pan, lightly oiled*

| ½ | head cabbage, cored | ½ |
| 2 tbsp | freshly squeezed lemon juice | 25 mL |

Chestnut Filling

3 tbsp	olive oil, divided	45 mL
1	small onion, finely chopped	1
3	cloves garlic, minced	3
1 to 2 tbsp	Madras Curry Paste (page 255) or curry powder	15 to 25 mL
1 cup	chopped shelled roasted chestnuts or Brazil nuts (see Tips, left)	250 mL
¼ cup	whole wheat bread crumbs	50 mL
¼ cup	chopped fresh mixed herbs (see Tips, left)	50 mL
	Sea salt and freshly ground pepper	

1. In a saucepan, cover cabbage with water. Add lemon juice and bring to a boil over high heat. Cover, reduce heat and boil gently for 12 minutes or until cabbage is almost tender (the tip of a knife should meet with some resistance when the cabbage is pierced). Drain, reserving cooking water for another use. Let cool and cut cabbage into 4 wedges.

2. *Chestnut Filling:* Meanwhile, in a skillet, heat 2 tbsp (25 mL) of the oil over medium heat. Add onion and cook, stirring occasionally, for 5 minutes or until slightly softened. Add garlic and curry paste to taste, and cook, stirring frequently, for 2 minutes or until onion is soft. Add chestnuts, bread crumbs, herbs, and salt and pepper to taste, and cook, stirring constantly, for 1 or 2 minutes or until crumbs are browned.

3. Arrange cabbage wedges in prepared pan, cut sides up. Divide filling into 4 portions and press between the leaf layers and on the top of each wedge. Drizzle with remaining oil and bake in preheated oven for 10 to 15 minutes or until the filling is crisp.

Red Rice and Lentil Curry

Use this fragrant rice mixture as a filling for wraps and to stuff roasted vegetables. It makes a very good accompaniment for greens and side dishes.

Tip

• I prefer Lundberg short-grain brown rice, which is soft and chewy when cooked, but long-grain brown rice, red rice or a blend of your favorites will also work.

½ cup	dried red lentils	125 mL
2 tbsp	olive oil	25 mL
1 cup	chopped red onion	250 mL
1 or 2 tbsp	Yellow Curry Paste (page 257) or curry powder	15 or 25 mL
1 cup	red or brown rice (see Tip, left)	250 mL
3¼ cups	water	800 mL
½ tsp	sea salt	2 mL
1 cup	cooked red kidney beans, drained and rinsed, optional	250 mL

1. In a strainer, pick over and remove any small stones or grit from lentils. Rinse under cool water. Drain and set aside.

2. In a saucepan, heat oil over medium heat. Add onion and cook, stirring frequently, for 6 to 8 minutes or until soft. Add curry paste, to taste, and stir until well mixed. Add rice and cook, stirring constantly, for 1 minute. Add water. Increase heat to high and bring to a boil.

3. Stir lentils and salt into saucepan. Cover, reduce heat to low and cook for 40 minutes, until rice and lentils are tender and liquid is absorbed. Fluff with a fork and stir in kidney beans, if using.

Spiced Winter Vegetables

Easy to prepare, this vegetable stew thickens as the kasha cooks. It's complete on its own and requires no other accompaniment. Replace any of the vegetables with an equal amount of your favorite winter vegetable.

2 tbsp	olive oil	25 mL
2 tsp	whole cumin seeds	10 mL
1 tsp	whole cardamom seeds	5 mL
1 tsp	whole coriander seeds	5 mL
½ tsp	whole fennel seeds	2 mL
2 tsp	grated fresh gingerroot	10 mL
1 to 2 tbsp	curry powder or paste	15 to 25 mL
2 cups	chopped onion	500 mL
2	carrots, cut into 1-inch (2.5 cm) pieces	2
2	parsnips, cut into 1-inch (2.5 cm) pieces	2
2 cups	fingerling or regular potatoes, cut into 2-inch (5 cm) cubes	500 mL
2 cups	cauliflower or broccoli florets	500 mL
3 cups	vegetable stock or water	750 mL
½ cup	kasha or millet seeds	125 mL
2 tbsp	mango chutney	25 mL

1. In a large saucepan, heat oil over medium heat. Add cumin, cardamom, coriander and fennel seeds and cook, stirring frequently, for 1 minute. Stir in ginger and curry powder to taste. Add onion and cook, stirring frequently, for 6 to 8 minutes or until soft.

2. Add carrots, parsnips, potatoes and cauliflower and stir well. Add stock. Increase heat and bring to a boil. Stir in kasha. Cover, reduce heat and simmer, stirring occasionally, for 25 minutes or until vegetables are tender. Stir in chutney and cook for 2 to 3 minutes to heat through.

The broccoli is tender-crisp and the whole dish is ready in less than half an hour. Serve as a side dish with rice and/or lentils. Use the Stir Sauce in other stir-fry dishes.

Almond and Curry Broccoli Stir-Fry

Stir Sauce

2 tbsp	rice vinegar	25 mL
1 tbsp	tamari or soy sauce	15 mL
2 tsp	sesame oil	10 mL
2 tsp	grated fresh gingerroot	10 mL
2 tbsp	olive oil	25 mL
¼ cup	chopped almonds	50 mL
1 to 2 tbsp	Green Curry Paste (page 256) or curry powder	15 to 25 mL
2 cups	broccoli florets	500 mL

1. *Stir Sauce:* In a bowl, combine rice vinegar, tamari, sesame oil and grated ginger.

2. In a wok or saucepan, heat oil over medium-high heat. Add almonds and toast, stirring frequently, for 1 or 2 minutes or until lightly browned. Add curry paste to taste and stir. Add broccoli and stir-fry for 2 minutes or until al dente. Toss with Stir Sauce and serve immediately.

Potato, Leek and Kale Curry

4	medium potatoes	4
1 tsp	whole cumin seeds	5 mL
1 tsp	whole fennel seeds	5 mL
1 tsp	whole mustard seeds	5 mL
2 tbsp	olive oil	25 mL
1	small onion, chopped	1
1	leek, white and green parts, sliced	1
¼ cup	chopped walnuts	50 mL
2 cups	shredded kale	500 mL

1. In a pot of boiling salted water, cook potatoes for 15 to 20 minutes or until tender when pierced with the tip of a knife. Drain and rinse with cold water and let cool. Peel and coarsely chop.

2. Meanwhile, in a large skillet or saucepan over medium-high heat, toast cumin, fennel and mustard seeds until the seeds begin to pop and their fragrance is released, about 2 minutes (do not let seeds smoke or burn). Reduce heat to medium. Add oil and swirl to coat pan. Add onion and leek and cook, stirring occasionally, for 6 or 8 minutes or until soft. Add walnuts and cook, stirring constantly, for 2 minutes. If necessary, set aside until potatoes are cooked and cooled.

3. Just before serving, heat onion mixture over medium-high heat. Add kale and cook, stirring frequently, about 3 minutes or until wilted. Stir in potatoes.

The mushrooms lend a rich and earthy flavor to this curry.

Sweet Potato and Black-Eyed Pea Curry

2 tbsp	vegetable oil	25 mL
1	onion, chopped	1
2	cloves garlic, finely chopped	2
2 cups	sliced mushrooms	500 mL
1	sweet potato, cut into 1-inch (2.5 cm) cubes	1
1 cup	Cashew Cream (page 144) or 1 can (14 oz/400 mL) coconut milk	250 mL
1 cup	vegetable stock or water	250 mL
1 tbsp	Green Curry Paste (page 256) or curry powder	15 mL
2 tsp	jaggery or brown sugar	10 mL
2 tbsp	freshly squeezed lime juice	25 mL
1	can (14 oz/398 mL) black-eyed peas, drained and rinsed	1

1. In a wok, heat oil over medium-high heat. Add onion and stir-fry for 3 minutes. Stir in garlic and mushrooms and stir-fry for 2 minutes. Stir in sweet potato, Cashew Cream, stock, curry paste and jaggery. Bring to a boil. Reduce heat and boil gently, stirring occasionally, for 15 minutes or until sweet potato is tender.

2. Stir in lime juice and black-eyed peas and cook for 1 or 2 minutes or until heated through.

Baked, Roasted and Stir-Fried Vegetables

Zucchini Moussaka

Serves 4 to 6

The baked shredded potatoes lend an unexpected crisp texture to this classic Greek dish.

Variations

- Use 1 large eggplant, cut lengthwise in $1/4$-inch (0.5 cm) slices in place of the zucchini.

- Substitute Creamy White Sauce (page 149) or Garlic White Sauce (page 150) for the Avocado Sauce

- Try mashed potatoes on top instead of the shredded potatoes.

- *Preheat oven to 400°F (200°C)*
- *2 rimmed baking sheets, lightly oiled*
- *8-cup (2 L) casserole dish, lightly oiled*

2	large zucchini, cut lengthwise into $1/4$-inch (0.5 cm) slices	1
3 tbsp	olive oil, divided	45 mL
	Sea salt and freshly ground pepper	
4	medium potatoes, shredded	4
1	onion, shredded	1
3 cups	tomato sauce	750 mL
2 cups	Avocado Sauce (page 148) or non-dairy sour cream	500 mL

1. Arrange zucchini slices in one layer on prepared baking sheet. Drizzle with $1\frac{1}{2}$ tbsp (22 mL) of the oil and season with salt and pepper to taste. Combine potatoes and onion on the other prepared baking sheet. Drizzle with remaining olive oil and season with salt and pepper to taste. Place both baking sheets in preheated oven and bake for 15 minutes or until zucchini slices are tender and edges are browned. Let cool. Stir potatoes and cook for another 30 minutes or until almost tender. Let cool in pan on a rack.

2. Reduce oven temperature to 375°F (190°C). Spread half of the tomato sauce over bottom of prepared dish. Spread half of the zucchini slices over tomato sauce. Spread avocado sauce over zucchini. Spread remaining zucchini slices over avocado sauce and top with remaining tomato sauce. Arrange potato mixture over top of dish and bake for 30 minutes or until potato is crisp and tomato sauce is bubbly.

Maple Baked Beans

An easy weekend recipe, this is a simple version of slow-cooked, fire-baked Boston beans. Freeze small batches to serve with salads, steamed vegetables, rice and breakfast dishes.

Tips

- *To use the oven:* Preheat oven to 325°F (160°C) and use a Dutch oven or stoneware casserole with a lid. Follow Steps 1 through 5, then bake in preheated oven for 6 to 8 hours. Halfway through the cooking time, stir and check that there is enough liquid in the pot. Add up to ¼ cup (50 mL) water as required.

- If substituting fresh portobello mushrooms for the dried Chinese black fungi (mushrooms), coarsely chop them and skip Step 2. You may need to add up to ½ cup (125 mL) of water in Step 4 if using fresh mushrooms.

- *Slow cooker (see Tips, left)*

2 cups	dried white or navy (pea) beans	500 mL
1 cup	wheat berries	250 mL
½ oz	dried wild mushrooms or ½ cup (125 mL) sliced cremini mushrooms	14 g
3	dried Chinese black fungi (mushrooms) or portobello mushrooms (see Tips, left)	3
1 cup	sun-dried tomatoes (3 oz/90 g)	250 mL
4	onions, chopped	4
1 cup	whole pitted dates	250 mL
½ cup	pure maple syrup	125 mL
¼ cup	brown rice syrup or packed brown sugar	50 mL
3 tbsp	tamari or soy sauce	45 mL
1 tbsp	hot pepper flakes or chipotle flakes	15 mL
1 tbsp	toasted sesame oil	15 mL
2 tsp	dry mustard	10 mL

1. Rinse beans and remove any debris. In a large pot, combine beans, wheat berries and 12 cups (3 L) boiling water. Bring to a boil over high heat and boil for 2 minutes. Remove from heat, cover and let stand for one hour. Drain and rinse.

2. Meanwhile, in a bowl, combine dried wild mushrooms, black fungi and 2 cups (500 mL) boiling water. Let stand for 30 minutes. Using a slotted spoon, remove wild mushrooms. Let black fungi stand for another 30 minutes. Drain and reserve liquor. Coarsely chop mushrooms and set aside.

3. In a bowl, combine sun-dried tomatoes with 2 cups (500 mL) boiling water. Let stand for 30 minutes. Drain and reserve liquor. Cut sun-dried tomatoes into thin slices and set aside.

4. In slow cooker stoneware, combine beans, wheat berries, mushrooms, sun-dried tomatoes and 6 cups (1.5 L) boiling water. Using a cheesecloth-lined strainer, strain tomato and mushroom liquors into stoneware.

5. Add onions, dates, maple syrup, rice syrup, tamari, hot pepper flakes, sesame oil and mustard powder. Cover and cook on Low for about 10 hours or until beans are tender and sauce is thick and dark.

Preparation time is significantly reduced if the tofu is prepared and marinated in the refrigerator the night before.

Tip

• Sambal oelek is a condiment used by Southeast Asians that is made from a variety of very hot chile peppers. As a precaution, check that no dried shrimp have been added, as some blends do contain that ingredient.

Baked Cranberry Tofu with Creamed Asparagus and Leeks

• *Preheat oven to 375°F (190°C)*
• *Rimmed baking sheet, lightly oiled*

Tofu Marinade

¼ cup	whole cranberry sauce	50 mL
2 tbsp	tamari or soy sauce	25 mL
1 tbsp	grated lime zest	15 mL
	Juice of 1 lime	
1 to 2 tbsp	chili paste or sambal oelek (see Tip, left)	15 to 25 mL
12 oz	extra-firm tofu	375 g

Creamed Asparagus and Leeks

3 tbsp	olive oil	45 mL
3	leeks, white and tender green parts, sliced	3
1	onion, halved and sliced	1
1 tbsp	grated fresh gingerroot	15 mL
½ cup	chopped fresh basil	125 mL
2 tbsp	chopped fresh tarragon or cilantro	25 mL
1	can (14 oz/400 mL) coconut milk	1
2 cups	1-inch (2.5 cm) asparagus pieces	500 mL
	Salt and freshly ground pepper	
8 oz	rice noodles, cooked, optional	250 g
4	fresh basil or cilantro sprigs, optional	4

1. *Tofu Marinade:* In a bowl, combine cranberry sauce, tamari, lime zest and juice and chili paste. Slice tofu into ¾-inch (2 cm) slices and add to bowl. Set aside for 15 to 20 minutes or cover and refrigerate overnight. On prepared baking sheet, arrange slices in one layer. Spoon half of the marinade over tofu slices. Bake in preheated oven for 5 minutes. Turn, spoon remaining marinade over tofu and bake for another 5 minutes.

2. *Creamed Asparagus and Leeks:* In a saucepan, heat oil over medium-high heat. Add leeks and onion. Cover, reduce heat to low and sweat vegetables for 15 minutes or until soft. Add ginger, basil and tarragon and cook, stirring constantly, for 1 minute. Add coconut milk and bring to a boil over high heat. Add asparagus. Reduce heat and simmer, stirring occasionally, for 10 minutes or until tender when pierced with the tip of a knife. Season to taste with salt and pepper.

3. *To serve:* You can either spoon the creamed asparagus and leek mixture into the center of a plate or flat soup bowl or pile cooked rice noodles, if using, in the center then top with the creamed mixture. Top with baked tofu slices. Garnish with fresh basil or cilantro sprigs, if using.

Cauliflower Gratin

Pure comfort food at its finest, this dish is great the next day — reheat for lunch or even breakfast.

- *Preheat oven to 375°F (190°C)*
- *8-cup (2 L) casserole dish, lightly oiled*

1	head cauliflower, trimmed	1
2	medium potatoes, halved	2
1 tbsp	olive oil	15 mL
1	onion, chopped	1
3	cloves garlic, finely chopped	3
1	leek, white and light green parts, sliced	1
1	zucchini, cut into 1-inch (2.5 cm) pieces	1
1½ cups	rice milk or soy milk	375 mL
1 tbsp	fresh rosemary leaves	15 mL
	Sea salt and freshly ground pepper	

Topping

1 cup	whole wheat bread crumbs	250 mL
¼ cup	chopped trail mix	50 mL
¼ cup	grated soy mozzarella	50 mL

1. In a saucepan, cover cauliflower and potatoes with water. Bring to a boil over high heat. Cover, reduce heat and simmer for 20 minutes or until cauliflower is tender when pierced with the tip of a knife. Remove cauliflower from pan. Rinse, drain and set aside until cool. Continue to cook potatoes until tender, about another 5 minutes. Remove potatoes. Rinse, drain and set aside until cool. Reserve cooking water for stock or discard.

2. Meanwhile, in another saucepan, heat oil over medium heat. Add onion and cook, stirring occasionally, for 5 minutes or until slightly softened. Add garlic, leek and zucchini. Reduce heat to low and cook, stirring occasionally, for 8 to 10 minutes or until vegetables are very soft.

3. In a blender, combine rice milk, rosemary and 2 potato halves. Add ½ cup (125 mL) of onion mixture. Season to taste with salt and pepper. Blend until smooth.

4. *Topping:* In a bowl, combine bread crumbs, trail mix and soy mozzarella. Set aside.

5. *Assemble gratin:* Slice cauliflower and arrange in bottom of prepared casserole dish. Spread remaining onion mixture over cauliflower. Slice remaining 2 potato halves and arrange over onion mixture. Pour potato sauce over vegetables. Sprinkle topping over top and bake in preheated oven for 30 minutes or until bubbly and slightly browned on top.

Leek, Kohlrabi, Garlic and Onion Tart

- *Preheat oven to 400°F (200°C)*
- *Rimmed baking sheet, lightly oiled*

½	kohlrabi, thinly sliced	½
2	onions, quartered	2
6	cloves garlic	6
3 tbsp	olive oil, divided	45 mL
2	leeks, white and light green parts, sliced	2
I tbsp	balsamic vinegar	15 mL
I	naan or 10-inch (25 cm) prepared pizza shell	I
½ cup	Basil Pesto (page 188), Romesco Tomato Tapenade (page 189) or store-bought pesto, tapenade or tomato sauce	125 mL
	Sea salt and freshly ground pepper	

1. On prepared baking sheet, toss kohlrabi, onions, garlic and 1 tbsp (15 mL) of the oil. Bake, stirring once or twice, in preheated oven for 20 minutes, until vegetables are tender. Transfer to a bowl and let cool. Do not turn oven off.

2. In a skillet, heat remaining oil over medium heat. Add leeks and cook, stirring frequently, for 8 to 10 minutes, until very soft. Stir in balsamic vinegar.

3. Arrange naan on baking sheet and spread pesto evenly over. Spread leeks over pesto and top with roasted kohlrabi, onions and garlic. Season to taste with salt and pepper. Bake in preheated oven for 6 to 10 minutes or until base is lightly browned.

Eggplant Wraps

Easy and fast, this dish makes an elegant starter or light lunch. Serve with pasta, rice or noodles for a main course.

- *Preheat oven to 400°F (200°C)*
- *2 rimmed baking sheets, lightly oiled*

2	large eggplants	2
3 tbsp	olive oil	45 mL
4 cups	fresh spinach, stems removed	1 L
1 cup	Romesco Tomato Tapenade (page 189) or tomato sauce	250 mL
1 cup	tomato sauce	250 mL

1. Cut tops of eggplants straight across to remove stem and leaves. Place each eggplant cut side down on cutting board and cut a thin lengthwise slice from two opposite sides to make sides flat. Discard cut-off pieces. Cut each eggplant lengthwise into ½-inch (1 cm) thick slices (you'll get 4 to 6 depending on the width of the eggplants). Arrange eggplant slices in one layer on prepared baking sheets and brush with oil. Bake in preheated oven for 15 minutes or until eggplant is lightly colored but shows some resistance when pierced with a knife. Let cool slightly on baking sheets. Do not turn oven off.

2. Meanwhile, bring a large saucepan of water to a boil over high heat. Add spinach and cook for 1 minute. Using a slotted spoon, transfer spinach to a colander and rinse with cold water until cool to the touch. Drain well and squeeze out any remaining water. Discard cooking liquid or reserve for another use. Coarsely chop spinach and transfer to a bowl. Add tapenade and mix well.

3. Slide a metal spatula under each slice of eggplant to loosen. Divide spinach mixture evenly among the eggplant slices and spread lengthwise along the left side of each slice. Fold over the other half of the eggplant like a book to cover the filling. Bake in preheated oven for 8 to 10 minutes or until filling is bubbly.

4. In a saucepan, heat tomato sauce, stirring occasionally, over medium-high heat. Divide eggplant wraps among serving plates and serve with ¼ cup (50 mL) tomato sauce on the side.

Corn, Beans and Squash Bake with Oat Nut Topping

A colorful dish, this one-pot meal is delicious on its own or served with greens or rice.

- *Preheat oven to 375°F (190°C)*
- *Dutch oven or flameproof baking dish*

2 tbsp	olive oil	25 mL
1 to 2 tbsp	Green Curry Paste (page 256) or curry powder	15 to 25 mL
1 tbsp	Garam Masala Spice Blend (page 254) or store-bought	15 mL
1 tbsp	grated fresh gingerroot	15 mL
1	onion, chopped	1
2 cups	cubed (1 inch/2.5 cm) butternut squash or sweet or pie pumpkin	500 mL
2 cups	1-inch (2.5 cm) green bean pieces	500 mL
1 cup	corn kernels	250 mL
1½ cups	vegetable stock or water	375 mL
1½ cups	Oat Nut Topping (page 158)	375 mL

1. In Dutch oven, heat oil over medium heat. Add curry paste to taste, and cook, stirring frequently, for 2 minutes. Add garam masala, ginger and onion. Cook, stirring frequently, for 6 to 8 minutes or until soft. Add butternut squash, green beans and corn and stir to coat vegetables.

2. Add stock and bring to a boil. Cover and bake in preheated oven for 45 minutes or until mixture is bubbly and vegetables are tender when pierced with the tip of a knife.

3. Spread Oat Nut Topping evenly over top of vegetables and bake for 10 minutes, until topping is browned and crisp.

In this very tasty breakfast or light lunch dish, the thin potato slices are seasoned with a garlic, onion and mushroom layer and cooked until tender.

Tip

- If using a food processor, use a 1 or 2 mm slicing blade to cut the potatoes into thin wafers.

Variation

- If you have 1 cup (250 mL) of the Creamy Mushroom and Leek Sauce (page 307) left over, use it in place of the sautéed onion, mushrooms and garlic and skip Step 1.

Potato Cake

- *Preheat oven to 375°F (190°C)*
- *9-inch (23 cm) springform pan, lightly oiled*

3 tbsp	olive oil	45 mL
1	onion, chopped	1
1 cup	chopped mushrooms	250 mL
2	cloves garlic, finely chopped	2
4	potatoes, thinly sliced (see Tip, left)	4
2 to 3 tbsp	rice milk or vegetable stock	25 to 45 mL
1 ½ cups	Crumb Nut Topping (page 157) or Oat Nut Topping (page 158)	375 mL

1. In a skillet, heat oil over medium heat. Add onion and cook, stirring occasionally, for 5 minutes or until slightly softened. Add mushrooms and garlic and cook, stirring frequently, for 3 minutes or until tender.

2. Arrange enough of the potato slices, overlapping slightly as necessary, to make one layer on bottom of prepared springform pan. Spread 2 or 3 tbsp (25 to 45 mL) of the mushroom mixture over potatoes. Keep layering potatoes and mushroom mixture, ending with a layer of potatoes. Press down on the layers to compact them. Drizzle rice milk over top and spread Crumb Nut Topping evenly over top. Bake in preheated oven for 1 hour or until potatoes are tender when pierced with the tip of a knife.

Winter greens— cabbage, beet tops, Swiss chard, kale, spinach — add important nutrients to a winter vegan diet and this easy dish is a tasty way to enjoy them.

Baked Winter Greens

- *Preheat oven to 350°F (180°C)*
- *8-inch (2 L) baking dish, lightly oiled*

2 cups	shredded green or Savoy cabbage	500 mL
2 cups	chopped kale leaves, thick ribs removed	500 mL
2 cups	chopped Swiss chard leaves	500 mL
2 cups	Garlic White Sauce (page 150)	500 mL

1. In a bowl, toss cabbage, kale and Swiss chard together. Pour about ¼ cup (50 mL) of the Garlic White Sauce into bottom of prepared baking dish. Pile greens on top and pour remaining white sauce over. Cover and bake in preheated oven for 30 minutes or until sauce is bubbly and greens are soft.

The coconut adds a tropical flavor to the winter root vegetables.

Winter Vegetable Bake with Coconut Nut Topping

- *Preheat oven to 400°F (200°C)*
- *13- by 9-inch (3 L) baking dish, lightly oiled*

2 cups	finely sliced green or Savoy cabbage	500 mL
I cup	cubed (I inch/2.5 cm) rutabaga	250 mL
3	carrots, cut into I-inch (2.5 cm) chunks	3
2	potatoes, cut into I-inch (2.5 cm) chunks	2
I	parsnip, cut into I-inch (2.5 cm) chunks	I
4 tbsp	olive oil, divided	60 mL
I	onion, chopped	I
2 tbsp	all-purpose flour	25 mL
I ½ cups	rice milk or vegetable stock	375 mL
½ tsp	ground nutmeg	2 mL
	Sea salt and freshly ground pepper	

Coconut Nut Topping

2 tbsp	coconut oil, at room temperature	25 mL
½ cup	fresh bread crumbs	125 mL
½ cup	chopped cashews	125 mL
¼ cup	unsweetened shredded coconut	50 mL

I. In a large saucepan, cover cabbage, rutabaga, carrots, potatoes and parsnip with water. Bring to a boil over high heat. Reduce heat and boil gently for 6 minutes. Drain well and arrange in prepared dish.

2. Meanwhile, in a saucepan, heat 2 tbsp (25 mL) of the oil over medium heat. Add onion and cook, stirring occasionally, for 6 to 8 minutes or until soft. Remove onion and spread evenly over vegetables in dish.

3. In same saucepan, heat remaining oil over medium-high heat. Stir in flour and cook, stirring constantly, for 1 minute. Whisk in rice milk and nutmeg. Bring almost to a boil, whisking constantly. Simmer, stirring constantly, for 3 minutes or until sauce is thickened. Season to taste with salt and pepper. Pour sauce over vegetables in dish.

4. *Coconut Nut Topping:* In a warm bowl, cream coconut oil by mashing against sides of bowl with the back of a spoon. Add bread crumbs, cashews and coconut and stir well to combine. Spread over vegetables and bake in preheated oven for 30 minutes or until topping is browned, sauce is bubbly and vegetables are tender when pierced with a knife.

Fragrant and creamy Coconut Rice with Cauliflower is perfect for this recipe, but any cooked rice may be used. If you have any of the mixture left over, purée it and use as a base for other vegetable main dishes or freeze and use in vegetable soups.

Tip

• Stainless steel baking rings are available at restaurant supply and kitchen specialty stores. Rings with a minimum 1-inch (2.5 cm) depth are the most popular. Handles are not easy to work with because they prevent the ring (and the food in it) from being flipped to brown the other side.

Roasted Squash in Cashew Curry Sauce

• *Preheat oven to 375°F (190°C)*
• *11- by 7-inch (2 L) baking dish, lightly oiled*
• *Rimmed baking sheet, lightly oiled*
• *Six 4-inch (10 cm) baking rings, lightly oiled (see Tip, left)*

1	small butternut or acorn squash (about 2 lbs/1 kg)	1
6	cloves garlic	6
2 tbsp	olive oil	25 mL
2 cups	Coconut Rice with Cauliflower (page 316) or cooked rice	500 mL
2 cups	Cashew Curry Sauce (page 156) or non-dairy sour cream	500 mL

1. Peel and cut squash into large chunks and toss with garlic and oil in prepared baking dish. Bake in preheated oven for 45 minutes or until soft and lightly colored. Do not turn oven off. Let squash cool slightly and chop further into small dice. Set aside.

2. In a bowl, combine rice, roasted squash and garlic and curry sauce.

3. Arrange baking rings on prepared baking sheet. Spoon squash mixture into each ring, pressing gently with the back of the spoon to pack it in tightly. Bake for 10 to 15 minutes or until browned.

Serving Suggestions
• Serve atop a green salad such as Citrus Greens with Fig Dressing (page 209) or warm Braised Greens with Cherries and Pine Nuts (page 223).
• Serve over a vegetable purée such as Gingered Carrot-Turnip Purée (page 218).
• Any of the salsas (see pages 187 to 190) make a delicious accompaniment to roasted squash.

Roasted Butternut Squash with Spiced Lima Beans

If you roast the squash and garlic the night before, this dish comes together in less than half an hour. The spicy onion sauce is finished in 10 minutes and then tossed with the beans and warmed.

Variations

- If like me, you always keep a tin of asparagus in the pantry, substitute it for the lima beans in this recipe.
- Sprinkle ½ cup (125 mL) toasted almonds, peanuts or cashews on top or add a topping (see pages 157 to 158) before returning the dish to the oven in Step 3.

- *Preheat oven to 375°F (190°C)*
- *11- by 7-inch (2 L) baking pan, lightly oiled*

1	head garlic	1
3 tbsp	olive oil, divided	45 mL
1	small butternut squash, halved (about 2 lbs/1 kg)	1
5	green onions, cut diagonally into 1-inch (2.5 cm) pieces	5
1 tsp	hot pepper flakes	5 mL
1 tsp	curry powder	5 mL
1 tsp	brown sugar	5 mL
1 tsp	cornstarch	5 mL
2 tbsp	freshly squeezed lemon juice	25 mL
1 tsp	prepared mustard	5 mL
1	can (14 oz/398 mL) lima or haricot beans with liquid	1

1. Remove loose, papery skin from garlic head. Slice off and discard ¼ inch (0.5 cm) from tops of the cloves in entire head. In prepared baking pan, arrange garlic, cut side up, and drizzle with 1 tbsp (15 mL) of the olive oil. Add squash halves, cut side down, and roast in preheated oven for 1 hour or until tender when pierced with the tip of a knife and garlic is soft. Do not turn oven off. Let squash cool enough to handle, then peel, remove seeds and cut into chunks and return to baking dish. Set garlic head aside to cool slightly.

2. In a skillet, heat remaining oil over medium heat. Add green onions and squeeze roasted garlic into the pan, discarding skins and mashing garlic with the back of a spoon. Cook, stirring occasionally, for 4 minutes or until onions are soft.

3. Meanwhile, in a bowl, combine hot pepper flakes, curry powder, brown sugar and cornstarch. Whisk in lemon juice and mustard. Add to onions and simmer gently for 3 minutes or until sauce is thickened.

4. Add lima beans with liquid and spiced onion sauce to squash in baking dish and toss together. Bake in preheated oven for 5 to 7 minutes or until sauce is bubbly.

Portobello Pot-au-feu

The French term *pot-au-feu* literally means "pot on fire" and is a dish of meat and vegetables slowly cooked in water. The broth is served as a first course and the meat and vegetables make up the entrée. This is a vegan take on the traditional dish, with two ways to serve it.

- *Preheat oven to 375°F (190°C)*
- *Rimmed baking sheet, lightly oiled*

4	carrots, halved lengthwise	4
4	white baby turnips, halved	4
8	asparagus spears	8
3 tbsp	olive oil, divided	45 mL
4	large portobello mushrooms, stems removed	4
	Sea salt and freshly ground pepper	
3 cups	Mushroom Broth (page 138), vegetable stock or water	750 mL
20	fresh fiddleheads or green beans	20
4	green onions, sliced	4
2 cups	packed baby spinach	500 mL
¼ cup	chopped fresh chives, optional	50 mL

1. On prepared baking sheet, combine carrots, turnips and asparagus. Toss with 2 tbsp (25 mL) of the oil. Roast in preheated oven for 10 minutes. Stir vegetables. Add mushrooms, gills facing down. Drizzle remaining oil over mushrooms. Season vegetables and mushrooms with salt and pepper to taste. Roast for 20 minutes or until vegetables are easily pierced with the tip of a knife.

2. Meanwhile, in a saucepan over high heat, bring broth to a gentle boil. Add fiddleheads. Reduce heat and simmer for 8 minutes. Add green onions and spinach and simmer for 2 minutes.

3. *To serve:* Divide roasted vegetables evenly among 4 large soup bowls. Spoon broth and simmered vegetables over roasted vegetables. Garnish each bowl with chives, if using.

Serving Suggestions
- Ladle broth into bowls and serve as a first course, garnished with chives, if using.
- For the entrée, serve roasted and simmered vegetables atop Garlic Mashed Potatoes (page 224) or Gingered Carrot-Turnip Purée (page 218).

When served over a green salad, cooked greens, puréed vegetables, rice or noodles, this makes a sophisticated main course. For entertaining, make and stuff the zucchini shells a day ahead and bring to room temperature before baking in Step 3.

Tip

- Use brown rice, quinoa, wheat berries, Kamut, bulgur, couscous or any other cooked grain for this stuffing.

Roasted Zucchini Shells with Almond Filling and Red Pepper Sauce

- *Preheat oven to 400°F (200°C)*
- *Rimmed baking sheet, lightly oiled*

4	medium zucchini, trimmed	4
2 tbsp	olive oil	25 mL

Almond Filling

2 tbsp	olive oil	25 mL
I	onion, chopped	I
2	cloves garlic, finely chopped	2
I	slice (I inch/2.5 cm) candied ginger, finely chopped	I
I tsp	ground cumin	5 mL
½ cup	cooked whole-grain or whole wheat bread crumbs (see Tip, left)	125 mL
⅓ cup	chopped almonds	75 mL
I ½ cups	Red Pepper Sauce (page 150)	375 mL

1. In a saucepan of boiling water, cook zucchini for 7 minutes. Immerse in cold water until cool, then drain. Cut in half lengthwise and remove the flesh, leaving a ¼-inch (0.5 cm) shell. Finely chop flesh and set aside. Brush shell inside and out with oil. Arrange, cut side up, on prepared baking sheet and set aside.

2. *Almond Filling:* Meanwhile, in a skillet, heat oil over medium heat. Add onion and cook, stirring occasionally, for 5 minutes or until slightly softened. Add garlic, ginger and cumin. Cook, stirring frequently, for 2 minutes or until onion is tender. Remove from heat and stir in reserved chopped zucchini flesh, cooked grain and almonds.

3. Divide filling into 8 portions and press into zucchini shells. Bake in preheated oven for 10 to 12 minutes or until filling is lightly browned and bubbly and zucchini are tender when pierced with the tip of a knife. Drizzle serving plates with Red Pepper Sauce and serve stuffed zucchini on top.

Make this dish seasonal
by using summer
vegetables as they
become available.

Roasted Vegetables with Garlic White Sauce

- *Preheat oven to 375°F (190°C)*
- *13- by 9-inch (3 L) baking pan, lightly oiled*

I	eggplant, peeled and cut into 1-inch (2.5 cm) cubes	I
3	parsnips, cut into ½-inch (I cm) pieces	3
3	carrots, cut into ½-inch (I cm) pieces	3
I	onion, cut into eighths	I
¼ cup	chopped fresh parsley	50 mL
2 tbsp	olive oil	25 mL

Garlic White Sauce

I tbsp	olive oil	15 mL
½	onion, finely chopped	½
3 tbsp	finely chopped fresh parsley	45 mL
I	head roasted garlic (page 132)	I
I ½ cups	rice milk or soy milk	375 mL
I to 2 tbsp	hot red pepper paste, optional	15 to 25 mL

I. In a bowl, toss eggplant, parsnips, carrots, onion and parsley with oil. Spread evenly in prepared baking pan. Bake in preheated oven for 40 minutes or until vegetables are tender when pierced with a knife. Set aside. Do not turn oven off.

2. *Garlic White Sauce:* Meanwhile, in a saucepan, heat oil over medium heat. Add onion and cook, stirring occasionally, for 5 minutes or until slightly softened. Add parsley and squeeze roasted garlic cloves into pan, mashing them against the side of the pan with the back of a spoon. Cook, stirring occasionally, for 4 minutes or until onion is soft. Remove from heat.

3. In a blender, combine onion mixture, rice milk, and red pepper paste, if using. Blend until liquefied.

4. Toss sauce with roasted vegetables in baking pan. Bake in preheated oven for 10 to 15 minutes or until lightly browned and bubbly.

Make this quick and easy dinner even easier by omitting the mashed potatoes and serving over cooked pasta or rice.

Tip

• You can use 2 cups (500 mL) cooked chickpeas, drained and rinsed, instead of canned.

Moroccan Roasted Vegetables with Garlic Mashed Potatoes

- *Preheat oven to 375°F (190°C)*
- *13- by 9-inch (3 L) baking pan, lightly oiled*

12	cloves garlic	12
3	onions, quartered	3
1	small eggplant (about 8 oz/250 g), peeled and cut lengthwise into eighths	1
¼ cup	olive oil	50 mL
3 tbsp	balsamic vinegar	45 mL
1	can (28 oz/796 mL) tomatoes with juice	1
1	can (14 to 19 oz/398 to 540 mL) chickpeas, drained and rinsed (see Tip, left)	1
1 tbsp	Garam Masala Spice Blend (page 254) or store-bought	15 mL
1 tsp	hot pepper flakes	5 mL
1 tsp	sea salt	5 mL
3 cups	Garlic Mashed Potatoes (page 224), optional	750 mL

1. In prepared pan, combine garlic, onions and eggplant. Drizzle with oil and vinegar and roast in preheated oven for 40 minutes.

2. Stir in tomatoes with juice and chickpeas. Add garam masala, hot pepper flakes and sea salt. Return to oven and bake for 30 minutes.

3. Meanwhile, make Garlic Mashed Potatoes, if using. Spread over roasted vegetables and bake for about 10 minutes, until heated through.

Mushroom Bean Loaf with Herbed Tomato-Leek Sauce

This loaf holds together for slicing but is delicate and tends to crumble easily if overhandled (see Serving Suggestion, below). Asian sticky rice is best for this recipe because it's gelatinous and helps to bind the ingredients together.

Tip

- You can use 2 cups (500 mL) cooked black-eyed peas, drained and rinsed, instead of canned.

Serving Suggestion

- Arrange a vegetable side dish, such as Braised Greens with Cherries and Pine Nuts (page 223), on heated plates. Spoon a serving of Mushroom Bean Loaf over, with Herbed Tomato-Leek Sauce over top.

- *Preheat oven to 350°F (180°C)*
- *9- by 5-inch (2 L) loaf pan, lightly oiled and bottom lined with parchment paper*
- *One piece of parchment paper, cut to fit top of loaf pan, one side lightly oiled*

2 tbsp	olive oil	25 mL
I	onion, chopped	I
4 cups	chopped mushrooms	I L
2	cloves garlic, minced	2
I	can (8 oz/227 mL) water chestnuts, drained	I
I cup	cashew nuts	250 mL
I	can (14 to 19 oz/398 to 540 mL) black-eyed peas, drained and rinsed (see Tip, left)	I
I cup	cooked sticky rice (see Intro, left)	250 mL
2 cups	Herbed Tomato-Leek Sauce (page 285)	500 mL

1. In a skillet, heat oil over medium heat. Add onion and cook, stirring occasionally, for 5 minutes or until slightly softened. Add mushrooms and cook, stirring frequently, for 5 minutes or until tender. Stir in garlic and cook, stirring frequently, for 2 minutes. Set aside.

2. Meanwhile, in a food processor or blender, process water chestnuts and cashews until coarsely chopped. Transfer to a large bowl. Add black-eyed peas to food processor and process until almost a paste. Add to nuts.

3. Stir in onion-mushroom mixture and rice and combine well. Press into prepared loaf pan and place parchment, oil side to loaf, over top. Bake for 45 minutes or until firm and pulling away slightly from sides of pan. Let stand for 10 minutes and turn out onto a plate. Slice and top with Tomato-Leek Sauce, or see alternative serving suggestion left.

Herbed Tomato-Leek Sauce

Use one herb or a mixture of all three fresh herbs listed. The longer this sauce simmers, the more the flavors meld.

Variation

• In winter, substitute 1 tsp (5 mL) each of dried herbs for 1 tbsp (15 mL) in total.

2 tbsp	olive oil	25 mL
2	leeks, white and light green parts, sliced	2
1	onion, chopped	1
1	clove garlic, minced	1
1	can (28 oz/796 mL) crushed tomatoes with juice	1
¼ cup	chopped fresh basil, parsley or oregano	50 mL

1. In a skillet or saucepan, heat oil over medium heat. Add leeks and onion and cook, stirring frequently, for 5 minutes or until slightly softened. Stir in garlic and cook, stirring frequently, for 3 minutes or until vegetables are tender. Add tomatoes with juice and simmer, stirring occasionally, for 15 minutes or for up to 1 hour, adding up to ¼ cup (50 mL) water as the sauce thickens. Stir in herbs and simmer for 1 minute.

Try this as a substitute for rice, pasta or noodles.

Tip
- Use one or a combination of basil, tarragon, sage, thyme, oregano, marjoram or rosemary.

Roast Potatoes, Fennel and Leeks

- *Preheat oven to 375°F (190°C)*
- *Rimmed baking sheet, lightly oiled*

2	medium potatoes, quartered	2
2	leeks, white and tender green parts, split lengthwise	2
½	fennel or kohlrabi, cut into 4 wedges	½
2 tbsp	olive oil	25 mL
2 tbsp	Basil Pesto (page 188) or chopped fresh herbs (see Tip, left)	25 mL

1. In a bowl, toss together potatoes, leeks, fennel, oil and pesto. Spread in one layer on prepared baking sheet. Bake in preheated oven for 20 minutes. Stir and continue baking for another 15 minutes or until vegetables are crisp on the outside and tender when pierced with the tip of a knife.

When cut into small squares, this open-style "pizza" makes a very nice appetizer. Larger squares, when served with a salad, are perfect for a light lunch.

Roast Vegetable and Polenta Pie

- *Preheat oven to 400°F (200°C)*
- *2 rimmed baking sheets, one lightly oiled, the other lined with parchment paper*

3	small carrots, halved lengthwise	3
3	cloves garlic	3
2	onions, quartered	2
2	small parsnips, halved lengthwise	2
I	sprig fresh rosemary	I
3 tbsp	olive oil, divided	45 mL
12	mushrooms, halved	12
4 cups	vegetable stock or water	I L
I tsp	sea salt, or to taste	5 mL
I ⅓ cups	cornmeal	325 mL
¼ cup	hummus or tomato sauce	50 mL
	Sea salt and freshly ground pepper	

1. On oiled baking sheet, arrange carrots, garlic, onions and parsnips in one layer. Strip leaves from rosemary sprig and sprinkle over top. Drizzle with 2 tbsp (25 mL) of the oil. Roast in preheated oven for 30 minutes. Stir and add mushrooms and drizzle with remaining oil. Bake for 20 minutes or until vegetables are lightly browned and tender.

2. Meanwhile, in a saucepan, combine stock and salt. Bring to a boil over high heat. Using a whisk, slowly and whisking constantly pour in cornmeal. Reduce heat but keep mixture bubbling and stir constantly with a wooden spoon for 4 minutes until very thick. Turn out onto parchment-lined baking sheet and spread evenly to about a 1-inch (2.5 cm) thickness. Spread hummus over cornmeal.

3. In a food processor, process roasted vegetables until coarsely chopped. Spread over hummus. Season with salt and pepper to taste. Bake for 10 minutes or until topping is heated through.

Bok Choy, Mushroom and Black Bean Stir-Fry

Serves 4

With just the right amount of crisp, chewy and soft textures, this stir-fry is perfectly balanced. It is a drier mixture than other stir-fry dishes and teams well with puréed vegetables.

2 tbsp	olive oil	25 mL
2	cloves garlic, finely chopped	2
1 tbsp	Asian Five-Spice Seasoning (page 133) or store-bought	15 mL
¼ cup	sunflower seeds or pine nuts	50 mL
1 cup	sliced shiitake mushroom caps	250 mL
6 tbsp	tamari or soy sauce, divided	90 mL
1	head bok choy, thinly sliced	1
1	can (6 oz/175 g) water chestnuts, drained and thinly sliced	1
2 tsp	toasted sesame oil	10 mL
4	green onions, thinly sliced	4
1 cup	cooked black beans	250 mL
¼ cup	shredded Thai basil	50 mL

1. In a wok or saucepan, heat oil over medium-high heat. Add garlic, five-spice seasoning and sunflower seeds. Stir-fry for 1 minute or until garlic begins to color. Increase heat to high, and add mushrooms and stir-fry for 2 minutes. Add 3 tbsp (45 mL) of the tamari, bok choy and water chestnuts and stir-fry for 1 to 2 minutes or until bok choy is wilted. Add remaining tamari, sesame oil, green onions and black beans. Stir-fry for 1 to 2 minutes or until onions are al dente. Toss basil with vegetables.

Sweet and Sour Tempeh and Eggplant Stir-Fry

Marinating the tempeh and eggplant is essential to the finished flavor of this dish. It's an easy entertaining dish or one that can be marinating all day and then cooked in less than half an hour after a long day at work. Add a cup (250 mL) of any fresh vegetable and the meal is complete.

12 oz	tempeh, cut into ½-inch (1 cm) cubes	375 g
1	medium eggplant, peeled and cut into 1-inch (2.5 cm) pieces	1
1½ cups	orange juice	375 mL
½ cup	rice vinegar	125 mL
¼ cup	tamari or soy sauce	50 mL
¼ cup	brown rice syrup or agave nectar	50 mL
2	cloves garlic, minced	2
1 to 2 tbsp	Madras Curry Paste (page 255) or curry powder	15 to 25 mL
2 tbsp	olive oil	25 mL
2 tsp	sesame oil	10 mL
1	onion, chopped	1
2 tbsp	cornstarch	25 mL

1. In a bowl, combine tempeh, eggplant, orange juice, rice vinegar, tamari, rice syrup, garlic, and curry paste to taste. Toss to mix well. Cover and marinate at room temperature for 1 hour or in the refrigerator overnight.

2. In a wok or large saucepan, heat olive oil over medium-high heat. Add sesame oil and onion and stir-fry for 2 minutes or until slightly colored. Increase heat to high. Using a slotted spoon, lift tempeh and eggplant from marinade and stir into onions. Stir-fry for 3 minutes or until eggplant is tender when pierced with the tip of a knife.

3. Measure half of the marinade into a bowl and whisk in cornstarch. Set aside remaining marinade for another use. Add marinade mixture to wok. Reduce heat to medium-high and stir-fry for about 4 minutes or until sauce is thickened.

Candied Nut Fried Rice

The candied nuts add a sweet perk to the fried rice but you may also use raw or toasted pecans, almonds or walnuts.

2 tbsp	olive oil	25 mL
2 tsp	sesame oil	10 mL
1 tbsp	Madras Curry Paste (page 255) or curry powder	15 mL
1 cup	chopped broccoli florets	250 mL
½ cup	shredded carrot	125 mL
2	green onions, sliced	2
1 tbsp	tamari or soy sauce	15 mL
4 cups	cooked brown or red rice	1 L
¾ cup	coarsely chopped Candied Nuts (page 157) (see Intro, left)	175 mL

1. In a wok or large, deep skillet, heat olive oil over medium-high heat. Add sesame oil and curry paste and stir-fry for 30 seconds. Add broccoli and stir-fry for 2 minutes. Add carrot and green onions and stir-fry for 1 minute. Add tamari and rice and stir-fry for 1 minute or until heated through. Stir in nuts.

Pad Thai

In Bangkok, pad Thai is the quintessential street food. Perfected by food-cart cooks, it is dry and easy to eat with chopsticks and has a balanced, fresh flavor. This version is close to being authentic but substitutes date molasses for the traditional fish sauce and uses chopped cabbage and tempeh in place of the popular shrimp.

¼ cup	Date Molasses (page 147) or blackstrap molasses	50 mL
1 tbsp	finely chopped pitted tamarind	15 mL
1 tbsp	brown rice syrup	15 mL
1 tsp	rice vinegar	5 mL
1 tsp	Thai red chile paste	5 mL
8 oz	tempeh, cut into ½-inch (1 cm) cubes	250 g
8 oz	rice noodles	250 g
2 tbsp	olive oil	25 mL
⅓ cup	unsalted raw peanuts	75 mL
1 tsp	toasted sesame oil	5 mL
5	green onions, thinly sliced on the diagonal, divided	5
3	cloves garlic, minced	3
2 cups	thinly sliced green cabbage	500 mL
5	slices (¼ inch/0.5 cm) rutabaga, cut into matchsticks (about 1 cup/250 mL)	5
1 cup	bean sprouts, optional	250 mL

1. In a pie plate or shallow bowl, combine molasses, tamarind, rice syrup, vinegar and chile paste. Add tempeh and set aside, stirring occasionally, for 15 minutes or for up to 1 hour.

2. In a bowl, cover rice noodles with boiling water. Let stand for 7 minutes or according to package directions. Drain, rinse with cold water and set aside.

3. Meanwhile, in a wok, heat olive oil over medium-high heat. Add peanuts and stir-fry for 2 to 3 minutes or until lightly browned. Using a slotted spoon, transfer to a small bowl and set aside.

4. Add sesame oil and half of the green onions and all of the garlic. Stir-fry for 1 minute. Add cabbage and rutabaga and stir-fry for 3 minutes. Add tempeh and marinade and stir-fry for 3 minutes. Add drained noodles and stir-fry for 2 to 3 minutes, until soft and tangled. Lift into bowls and garnish with remaining green onions, toasted peanuts and bean sprouts, if using.

The filling for these tasty quesadillas may also be used to stuff baked vegetable shells and with pasta.

Tips

• You can use 2 cups (500 mL) cooked black beans, drained and rinsed, instead of canned.

• While Roasted Corn Salsa makes a great garnish, any of the pestos or salsas (see pages 157 to 158) will also work.

Sweet Potato, Bean and Wild Rice Quesadillas

Sweet Potato-Bean Filling

2 cups	cubed sweet potato	500 mL
1 ¼ cups	vegetable stock or water	300 mL
½ cup	wild rice	125 mL
2 tbsp	olive oil	25 mL
1	onion, chopped	1
2	cloves garlic, chopped	2
1	can (14 to 19 oz/398 to 540 mL) black beans, drained and rinsed (see Tips, left)	1
1	ripe banana	1
1 tsp	hot pepper flakes	5 mL
	Sea salt and freshly ground pepper	
4 tsp	olive oil, divided	20 mL
8	large (10-inch/25 cm) whole-grain flour tortillas	8
1 cup	Roasted Corn Salsa (page 190), optional (see Tips, left)	250 mL

1. *Sweet Potato-Bean Filling:* In a saucepan, cover sweet potato with stock. Bring to a boil over high heat. Cover, reduce heat and simmer for 10 minutes or until soft. Using a slotted spoon, transfer sweet potato to a bowl and set aside.

2. Add rice to hot stock in the saucepan. Bring to a boil over high heat. Cover, reduce heat and simmer for 40 minutes or until rice is tender and most or all of the liquid is absorbed.

3. Meanwhile, in a skillet, heat oil over medium heat. Add onion and cook, stirring occasionally, for 6 to 8 minutes or until soft. Stir in garlic and cook, stirring frequently, for 2 minutes. Remove from heat. Add black beans and coarsely mash with a potato masher.

4. In a large mixing bowl, mash banana with reserved sweet potato. Add onion-bean mixture, cooked wild rice, hot pepper flakes and salt and pepper, to taste. Recipe can be made up until this point. Filling will keep tightly covered in the refrigerator for up to 2 days. Bring to room temperature before proceeding with Step 5. Divide into 4 equal portions.

5. Just before serving, preheat oven to 300°F (150°C).

6. *Assemble quesadillas:* In a large skillet, heat 1 tsp (5 mL) oil over medium-high heat. Place one tortilla in the skillet. Spread 1 portion of bean filling over tortilla, leaving a ½-inch (1 cm) border all around. Moisten edges of another tortilla with water and place, wet side down, over top of filled tortilla. Seal edges by pressing with a fork. Cook for 1 to 2 minutes per side, flipping once, or until crisp and lightly browned. Transfer to an ovenproof platter and keep warm in preheated oven. Repeat with remaining oil, tortillas and filling. Cut into wedges and garnish with Roasted Corn Salsa, if using.

Both the ginger marinade and the tempeh and vegetable filling for this dish are exceptionally versatile. Use the marinade for tofu and as a dressing on salads, or drizzle over roasted vegetables. Serve the filling over rice or stuff it into pitas, soft tortillas or roasted vegetables.

Tip

• To separate the iceberg lettuce into cups, core the lettuce and rinse under cold water, then lift off whole leaves. Drain on a clean towel until ready to fill with tempeh and vegetable filling.

Variation

• Use blanched fresh grape leaves or rice paper wrappers in place of the lettuce cups.

Rainbow Tempeh Lettuce Cups

Ginger Marinade

2 tbsp	grapeseed oil	25 mL
2 tbsp	rice vinegar	25 mL
I tbsp	tamari or soy sauce	15 mL
2 tsp	grated fresh gingerroot	10 mL
I tsp	toasted sesame oil	5 mL
I tsp	brown rice syrup	5 mL
¼ tsp	hot pepper flakes	I mL
8 oz	tempeh, cut into ½-inch (I cm) cubes	250 g

Filling

2 tbsp	olive oil	25 mL
I	onion, chopped	I
4	cloves garlic, finely chopped	4
½	red bell pepper, diced	½
I cup	chopped shiitake mushroom caps	250 mL
I	carrot, chopped	I
¼	head green cabbage, coarsely chopped or shredded	¼
6	iceberg lettuce cups (see Tip, left)	6
6	toothpicks	6

1. *Ginger Marinade:* In a bowl, whisk together grapeseed oil, vinegar, tamari, ginger, sesame oil, rice syrup and hot pepper flakes. Toss tempeh cubes in marinade. Cover and marinate at room temperature for 30 minutes or overnight in the refrigerator.

2. *Filling:* In a wok or large skillet, heat olive oil over medium-high heat. Add onion and stir-fry for 3 minutes. Add garlic and red pepper and stir-fry for 3 minutes. Add mushrooms, carrot, cabbage and tempeh with marinade. Stir and cover with a lid. Reduce heat and simmer, stirring occasionally, for 5 minutes or until cabbage is tender when pierced with the tip of a knife.

3. *Assemble lettuce cups:* Scoop about ⅓ cup (75 mL) of the tempeh and vegetable filling into each lettuce cup. Fold into a neat packet and secure with a toothpick.

Vegetable Paella

Traditional Spanish paella dishes feature saffron-flavored rice combined with a variety of meats and shellfish, garlic, onions, peas, artichoke hearts and tomatoes. Our vegetable version has all the color and flavor without the fuss, meats or lengthy preparation. Saffron adds a definite flowery taste and distinct orange colour. It may be omitted if desired.

Tip

• I prefer Lundberg short-grain brown rice, which is soft and chewy when cooked, but long-grain brown rice, red rice or a blend of your favorites will also work.

1	sweet potato, cut into 1-inch (2.5 cm) cubes	1
2½ cups	vegetable stock or water	625 mL
1 cup	mixed long- or short-grain brown and wild rice (see Tip, left)	250 mL
2 tbsp	olive oil	25 mL
1	onion, chopped	1
1	red bell pepper, chopped	1
4	cloves garlic, finely chopped	4
2 tsp	ground turmeric	10 mL
1 tsp	ground cumin	5 mL
1	can (14 oz/398 mL) lima beans, drained	1
4 to 6	saffron filaments, soaked in 2 tbsp (25 mL) warm water, optional	4 to 6

1. In a saucepan, combine sweet potato and stock. Bring to a boil over high heat and stir in rice. Cover, reduce heat to low and cook for 40 minutes or until rice is tender and most or all of the liquid is absorbed.

2. About 10 minutes before the rice is finished, heat oil over medium-high heat in a wok or large, deep skillet. Add onion and red pepper and stir-fry for 7 minutes or until soft. Add garlic, turmeric and cumin and stir-fry for 2 minutes.

3. Add cooked sweet potato and rice, lima beans and saffron filaments in their soaking water, if using. Stir-fry for 1 minute or until beans are heated through.

Stir-Fried Chipotle Chili

Quick, easy and satisfying, this chili makes use of both seasonal and pantry ingredients.

Tip

• You can use 2 cups (500 mL) cooked red or black kidney beans, drained and rinsed, instead of canned.

2 tbsp	olive oil	25 mL
1	onion, chopped	1
1	red or green bell pepper, chopped	1
2	cloves garlic, chopped	2
1 tbsp	ground coriander	15 mL
1 tsp	ground cumin	5 mL
2 cups	sliced mushrooms	500 mL
1	small zucchini, diced	1
1	carrot, diced	1
1	can (28 oz/796 mL) diced tomatoes with juice	1
1	can (14 to 19 oz/398 to 540 mL) red kidney or black beans, drained and rinsed (see Tip, left)	1
½	can (6 oz/175 g) chipotle peppers in adobo sauce, or to taste	½

1. In a wok or large, deep saucepan, heat oil over medium-high heat. Add onion and bell pepper and stir-fry for 2 minutes. Add garlic, coriander and cumin and stir-fry for 1 minute. Add mushrooms, zucchini and carrot and stir-fry for 2 minutes or until almost tender when pierced with the tip of a knife.

2. Add tomatoes with juice and simmer for 3 to 5 minutes. Add beans and chipotle peppers with ½ of the adobo sauce and heat through.

Pasta, Rice and Whole Grains

This dish makes its own sauce, so the noodles are not as crispy as they would be if they were simply roasted with oil.

Rice Noodles with Roasted Mediterranean Vegetables

- *Preheat oven to 375°F (190°C)*
- *Roasting pan, lightly oiled*

2	zucchini, trimmed and cut into 1-inch (2.5 cm) pieces	2
2	large tomatoes, halved	2
2	onions, quartered	2
1	eggplant, trimmed and cut into 1-inch (2.5 cm) pieces	1
1	red bell pepper, thickly sliced	1
2	cloves garlic	2
¼ cup	tamari or soy sauce	50 mL
2 tbsp	olive oil	25 mL
2 tbsp	freshly squeezed lime or lemon juice	25 mL
1 tbsp	toasted sesame oil	15 mL
8 oz	dried wide rice noodles	250 g

1. In prepared roasting pan, combine zucchini, tomatoes, onions, eggplant, red pepper and garlic.

2. In a bowl, whisk together tamari, olive oil, lime juice and sesame oil. Toss with vegetables in roasting pan. Bake in preheated oven, stirring once or twice, for 30 to 40 minutes or until vegetables are tender when pierced with the tip of a knife. Do not turn the oven off.

3. Meanwhile, in a bowl, cover rice noodles with hot water. Soak for 15 to 20 minutes or according to package directions, until al dente. Drain and set aside. When vegetables are cooked, toss drained noodles with roasted vegetables. Return to the oven for 10 minutes to heat through.

Mushroom Lasagna

Because they impart a heartier mushroom essence, I prefer a mixture of wild and cultivated mushrooms in this dish. Even reconstituted dried mushrooms may be used.

Tip

• Make lasagna up to 1 day ahead, cover and store in refrigerator. Return to room temperature and bake in preheated oven for 40 minutes.

- *Preheat oven to 375°F (190°C)*
- *13- by 9-inch (3 L) baking dish, oiled*

9 or 10	whole wheat lasagna noodles (6 to 8 oz/175 to 250 g)	9 or 10
1 tsp	sea salt	5 mL
2 tbsp	olive oil	25 mL
2	onions, sliced and separated into rings	2
2	cloves garlic, finely chopped	2
8 oz	cremini mushrooms, sliced	250 g
8 oz	shiitake mushroom caps, sliced	250 g
2	small zucchini, coarsely chopped	2
½ cup	chopped fresh parsley	125 mL
2 tbsp	chopped fresh basil	25 mL
1 tbsp	fresh thyme leaves	15 mL
10 oz	extra-firm tofu, drained and diced	300 g
4 cups	Creamy White Sauce (page 149) or non-dairy sour cream	1 L
¼ cup	rice milk	50 mL
2 cups	Crumb Nut Topping (page 157)	500 mL

1. In a large pot of boiling salted water, cook noodles for about 10 minutes or according to package directions, until al dente. Using tongs, transfer noodles to a bowl filled with cold water. When cool, drain and lay flat on clean lint-free kitchen towels (not paper towels).

2. Meanwhile, in a skillet or saucepan, heat oil over medium heat. Add onions and cook, stirring occasionally, for about 5 minutes or until slightly softened. Add garlic, cremini and shiitake mushrooms and zucchini and cook, stirring frequently, for 7 minutes or until mushrooms are reduced in size and tender.

3. In a bowl, combine onion-mushroom mixture, parsley, basil, thyme and tofu. Set aside.

4. *Assemble lasagna:* Arrange one-third of the noodles in a single layer on bottom of prepared dish. Spread half of the onion-mushroom mixture over noodles. Pour half of the white sauce over filling. Repeat with another layer of noodles, onion-mushroom mixture and remaining sauce. Spread remaining noodles in one layer over top. Drizzle rice milk over lasagna and sprinkle Crumb Nut Topping over top. Bake in preheated oven for 40 minutes or until sauce is bubbly and top is crisp and brown.

Penne with Spinach-Artichoke Cream Sauce

The sauce for this dish is easy to make for a heavenly light lunch or brunch dish. Keep all the ingredients in the pantry for last-minute dinners.

Spinach-Artichoke Cream Sauce

3 tbsp	olive oil	45 mL
I cup	chopped onion	250 mL
2	cloves garlic, finely chopped	2
I	can (6 oz/175 g) marinated artichokes with liquid	I
I	package (10 oz/300 g) frozen spinach, thawed and drained	I
I cup	Soy Sour Cream (page 145) or non-dairy sour cream	250 mL
2½ cups	whole wheat penne	625 mL

1. *Spinach-Artichoke Cream Sauce:* In a saucepan, heat oil over medium heat. Add onion and garlic and cook, stirring occasionally, for 6 to 8 minutes or until soft. Add artichokes with liquid and spinach. Reduce heat and simmer, stirring frequently, for 10 minutes or until most of the liquid is evaporated. Stir in Soy Sour Cream and heat through.

2. Meanwhile, in a large pot of boiling salted water, cook penne for about 10 minutes or according to package directions, until al dente. Drain and return to the pot. Add sauce and toss gently to combine.

Spaghetti with Red Pepper Sauce

When red peppers are in season, one of the tastiest ways to preserve them is to roast and freeze them or make a large quantity of Red Pepper Sauce and freeze it. If you have the sauce already made, this recipe is easy and fabulous.

8 oz	spaghetti	250 g
1½ cups	Red Pepper Sauce (page 150) or tomato sauce	375 mL
¼ cup	Basil Pesto (page 188) or shredded fresh basil, optional	50 mL

1. In a large pot of boiling salted water, cook spaghetti for 6 minutes or according to package directions, until al dente. Drain and rinse with hot water.

2. Meanwhile, in a saucepan over high heat, bring sauce to a boil. Reduce heat and simmer until spaghetti is ready. Toss spaghetti with sauce. Garnish with pesto, if using.

Rice Noodles with Spicy Spaghetti Sauce

Rice noodles are used extensively in Thai and other Asian cuisines. Because dried rice noodles are widely available, store easily and are simple to prepare, they are an essential item for a vegan pantry.

Tip

• You can use 2 cups (500 mL) cooked kidney beans, drained and rinsed, instead of canned.

Spicy Spaghetti Sauce

1 tbsp	olive oil	15 mL
2	onions, coarsely chopped	2
3	cloves garlic, finely chopped	3
1	red or green bell pepper, chopped	1
1	stalk celery, chopped	1
1	eggplant, coarsely chopped	1
1	can (28 oz/796 mL) crushed tomatoes with juice	1
3 tbsp	Date Molasses (page 147), Pomegranate Molasses (page 146) or blackstrap molasses	45 mL
1 tbsp	tamari or soy sauce	15 mL
	Sea salt and freshly ground pepper	
1	can (14 to 19 oz/398 to 540 mL) red kidney beans, drained, rinsed and coarsely chopped (see Tip, left)	1
3 tbsp	chopped fresh parsley	45 mL
1 tbsp	chopped fresh oregano	15 mL
1 tsp	fresh thyme leaves	5 mL
1 tsp	chipotle flakes, optional	5 mL
12 oz	dried wide rice noodles	375 g

1. *Spicy Spaghetti Sauce:* In a large saucepan, heat oil over medium heat. Add onions and garlic and cook, stirring occasionally, for 5 minutes or until slightly softened. Add bell pepper and celery and cook, stirring frequently, for 3 minutes. Add eggplant and cook, stirring occasionally, for about 5 minutes or until eggplant is almost tender when pierced with the tip of a knife.

2. Stir in tomatoes with juice, molasses, tamari, and salt and pepper to taste. Increase heat to high and bring to a boil. Partially cover, reduce heat and simmer, stirring occasionally, for 20 minutes. Stir in beans, parsley, oregano, thyme and chipotle flakes, if using. Cover and cook about 5 minutes to heat through.

3. *Rice noodles:* Meanwhile, in a bowl, cover rice noodles with hot water. Soak for 15 to 20 minutes or according to package directions, until al dente. Drain and toss with spaghetti sauce.

Roasted Squash Gnocchi

I like the soft buttery color of this pasta and the texture, which is velvety smooth. See Serving Suggestion (right) for ways to sauce this dish.

Tips

- If using all-purpose flour, you may find that less is needed in order to form the dough. The type of squash used will also influence how much flour needs to be used.

- Rolling the dough into hollow dumplings allows them to cook through, preventing an uncooked doughy mass in the center.

- *Preheat oven to 375°F (190°C)*
- *Rimmed baking sheet*
- *11- by-7-inch (2 L) baking dish, lightly oiled*

I	small acorn or butternut squash (about 1½ lbs/750 g)	I
2 to 3 cups	spelt flour (see Tips, left)	500 to 750 mL
	Sea salt and freshly ground pepper	
I tbsp	chopped fresh rosemary	15 mL
¼ tsp	ground nutmeg	I mL
2 tbsp	olive oil, divided	25 mL

1. Using a fork, prick squash all over and place on baking sheet. Roast in preheated oven for 60 to 70 minutes or until tender when pierced with the tip of a knife. Remove from oven and reduce temperature to 300°F (150°C). When squash is cool enough to handle, cut in half and scoop out seeds. Scoop flesh into a bowl, discarding skin.

2. Using a potato masher or fork, mash squash (it should still be warm). Place 2 cups (500 mL) of the flour on a work surface and sprinkle with salt and pepper. Make a well in center of flour and drop in squash. Sprinkle rosemary and nutmeg over squash. Using your hands, gradually draw flour into the well, mixing it with the squash as you work everything into a soft dough. Knead the dough for 5 minutes, until smooth and pliant, adding more flour if it's too sticky.

3. Bring a large pot of salted water to a boil over high heat. Reduce heat and keep gently boiling.

4. Divide dough into 4 pieces. Wrap 3 pieces in plastic wrap and refrigerate while you work on one piece. Using the palms of your hands, roll dough on a lightly floured surface until it forms a long rope about ½ inch (1 cm) in diameter. Cut rope into ¾-inch (2 cm) long pieces. Holding a piece of dough between thumb and forefinger, roll it against the work surface or the rough side of a grater to form a hollow, concave dumpling. When all the gnocchi have been formed from one piece of dough, drop them all at once into the boiling water and cook for about 2 minutes or until they float to the surface. Using a slotted spoon, transfer to a colander to drain. When water has evaporated from gnocchi, tip them into the prepared baking dish. Drizzle with 1 tsp (5 mL) of the oil and keep warm in the oven while shaping and cooking the remaining dumplings.

5. Repeat Step 4 with the remaining 3 pieces of dough, keeping unused pieces in the refrigerator until ready to shape and cook.

Serving Suggestion
* Serve with Gingered Carrot-Turnip Purée (page 218), Mushroom Sauce (page 154), Basil Pesto (page 188) or Tomato Sauce (page 151).

Udon Noodles with Tofu and Gingered Peanut Sauce

The tofu in this dish makes it a complete meal. This is intended to be served slightly warmer than room temperature, but if a piping hot dish is preferred, cook the noodles after the tofu and greens have been cooked in the peanut sauce.

8 oz	udon or soba noodles	250 g
8 oz	firm tofu, drained and cut into ½-inch (1 cm) cubes	250 g
2	cloves garlic, crushed	2
1 tbsp	grated fresh gingerroot	15 mL
1 or 2	dried cayenne peppers, crushed	1 or 2
⅓ cup	tamari or soy sauce	75 mL
2 tbsp	organic cane sugar or packed brown sugar	25 mL
⅓ cup	coarsely ground peanuts or natural peanut butter	75 mL
⅓ cup	warm water	75 mL
4 tbsp	olive oil, divided	60 mL
1	onion, chopped	1
2 cups	broccoli florets	500 mL
2 cups	shredded kale or spinach	500 mL

1. In a large pot of boiling salted water, cook noodles for 6 to 8 minutes or according to package directions, until al dente. Drain and rinse with cool water. Set aside.

2. Meanwhile, in a bowl, combine tofu, garlic, ginger, cayenne pepper to taste, tamari and sugar. Set aside. In another bowl, combine peanuts and warm water. Set aside.

3. In a wok or large, deep saucepan, heat 2 tbsp (25 mL) of the oil over medium-high heat. Add onion and stir-fry for 3 minutes. Using a slotted spoon, lift tofu from marinade, reserving marinade, and add to wok. Stir-fry for 2 to 3 minutes, until lightly colored. Scrape tofu and onions into marinade, stir in peanuts with water and set aside.

4. Add remaining oil to wok and heat. Add broccoli and stir-fry for 3 minutes or until tender-crisp. Stir in tofu mixture and kale. Simmer, stirring frequently, for 1 or 2 minutes, until kale is tender. Serve over cooked udon noodles.

Middle Eastern Noodle Pilaf

Capellini, vermicelli or angel hair pasta may be used in this dish. Toasting the pasta before adding to the pilaf gives a nutty flavor to the noodles.

2 tbsp	olive oil	25 mL
I cup	chopped onion	250 mL
I cup	chopped red bell pepper	250 mL
I tsp	ground turmeric	5 mL
½ tsp	ground cumin	2 mL
½ tsp	ground cinnamon	2 mL
10 oz	capellini pasta, broken into 1- or 2-inch (2.5 or 5 cm) pieces (see Intro, left)	300 g
2 cups	vegetable stock or water	500 mL

1. In a wok or large, deep saucepan, heat oil over medium-high heat. Add onion and red pepper and stir-fry for 4 minutes. Add turmeric, cumin, cinnamon and pasta and cook, stirring frequently, for 2 to 3 minutes or until noodles are lightly browned and onions and peppers are tender.

2. Add stock and bring to a boil. Cover, reduce heat to medium-low and simmer, stirring occasionally, for 3 to 5 minutes or until noodles are tender and most of the liquid is absorbed.

Asian Primavera

Serves 4

Fresh Asian vegetables are teamed with ginger, sesame and soy for a light yet satisfying pasta dish

8 oz	udon or soba noodles	250 g

Asian Vegetable Sauce

⅓ cup	Mushroom Broth (page 138) or water	75 mL
¼ cup	tamari or soy sauce	50 mL
1 tbsp	rice vinegar	15 mL
1 tbsp	tahini or peanut butter	15 mL
2 tsp	grated fresh gingerroot	10 mL
1 tsp	toasted sesame oil	5 mL
1 tbsp	cornstarch	15 mL
2 tbsp	olive oil	25 mL
1	red bell pepper, cut into matchsticks	1
6	shiitake mushrooms, caps thinly sliced	6
1 cup	snow or sugar snap peas, trimmed	250 mL
1	bunch bok choy, thinly sliced	1
1	can (8 oz/227 mL) water chestnuts, drained and thinly sliced	1

1. In a large saucepan of boiling salted water, cook noodles for 4 to 5 minutes or according to package directions, until al dente. Drain and rinse with cool water.

2. *Asian Vegetable Sauce:* Meanwhile, in a bowl, combine broth, tamari, rice vinegar, tahini, ginger and sesame oil. Whisk in cornstarch. Set aside.

3. In a wok or large, deep saucepan, heat olive oil over medium-high heat. Add red pepper and stir-fry for 2 minutes. Add mushrooms and stir-fry for 2 minutes. Add snow peas and bok choy and stir-fry for 2 minutes. Add broth mixture and bring to a simmer. Simmer, stirring occasionally, for 1 or 2 minutes or until mixture is thickened. Toss with cooked noodles and water chestnuts and heat through.

This mushroom, leek and kohlrabi combination makes an earthy and satisfying winter meal.

Variation

• The kohlrabi is a good winter choice, but 1 cup (250 mL) chopped green cabbage can always be substituted.

Kamut Spaghetti with Creamy Mushroom and Leek Sauce

4 tbsp	olive oil, divided	60 mL
I	onion, chopped	I
I	leek, white and light green parts, sliced	I
4	cloves garlic, finely chopped	4
I cup	chopped mushrooms	250 mL
I	kohlrabi bulb, chopped	I
3 tbsp	all-purpose flour	45 mL
2 cups	rice milk or soy milk	500 mL
I tbsp	miso, optional	15 mL
14 oz	Kamut spaghetti	420 g

1. In a skillet, heat 2 tbsp (25 mL) oil over medium heat. Add onion and leek and cook, stirring occasionally, for 5 minutes or until slightly softened. Add garlic, mushrooms and kohlrabi and cook, stirring often, for 10 minutes or until vegetables are tender. Transfer to a bowl and set aside.

2. Add remaining oil to skillet and heat. Stir in flour and cook, stirring constantly, for 1 minute. Whisk in rice milk and cook, stirring constantly, for 3 minutes or until the sauce is thickened. Return cooked vegetables to sauce and add miso, if using. Keep warm over low heat.

3. Meanwhile, in a large pot of boiling salted water, cook spaghetti for 10 to 12 minutes or according to package directions, until al dente. Drain and toss with sauce.

Makes eight 4-inch (10 cm) cakes

Sweet Potato Wild Rice Cakes

These cakes are so delicious they become the focus of the meal. Wild rice gives a chewy texture to the cakes and the gelatinous sticky rice helps to bind the ingredients together. The sticky rice should be moist and very sticky.

- *Eight 4-inch (10 cm) baking rings, lightly oiled (see Tip, page 278)*

1⅓ cups	vegetable stock or water	325 mL
⅓ cup	wild rice	75 mL
⅓ cup	sticky rice	75 mL
1	medium-large sweet potato, peeled and cut into large chunks	1
1 cup	shredded rutabaga or carrot	250 mL
2	sprigs fresh thyme	2
1	sprig fresh rosemary	1
3 tbsp	olive oil, divided	45 mL
1 tbsp	toasted sesame oil	15 mL
	Sea salt and freshly ground pepper	

Serving Suggestions

- Serve atop a green salad such as Citrus Greens with Fig Dressing (page 209) or warm Braised Greens with Cherries and Pine Nuts (page 223).

- Serve atop a vegetable purée such as Gingered Carrot-Turnip Purée (page 218).

- Apricot Tamarind Marmalade (page 183) or any of the salsas (pages 187 to 190) make a delicious accompaniment to the rice cakes.

1. In a saucepan over high heat, bring stock to a boil. Add wild rice, stir and cover. Reduce heat to low and cook for 10 minutes. Quickly stir in sticky rice. Cover and cook for 30 minutes. Remove from heat and fluff with a fork. Cover and set aside.

2. Meanwhile, in a steamer basket set over a pot of boiling water, steam sweet potato, covered, for 15 to 20 minutes, until tender. Let cool. Coarsely chop and place in a large bowl. Add rutabaga, thyme, rosemary and 1 tbsp (15 mL) of the olive oil. Add rice and stir gently to combine. Drizzle with sesame oil and add salt and pepper to taste. Stir well.

3. In one large or two medium skillets, heat remaining olive oil over medium heat. Arrange metal rings in the skillet and reduce heat to low. Press sweet potato-rice mixture into rings and cook for 5 minutes. Flip cakes and cook for 5 minutes. Flip and cook for about 5 minutes on each side one more time or until cakes are lightly browned on both sides and cooked through.

Lentil and Rice Bowl

This is very nice without the Yellow Coconut Curry Sauce, but the sauce makes it an exceptional side dish or salad. Ideally the rice and lentils should be hot, but if using leftovers, bring to room temperature before tossing with the sauce.

2 cups	cooked red or brown rice	500 mL
I tsp	toasted sesame oil	5 mL
2 cups	cooked yellow or red lentils (see Instructions, below)	500 mL
½ cup	Yellow Coconut Curry Sauce (page 155), optional	125 mL
2	green onions, thinly sliced, optional	2

I. In a bowl, toss rice with sesame oil. Add lentils and Yellow Coconut Curry Sauce, if using, and stir well. Garnish with green onion, if desired.

How to Cook Lentils

Makes 3 cups (750 mL)

Lentils (aka dal) are seeds from the legume or pulse family of plants. The seeds look like lenses; hence their Latin name, *Lens culinaris*. The dried form is widely available and popular in vegan dishes because lentils cook in less time than dried beans and do not require soaking. Lentils add protein, vitamin B1, minerals and healthy fiber to the diet. When they are combined with grains, a complete protein dish is the result. As with all legumes, adding salt during the cooking prevents the lentils from cooking properly and they will be tough. If using vegetable stock, be sure that it is not salted.

I cup	lentils	250 mL
2 cups	unsalted vegetable stock or water	500 mL

I. In a strainer, pick over and remove any small stones or grit from lentils. Rinse under cool water and drain.

2. In a saucepan, combine lentils and stock. Bring to a boil over medium-high heat. Cover, reduce heat and simmer for 30 to 40 minutes, until tender.

Variation: Cook mung beans using the same method.

Green Risotto

Rich and earthy, this
risotto takes advantage
of seasonal greens
throughout the year.

Tips

- Use any combination
  of fresh greens such
  as spinach, kale,
  Swiss chard or beet
  tops. You can add up
  to twice the amount
  of both greens and
  herbs.

- For the herbs, use
  parsley, oregano,
  thyme or marjoram
  alone or in
  combination.

8 cups	vegetable stock or Mushroom Broth (page 138)	2 L
3 tbsp	olive oil	45 mL
1 tsp	fennel seeds	5 mL
1	leek, white and light green parts, thinly sliced	1
3	cloves garlic, finely chopped	3
2	green onions, thinly sliced	2
¼ cup	chopped fresh herbs (see Tips, left)	50 mL
1½ cups	basmati rice	375 mL
2 cups	chopped fresh greens (see Tips, left)	500 mL

1. In a saucepan over high heat, bring stock to a boil. Reduce heat and keep simmering.

2. In a deep skillet, heat oil over medium heat. Add fennel seeds and leek and cook, stirring frequently, for 5 minutes or until slightly softened. Add garlic, green onions and herbs and cook, stirring constantly, for 3 minutes or until onions are soft. Add rice and stir-fry for 1 or 2 minutes or until rice is translucent and glass-like.

3. Increase heat to medium-high. Ladle ½ cup (125 mL) of the simmering stock into skillet, stirring constantly. When the liquid has been absorbed, keep adding stock, ½ cup (125 mL) at a time, stirring until absorbed and all but 2 cups (500 mL) have been added.

4. Add greens to remaining simmering stock and cook, stirring, for 1 or 2 minutes, until wilted. Test the risotto. If rice is tender, using a slotted spoon, transfer greens to skillet. If rice is not quite tender, add ½ cup (125 mL) of hot stock and some greens and stir until absorbed. Test again and add remaining greens and herbs when rice is tender.

Yellow Barley Risotto

Barley is a nice change from rice in this twist on traditional risotto.

8 cups	vegetable stock or Mushroom Broth (page 138)	2 L
3 tbsp	olive oil, divided	45 mL
1	onion, chopped	1
4	cloves garlic, finely chopped	4
2	tomatoes, peeled and chopped	2
2 cups	cubed butternut squash or sweet or pie pumpkin	500 mL
1 ¼ cups	pot barley	300 mL
	Sea salt and freshly ground pepper	

1. In a saucepan over high heat, bring stock to a boil. Reduce heat and keep simmering.

2. In a deep skillet, heat 2 tbsp (25 mL) of the oil over medium heat. Add onion and cook, stirring frequently, for 5 minutes or until slightly softened. Add garlic, tomatoes and squash and cook, stirring frequently, for 3 minutes or until onion is soft. Add remaining oil and barley to skillet. Cook, stirring constantly, for 2 minutes. Add 4 cups (1 L) of the hot stock and bring to a boil. Cover, reduce heat and simmer for 10 minutes or until squash is almost tender and flesh shows some resistance when pierced with the tip of a knife.

3. Remove lid, increase heat to keep liquid simmering and stir until any remaining liquid is absorbed. Ladle ½ cup (125 mL) of simmering stock into skillet, stirring constantly. When the liquid has been absorbed, add another ½ cup (125 mL) of stock, and keep adding, stirring often, until barley is tender and most or all of the stock has been used. Season to taste with salt and pepper.

Candied Nut Dirty Rice

The nuts and the hearty red and brown rice combine to make this a chewy underpinning for root vegetables and other hearty dishes.

Tips

• If candied nuts are not available, use any favorite nuts or seeds.

• I prefer Lundberg short-grain brown rice, which is soft and chewy when cooked, but long-grain brown rice, red rice or a blend of your favorites will also work.

1 tbsp	olive oil	15 mL
1	small onion, chopped	1
1	clove garlic, minced	1
1 tsp	Garam Masala Spice Blend (page 254) or store-bought	5 mL
	Sea salt and freshly ground pepper	
½ cup	red rice	125 mL
½ cup	short-grain brown or wild rice (see Tips, left)	125 mL
1¾ cups	vegetable stock or water	425 mL
½ cup	Candied Nuts (page 157), chopped (see Tips, left)	125 mL

1. In a saucepan, heat oil over medium heat. Add onion and cook, stirring frequently, for 5 minutes or until slightly softened. Stir in garlic, garam masala, salt and pepper to taste, and cook, stirring constantly, for 2 minutes or until onion is soft. Add red and brown rice and cook, stirring constantly, for 1 minute.

2. Add stock and bring to a boil over high heat. Cover, reduce heat to low and cook for 40 minutes or until rice is tender and liquid is absorbed. Do not remove the lid during cooking. Fluff with a fork and stir in Candied Nuts.

Fresh young spring
vegetables are
combined with rice for
this light main course.

Tip

- If using leftover rice,
  bring to room
  temperature before
  adding in Step 2.

Variation

- Use fresh green
  beans or bean sprouts
  in this dish once
  asparagus is no
  longer in season.

Spring Vegetable Fried Rice

3 tbsp	tamari or soy sauce	45 mL
1 tbsp	grated fresh gingerroot	15 mL
2 tbsp	olive oil	25 mL
2	green onions, thinly sliced	2
1	clove garlic, minced	1
1	carrot, julienned	1
1	turnip, julienned	1
1 cup	pieces (1 inch/2.5 cm) asparagus	250 mL
½ cup	fresh or frozen green peas	125 mL
4 cups	cooked brown rice (see Tip, left)	1 L

1. In a bowl, combine tamari and ginger. Set aside.

2. In a wok or large, deep skillet, heat oil over medium-high
   heat. Add green onions and garlic and stir-fry for 2 minutes.
   Add carrot and turnip and stir-fry for 3 minutes. Add
   asparagus and peas and stir-fry for 2 minutes. Add rice and
   stir-fry for 1 minute or until heated through. Drizzle with
   tamari-ginger mixture and stir until combined.

Tomato and Curry–Sauced Rice

This rice makes a nice side dish or you can use it as stuffing for peppers or other "pocket" vegetables.

Tip

• Double the recipe and freeze half in an airtight container for up to 2 months.

3 tbsp	olive oil, divided	45 mL
½	onion, finely chopped	½
I	clove garlic, finely chopped	I
I	small zucchini, finely chopped	I
I cup	chopped tomato or drained, diced canned tomato	250 mL
I cup	vegetable stock or water	250 mL
I tbsp	Pomegranate Molasses (page 146) or store-bought or blackstrap molasses	15 mL
¼ tsp	Red Curry Spice (page 252) or curry powder	I mL
¼ tsp	hot pepper flakes	I mL
I cup	red or short-grain brown rice	250 mL

I. In a saucepan, heat 2 tbsp (25 mL) of the oil over medium heat. Add onion and cook, stirring occasionally, for 5 minutes or until slightly softened. Add remaining oil. Stir in garlic and zucchini and cook, stirring occasionally, for 5 minutes, until vegetables are tender.

2. Add tomato and stock. Increase heat to high and bring to a gentle boil. Stir in molasses, curry, hot pepper flakes and rice. Cover, reduce heat to low and simmer for 1 hour or until rice is tender and sauce is thick. Do not remove lid during cooking.

Spiced Lemon Rice

Lemon and cinnamon lend a fresh and slightly exotic essence to the basmati rice.

Variation

- *Dessert Rice:* Omit onion and garlic. In a bowl, combine lemon rice with $1/2$ cup (125 mL) raisins and about $1/3$ cup (75 mL) rice milk. Drizzle each serving with 1 tbsp (15 mL) brown rice syrup.

2 tbsp	olive oil	25 mL
I tsp	cumin seeds	5 mL
2	whole cloves	2
I	stick cinnamon, about 2 inches (5 cm), broken into pieces	I
I	onion, chopped	I
2	cloves garlic, finely chopped	2
I	carrot, grated	I
I $1/2$ cups	basmati rice, rinsed	375 mL
3 cups	vegetable stock or water	750 mL
I tsp	grated lemon zest	5 mL
$1/4$ cup	freshly squeezed lemon juice	50 mL

1. In a saucepan, heat oil over medium heat. Stir in cumin seeds, cloves and cinnamon pieces and cook for 30 seconds. Add onion. Reduce heat to medium-low and cook, stirring once or twice, for about 10 minutes or until soft. Add garlic and carrot and cook, stirring occasionally, for 3 minutes. Add rice and cook, stirring occasionally, for 2 minutes.

2. Add stock and lemon juice. Increase heat to high and bring to a gentle boil. Cover, reduce heat to low and cook for 20 minutes or until rice is tender and liquid is absorbed. Do not remove lid during cooking. Fluff rice with a fork. Remove cloves and cinnamon pieces and stir in lemon zest.

With the texture of
a creamy risotto,
but without the
time-consuming
stirring, this creamy
rice is delicious
served with roasted
and baked main dishes.

Tip

• I prefer Lundberg
short-grain brown rice,
which is soft and
chewy when cooked,
but long-grain brown
rice, red rice or a
blend of your favorites
will also work.

Variations

• Use 1 to 2 cups
(250 to 500 mL)
grated parsnips,
turnip or carrot
in place of the
cauliflower.

Coconut Rice with Cauliflower

1	can (14 oz/400 mL) coconut milk	1
1 cup	short-grain brown rice (see Tip, left)	250 mL
2 tbsp	olive oil	25 mL
1	small onion, chopped	1
1	clove garlic, finely chopped	1
1	piece (1 inch/2.5 cm) candied ginger, finely chopped	1
2 cups	finely chopped cauliflower	500 mL
½ cup	fresh whole wheat bread crumbs	125 mL
	Sea salt and freshly ground pepper	

1. In a saucepan over high heat, bring coconut milk to a gentle
boil. Stir in rice. Cover and reduce heat to low and cook for
40 minutes. Do not remove lid during cooking. Stir rice,
which will be very wet and soupy. Increase heat and simmer
uncovered, stirring frequently, for 10 minutes or until rice is
tender and creamy.

2. Meanwhile, in a deep skillet, heat oil over high heat. Stir
in onion. Reduce heat to medium-low and cook, stirring
occasionally, for 5 minutes or until slightly softened. Add
garlic and ginger and cook, stirring frequently, for 2 minutes.
Stir in cauliflower and cook, stirring frequently, for 10 minutes
or until tender and fairly dry. Stir in bread crumbs.

3. Add cauliflower mixture to rice and season to taste with salt
and pepper.

Broccoli Lemon Rice

The lemon is subtle yet its presence is fresh and complements that of the broccoli. For a more pronounced lemon flavor, add 1 tsp (5 mL) grated lemon zest in Step 2.

2 cups	broccoli florets	500 mL
2½ cups	water	625 mL
½ tsp	sea salt	2 mL
1 tbsp	freshly squeezed lemon juice	15 mL
1 cup	short-grain brown rice (see Tip, page 316)	250 mL

1. In a saucepan, combine broccoli, water and salt. Bring to a boil over high heat. Cover, reduce heat and simmer for 5 minutes. Using a slotted spoon, lift broccoli from saucepan, rinse under cold water, drain and set aside.

2. Add lemon juice to broccoli water. Increase heat to high and bring to a boil. Stir in rice. Cover and simmer for 40 minutes or until rice is tender and liquid is absorbed. Do not remove lid during cooking. Fluff rice with a fork and stir in broccoli.

Refried Rice and Beans

This recipe is based on a traditional Latino or Mexican dish in which black or pinto beans are cooked until soft and then fried, along with lard and garlic and some spices. This is a hearty vegan version with rice and some extra vegetables added.

Tip

- Any type of cooked rice will work in this recipe. Use long- or short-grain brown rice, red rice or a blend of your favorites.

- *Baking sheet, lined with parchment*

2 cups	cooked pinto or black beans, rinsed and drained, or 1 can (14 to 19 oz/ 398 to 540 mL) pinto or black beans, drained and rinsed	500 mL
2 cups	cooked rice (see Tip, left)	500 mL
3 tbsp	olive oil, divided	45 mL
1 cup	finely chopped red onion	250 mL
¼ cup	finely chopped red bell pepper	50 mL
1	stalk celery, finely chopped	1
1 to 2 tbsp	tamari or soy sauce	15 to 25 mL

1. In a bowl, mash pinto beans. Add cooked rice and stir well to combine. Set aside.

2. In a skillet, heat 1 tbsp (15 mL) of the oil over medium heat. Add onion, red pepper and celery and cook, stirring frequently, for 6 to 8 minutes or until soft. Add to rice-bean mixture and mix well. If it is too dry to shape, gradually add just enough of the tamari to moisten. Divide into 12 portions and shape into ½-inch (1 cm) thick patties. Arrange patties in one layer on prepared baking sheet. Cover and chill for at least 1 hour or overnight.

3. Add 1 tbsp (15 mL) of the remaining oil to the skillet and heat over medium-high heat. Add one or two patties and cook, turning once, for 2 to 3 minutes per side or until golden and crisp. Repeat with remaining patties, adding remaining oil to skillet as needed.

Moroccan Couscous

I like couscous as a light accompaniment for hearty curry dishes and winter vegetable casseroles. It's fast and the addition of vegetables and herbs makes it nutritious.

1 tbsp	olive oil	15 mL
½	onion, finely chopped	½
¼ cup	finely chopped carrot	50 mL
¼ cup	finely chopped celery or fennel	50 mL
1	clove garlic, minced	1
1 tsp	Red Curry Spice (page 252) or curry powder	5 mL
½ cup	couscous	125 mL
¾ cup	vegetable stock or water	175 mL
2 tbsp	chopped fresh parsley	25 mL
2 tbsp	chopped fresh mint	25 mL

1. In a skillet, heat oil over medium heat. Stir in onion, carrot and celery and cook, stirring frequently, for 5 minutes or until slightly softened. Add garlic, curry and couscous and cook, stirring constantly, for 2 minutes. Stir in stock. Cover, remove from heat and let stand for 10 minutes or until all of the liquid is absorbed. Fluff with a fork and add parsley and mint.

The neutral flavor of the millet and the squash is pumped up by using herbs and spices. This is delicious cold or reheated for breakfast.

Tip

• If using precooked millet, bring to room temperature before adding in Step 2.

Herbed Millet and Spaghetti Squash

• *Preheat oven to 375°F (190°C)*
• *Rimmed baking sheet, lightly oiled*

I	medium spaghetti squash, cut in half lengthwise	I
I tbsp	toasted sesame oil	15 mL
3 tbsp	olive oil	45 mL
I	small red onion, halved and thinly sliced	I
I to 2 tbsp	Madras Curry Paste (page 255) or curry powder	15 to 25 mL
½ tsp	sea salt	2 mL
3 cups	cooked millet (see Instructions, right)	750 mL
¼ cup	shredded fresh basil	50 mL
2 tbsp	chopped fresh parsley	25 mL
2 tbsp	freshly squeezed lemon juice	25 mL
I tbsp	tamari or soy sauce	15 mL
3 tbsp	toasted sesame seeds, optional	45 mL

1. Arrange spaghetti squash, cut side down, on prepared baking sheet. Bake in preheated oven for 30 to 40 minutes, until tender when pierced with the tip of a knife. Using a long-handled spoon, scoop out and discard seeds and fibers. Separate squash spaghetti strands by running a fork from stem to blossom end. Using a long-handled spoon, scoop out squash spaghetti strands and place in a bowl. Toss with sesame oil and set aside.

2. In a wok or deep-sided saucepan, heat olive oil over medium-high heat. Add onion and stir-fry for 3 minutes. Add curry paste and salt and stir-fry for 1 minute. Add millet and stir-fry for 1 minute. Add basil, parsley, lemon juice and tamari and stir-fry for 1 minute. Toss with spaghetti squash. Garnish with sesame seeds, if using.

How to Cook Millet

Makes 3 cups (750 mL)

Millet, also known as proso, can be cooked, if desired, to a creamy texture by using slightly more liquid.

1 cup	millet	250 mL
2 cups	vegetable stock, water or fruit juice	500 mL
2 tsp	grapeseed or olive oil	10 mL

1. In a wok or saucepan over medium-high heat, toast millet, stirring constantly, about 4 minutes or until it begins to pop. Transfer to a bowl. Fill bowl with cold water and rub grains of millet between the palms of your hands for a few seconds. Pour into a fine mesh strainer and rinse under cold water for 1 minute or until the water runs clear. Drain well.

2. In a saucepan over medium-high heat, bring stock to a boil. Add millet. Cover, reduce heat to low and simmer for 15 to 20 minutes, until tender and all or most of the liquid has been absorbed. Remove from heat and let stand, covered, for 5 minutes. Drizzle with oil and fluff with a fork. Store cooked millet tightly covered in the refrigerator for up to 24 hours.

Red Lentil and Buckwheat Waffles

These savory waffles are great at breakfast with maple syrup or fruit, but they are also a quick-and-easy dinner item.

Tip

- Red lentils give the waffles a dark red tinge but any colour lentil may be used.

Variation

- *To use as pancake batter*: In a heavy skillet over medium-high heat, heat 2 tbsp (25 mL) vegetable oil. Ladle or pour into skillet about ¼ cup (50 mL) of batter for each pancake. Cook for 2 to 3 minutes or until edges are beginning to brown. Turn and cook on the other side for 2 minutes or until lightly browned.

- *Preheat oven to 300°F (150°C)*
- *Waffle iron, preheated*

¾ cup	all-purpose flour	175 mL
¼ cup	buckwheat flour	50 mL
1 tbsp	chia or poppy seeds	15 mL
1 tsp	baking powder	5 mL
¼ tsp	baking soda	1 mL
¼ tsp	sea salt	1 mL
1½ cups	cooked red lentils, rinsed and drained (see Instructions, page 309) (see Tip, left)	375 mL
1	ripe banana	1
½ cup	rice milk	125 mL
2 tbsp	grapeseed oil	25 mL
	Vegetable oil	

1. In a bowl, whisk together all-purpose flour, buckwheat flour, chia seeds, baking powder, baking soda and salt. Stir in lentils.

2. In another bowl, mash banana with a fork. Stir in rice milk and grapeseed oil. Pour over dry ingredients and stir until almost smooth. Some small lumps should remain.

3. Meanwhile, lightly oil hot waffle iron. In batches, pour or ladle batter into waffle iron and cook for 4 to 5 minutes or until waffles are golden and crisp. Transfer waffles to a platter, cover and keep warm in preheated oven. Repeat with remaining batter.

Citrus Wheat Berries and Greens

The chewy texture of the wheat berries is exceptional in this side dish or salad. Make lots and serve it hot or cold — it lasts through the workweek and just keeps getting better.

Citrus Dressing

⅓ cup	grapeseed oil	75 mL
	Grated zest and juice of 1 orange	
1 tbsp	freshly squeezed lemon juice	15 mL
1 tbsp	lemon thyme or regular thyme leaves	15 mL
1	clove garlic, minced	1
3 cups	hot or cold cooked wheat berries (see Instructions, 324)	750 mL
3 cups	coarsely chopped spinach or shredded greens	750 mL
1	carrot, shredded	1
½	red onion, thinly sliced	½
1 cup	toasted pine nuts or sunflower seeds	250 mL
½ cup	chopped dried cherries or apricots	125 mL

1. *Citrus Dressing:* In a jar or bowl with a tight-fitting lid, combine oil, orange zest and juice, lemon juice, thyme and garlic. Shake well.

2. In a bowl, combine wheat berries, spinach, carrot, onion, pine nuts and cherries. Toss with Citrus Dressing.

How to Cook Wheat Berries

Makes 3 cups (750 mL)

It is possible to simply cover wheat berries with water, bring to a boil and simmer for
1 hour or slightly more, but they will be very chewy. Toasting and soaking the berries
before cooking softens them so that the texture is more like that of brown rice.

1 cup	whole wheat berries	250 mL
½ tsp	sea salt	2 mL

1. In a wok or saucepan over medium-high heat, toast wheat berries, stirring
   constantly, for about 4 minutes or until berries begin to pop and emit a nutty
   aroma. Transfer to a bowl. Cover berries with cold water and stir. Cover and let
   soak for 1 hour or overnight in the refrigerator.

2. Drain and rinse berries. In a saucepan over medium-high heat, bring 2½ cups
   (625 mL) water and salt to a boil. Add rinsed berries. Cover, reduce heat to low
   and simmer gently for 1 hour or until chewy-tender and all or most of the liquid
   has been absorbed. Remove from heat and let stand, covered, for 5 minutes. Fluff
   with a fork. Store cooked wheat berries tightly covered in the refrigerator for up to
   24 hours.

Quinoa Beet Potato Salad

Serves 6

The beet stains the other ingredients, but the taste is worth the pink food.

1 ½ lbs	small potatoes	750 g
1	large carrot, shredded	1
1	medium beet, shredded	1
¼	fennel bulb, shredded	¼
2 cups	cold or room-temperature cooked quinoa (see Instructions, 326)	500 mL
½ cup	diced red onion	125 mL
¼ cup	chopped fresh parsley	50 mL
2 tbsp	chopped fresh tarragon	25 mL
½ cup	Tofu Mayonnaise (page 178) or store-bought	125 mL
	Sea salt and freshly ground pepper	

1. In a large saucepan, cover potatoes with water and bring to a boil over high heat. Cover, reduce heat to medium-low and simmer for 20 minutes or until potatoes are almost tender and show some resistance when pierced with the tip of a knife. Drain and rinse under cold water. Let stand, and when cool enough to handle, cut into ½-inch (1 cm) cubes.

2. Meanwhile, in a bowl, combine carrot, beet, fennel, quinoa, onion, parsley and tarragon. Add potatoes and mayonnaise. Stir to mix well. Season to taste with salt and pepper.

How to Cook Quinoa

Makes 3½ cups (875 mL)

Quinoa is a tiny grain that is naturally coated with a bitter substance called saponin, which imparts a bitter flavor unless it is washed off before cooking. Follow the instructions below to be sure that the resulting cooked quinoa is free of saponin's piney, resin-like taste.

1 cup	quinoa	250 mL
2 cups	vegetable stock or water	500 mL
½ tsp	sea salt	2 mL

1. In a deep bowl, cover quinoa with lukewarm water. Rub grains between your palms for 6 to 8 seconds. Drain through a fine mesh sieve and repeat the process with fresh water. In the sieve, rinse quinoa under cool running water until the water runs clear. Drain well.

2. In a saucepan over medium-high heat, bring stock and salt to a boil. Add rinsed and drained quinoa. Cover and reduce heat to medium-low. Simmer for 12 to 15 minutes or until liquid is absorbed and grains are translucent and tender. Let stand, covered, for 5 minutes. Fluff with a fork.

Serves 4

This is a great salad to team with other vegetables and leftover dishes. It stores for the whole workweek so lunchtime food is ready when you want it. The vinegar may seem out of proportion to the oil, but marinades for grains require more of a "hit" of the acid ingredient than the oil.

Minted Raspberry-Marinated Oats

2 cups	cold or room-temperature cooked whole oats (see Instructions, 328)	500 mL
½	red onion, thinly sliced	½
½ cup	chopped walnuts or almonds	125 mL

Minted Raspberry Marinade

½ cup	raspberry vinegar	125 mL
¼ cup	grapeseed or hemp oil	50 mL
¼ cup	chopped fresh mint	50 mL
½ tsp	sea salt	2 mL

1. In a bowl, combine oats, onion and walnuts and toss well to combine.

2. *Minted Raspberry Marinade:* In a jar or bowl with a tight-fitting lid, combine raspberry vinegar, oil, mint and salt. Shake vigorously to combine and pour over grains. Toss well to combine and let stand for at least 30 minutes. For best results, cover and refrigerate overnight or longer. Store marinated oats tightly covered in the refrigerator for up to 5 days.

How to Cook Whole Oats

Makes 3 cups (750 mL)

Sometimes called groats, whole oats are found in most health food stores. They require a longer cooking time than steel-cut or rolled oats, which lose their texture and cannot be substituted for whole grains in dishes.

I cup	whole oat groats	250 mL
I ¼ cups	vegetable stock, water or fruit juice	300 mL
½ tsp	sea salt	2 mL
2 tsp	olive oil	I0 mL

1. In a wok or saucepan over medium-high heat, toast oat groats, stirring constantly, for about 4 minutes or until they darken and become aromatic. Transfer to a bowl.

2. In a saucepan, bring stock to a boil over medium-high heat. Add oats, salt and oil. Cover, reduce heat to low and simmer for 40 to 50 minutes, until chewy-tender and oats have swelled to twice their size and absorbed all or most of the liquid (see Tip, below). Store cooked oat groats tightly covered in the refrigerator for up to 24 hours.

Tip: For a softer texture, increase the liquid by ¼ cup (50 mL). The grains will open more but will still be somewhat chewy in texture.

Amaranth Vegetable Pilaf

Fast and easy, this grain dish makes a light lunch when paired with greens or a fruit salad.

2 tbsp	olive oil	25 mL
1 cup	finely chopped red bell pepper	250 mL
½ cup	sliced red onion	125 mL
2	cloves garlic, finely chopped	2
2	green onions, chopped	2
1 cup	sliced white mushrooms	250 mL
2 cups	cooked amaranth (see Instructions, below)	500 mL
2 tsp	toasted sesame oil	10 mL
	Tamari or soy sauce	

1. In a wok or skillet, heat olive oil over medium-high heat. Add red pepper and onion and stir-fry for 2 minutes. Add garlic, green onions and mushrooms and stir-fry for 2 minutes. Add amaranth and stir-fry for 2 minutes or until heated through. Toss with sesame oil and season to taste with tamari or pass tamari at the table.

How to Cook Amaranth

Makes 1½ cups (375 mL)

Because amaranth may be slightly bitter, often a teaspoon (5 mL) of sweet syrup such as pure maple syrup, brown rice syrup or agave nectar is added to the cooking liquid. The tiny seeds are best if organic.

1 cup	amaranth seeds	250 mL
1½ cups	vegetable stock, water or fruit juice	375 mL
1 tsp	pure maple syrup (see Intro, above)	5 mL

1. In a wok or saucepan over medium-high heat, toast amaranth seeds, stirring constantly, until seeds start to pop and give off a nutty aroma, about 2 minutes. Transfer to a bowl.

2. In a saucepan, bring stock and maple syrup to a boil over medium-high heat. Add amaranth. Cover, reduce heat to low and simmer for 20 minutes or until all the liquid has been absorbed. Store cooked amaranth tightly covered in the refrigerator for up to 24 hours.

This Middle East-inspired salad is very good the next day. Serve it with a hearty whole-grain bread or with a creamy soup for a complete meal.

Tip

• You can use 2 cups (500 mL) cooked chickpeas, drained and rinsed, instead of canned.

Marinated Chickpea and Spelt Salad with Cilantro Dressing

Cilantro Dressing

I tbsp	whole cumin seeds	15 mL
2 tbsp	sunflower seeds	25 mL
I	clove garlic	I
I cup	fresh cilantro or parsley leaves	250 mL
3 tbsp	freshly squeezed lemon juice	45 mL
⅓ cup	grapeseed oil	75 mL
	Sea salt and freshly ground pepper	
2 cups	cold or room-temperature cooked spelt or Kamut (see Instructions, right)	500 mL
I	small cucumber, trimmed and cut into 1-inch (2.5 cm) chunks	I
I	medium tomato, chopped	I
½	red bell pepper, cut into thin strips	½
½	red onion, thinly sliced	½
½ cup	sliced pitted black olives	125 mL
I	can (14 to 19 oz/398 to 540 mL) chickpeas, drained and rinsed (see Tip, left)	I

1. *Cilantro Dressing:* In a small saucepan, toast cumin seeds over medium heat, stirring, until they begin to pop and fragrance is released, about 1 minute. Let cool.

2. In a blender, combine cumin seeds, sunflower seeds and garlic. Blend until finely chopped. Add cilantro. With the motor running, add lemon juice through the hole in the lid. Slowly add oil through the opening and blend until desired consistency is reached. Season to taste with salt and pepper.

3. In a bowl, combine spelt, cucumber, tomato, red pepper, onion, olives and chickpeas. Toss with Cilantro Dressing.

How to Cook Spelt and Kamut

Makes 2 cups (500 mL)

Spelt (*Triticum spelta*) is a durable, red wheat that has survived in its original form for thousands of years. Kamut (*Triticum durum*) is a variety of durum wheat with a very large grain that has its origins in the fertile Euphrates Valley. Both are cooked in the same way.

1 cup	spelt or Kamut berries	250 mL
1 ½ cups	vegetable stock or water	375 mL
2 tsp	toasted sesame oil	10 mL
½ tsp	sea salt	2 mL

1. In a wok or saucepan over medium-high heat, toast berries, stirring constantly, for about 4 minutes or until grains start to pop and turn a shade darker. Transfer to a strainer and rinse under cool running water for 5 seconds. Drain well.

2. In a saucepan, combine stock and rinsed berries. Cover and let soak for at least 1 hour or overnight. Add sesame oil and salt and bring to a boil, uncovered, over medium-high heat. Cover, reduce heat to medium-low and simmer for 45 minutes or until chewy-tender. Store cooked berries tightly covered in the refrigerator for up to 24 hours.

Tomato and Zucchini Bulgur

Bulgur is a processed grain made from wheat berries that have been steamed, dried and crushed. It cooks very quickly because of the processing. Tabbouleh is a well-known Middle Eastern dish that is made with bulgur, fresh chopped herbs and tomatoes. Cracked wheat is similar to bulgur but is uncooked and cracked apart rather than crushed. It is easier to cook than whole wheat berries, but it still takes longer than bulgur.

2 tbsp	olive oil	25 mL
I	onion, chopped	I
I	zucchini, chopped	I
2	cloves garlic, finely chopped	2
I	can (28 oz/796 mL) stewed tomatoes with juice, chopped	I
I cup	vegetable stock or water	250 mL
2 tbsp	chopped fresh oregano	25 mL
I tbsp	chopped fresh thyme	15 mL
I tsp	Garam Masala Spice Blend (page 254) or store-bought	5 mL
⅔ cup	medium-textured bulgur	150 mL
	Sea salt and freshly ground pepper	

1. In a saucepan, heat oil over medium-high heat. Add onion and cook, stirring occasionally, for 3 minutes or until slightly softened. Add zucchini and cook, stirring frequently, for 2 minutes. Add garlic and cook, stirring constantly, for 1 minute. Add tomatoes with juice and stock and bring to a boil. Stir in oregano, thyme, garam masala and bulgur. Cover, reduce heat and simmer for 20 to 25 minutes or until bulgur is tender and all or most of the liquid has been absorbed. Season to taste with salt and pepper.

Beverages and Snacks

Tropical Nog

A healthy version of the traditional holiday drink, this "nog" offers up creamy goodness all year long. If you are using canned pineapple, drain well. Add another banana for a thicker drink.

Variation
• Use cantaloupe in place of the mango.

2 cups	vanilla rice milk or soy milk	500 mL
1	mango, cut into chunks	1
1	banana	1
1 cup	fresh or drained canned pineapple chunks	250 mL
2 tbsp	Date Molasses (page 147) or molasses	25 mL
1 tsp	vanilla extract	5 mL
½ tsp	ground nutmeg	2 mL

1. In a blender, combine rice milk, mango, banana, pineapple, molasses, vanilla and nutmeg. Blend until thick and smooth.

Choco-Cappuccino

A great drink for frosty nights, this rich and creamy beverage is brimming with the comfort of chocolate and the heat of chiles.

• *Milk frother, optional*

3 cups	rice milk or soy milk	750 mL
15	semisweet vegan chocolate baking wafers or 3 or 4 tbsp (45 to 60 mL) vegan chocolate chips, to taste	15
1 or 2 tbsp	organic cane sugar	15 or 25 mL
1 tsp	vanilla extract	5 mL
½ tsp	ground cinnamon	2 mL
Pinch	ground cayenne or hot chile pepper	Pinch

1. In a saucepan, heat rice milk over high heat until small bubbles appear around the outside of the pan. Remove from heat and pour off half the hot milk into a frother or deep bowl. Add chocolate to the hot milk remaining in the pan and melt, stirring occasionally, over low heat.

2. Meanwhile, froth milk using a hand frother or immersion blender. Stir sugar, vanilla, cinnamon and cayenne into chocolate milk. Divide chocolate milk between two mugs and top with frothed milk.

Chilled Chia Chai

½ cup	cashews	125 mL
2 tbsp	whole chia seeds	25 mL
2 cups	rice milk	500 mL
1	can (14 oz/400 mL) coconut milk	1
¼ cup	sweetened shredded coconut	50 mL
6 to 8	pitted dates	6 to 8
½ tsp	vanilla extract	2 mL
¼ tsp	ground cinnamon	1 mL
¼ tsp	ground black pepper	1 mL
Pinch	Garam Masala Spice Blend (page 254) or store-bought	Pinch
4 to 6	sticks cinnamon, about 2 inches (5 cm), optional	4 to 6

1. In a bowl, combine cashews and chia seeds. Cover with water and let stand for 30 minutes. Drain.

2. In a blender or food processor, combine rice milk, coconut milk, coconut, dates to taste, vanilla, cinnamon, pepper, garam masala and cashew and chia seeds mixture. Blend until smooth. Pour into iced glasses and garnish with cinnamon sticks, if using.

Mango Pineapple Mocktail

1 cup	vanilla rice milk or soy milk	250 mL
1	ripe mango, cut into chunks	1
½ cup	pineapple juice	125 mL
2 tbsp	freshly squeezed lemon juice	25 mL
2 cups	Soy Ice Cream (page 346) or store-bought	500 mL
¼ cup	crushed ice	50 mL
	Crushed cardamom seeds	

1. In a blender, combine rice milk, mango, pineapple juice and lemon juice. Blend until smooth.

2. Add ice cream and process just until blended and thick. Place crushed ice in 4 glasses and spoon in mixture. Garnish with a pinch of crushed cardamom seeds.

Mango offers a fresh and fruity foil for the astringent green tea taste.

Green Tea Mocktail

2 cups	chilled brewed green tea	500 mL
2 tbsp	Spiced Sweet Glaze (page 147) or Green Tea Molasses (page 146)	25 mL
1	ripe mango, cut into chunks	1
¼ cup	crushed ice	50 mL

1. In a blender, combine green tea, Spiced Sweet Glaze, mango and ice. Blend until smooth. Strain into cocktail glasses.

Flaxseed oil delivers essential fatty acids and the orange-flavored flax oil makes drinks taste like orange cream soda.

Orange Creamsicle

1 cup	vanilla rice milk or soy milk	250 mL
½ cup	freshly squeezed orange juice	125 mL
1	orange, sectioned	1
1	banana	1
1 tbsp	orange-flavored (see Sources, 368) or regular flaxseed oil	15 mL

1. In a blender, combine rice milk, orange juice, orange sections, banana and flaxseed oil. Blend until smooth.

The Brazilian açai berry is high in antioxidant power. This mocktail includes other antioxidant-rich ingredients as well.

Açai Mocktail

½ cup	cranberry juice	125 mL
2	ice cubes	2
1 cup	frozen açai berries	250 mL
1 cup	blueberries or blackberries	250 mL
½ cup	raspberries	125 mL
1 tsp	fresh thyme leaves	5 mL

1. In a blender, combine cranberry juice, ice cubes, açai berries, blueberries, raspberries and thyme. Blend for 1 minute or until smooth.

Berry Chia Smoothie

Serves 2

With raspberries and açai berries for antioxidants, cashews for oleic acid, chia seeds for both of those benefits and soy for protein, this drink is good for people of all ages.

½ cup	cashews	125 mL
1 tbsp	whole chia seeds	15 mL
2 cups	vanilla rice milk or soy milk	500 mL
1 cup	frozen açai berries	250 mL
1 cup	frozen raspberries	250 mL
6 to 8	pitted dates	6 to 8

1. In a bowl, combine cashews and chia seeds. Cover with water and let stand for 30 minutes. Drain.

2. In a blender or food processor, combine rice milk, açai berries, raspberries, dates to taste, and cashew and chia seeds mixture. Blend until smooth.

Tropical Banana Tahini Smoothie

Serves 2

One taste of this smoothie transports you to a tropical isle for a few minutes. Take a break and enjoy this drink in the middle of the day.

2 cups	vanilla rice milk or soy milk	500 mL
1 cup	fresh or drained canned pineapple chunks	250 mL
1	banana	1
¼ cup	pineapple juice	50 mL
2 tbsp	freshly squeezed lemon juice	25 mL

1. In a blender, combine rice milk, pineapple, banana, pineapple juice and lemon juice. Blend until smooth.

Pomegranate Smoothie

Serves 2

Ruby-red pomegranate offers up its powerhouse of nutritional goodness in this not-too-sweet drink.

½ cup	pomegranate juice	125 mL
1 cup	fresh or canned raspberries, drained	250 mL
1	banana	1
½ cup	fresh or frozen blueberries	125 mL
2 tbsp	Pomegranate Molasses (page 146) or store-bought, or molasses	25 mL
1 tbsp	freshly squeezed lemon juice	15 mL

1. In a blender, combine pomegranate juice, raspberries, banana, blueberries, molasses and lemon juice. Blend until smooth.

Spiced and baked until crunchy, this salty snack is a healthy version of the ubiquitous potato chip.

Tips

- You can use 2 cups (500 mL) cooked chickpeas, drained and rinsed, instead of canned.

- Add another teaspoon (5 mL) of hot pepper flakes if you like heat.

Variation

- Use your favorite spice blend in place of the garam masala.

Seasoned Chickpeas and Almonds

- *Preheat oven to 400°F (200°C)*
- *Rimmed baking sheet, lightly oiled*

2 cups	whole almonds (unblanched)	500 mL
1	can (14 to 19 oz/398 to 540 mL) chickpeas, drained and rinsed (see Tips, left)	1
3	cloves garlic, coarsely chopped	3
2 tbsp	olive oil	25 mL
1 tbsp	freshly squeezed lime juice	15 mL
1 tbsp	Garam Masala Spice Blend (page 254) or store-bought	15 mL
1 tsp	hot pepper flakes (see Tips, left)	5 mL
	Sea salt and freshly ground pepper	

1. In a bowl, combine almonds, chickpeas, garlic, oil, lime juice, garam masala, hot pepper flakes and salt and pepper to taste. Spread evenly on prepared baking sheet. Bake in preheated oven, stirring once, for 30 minutes. Test for crunchiness and return to the oven, testing every 5 minutes until the desired dryness is achieved. Let cool.

2. Store mixture in an airtight container in the refrigerator for up to 2 weeks.

This loose, dry mixture of chopped nuts and spices is crushed, not powdered or ground to a paste. In the Middle East, it is usually eaten as a snack with bread dipped in olive oil, or served at breakfast or any other time throughout the day. Each family has a slightly different version. The amounts here may be doubled or tripled.

Dukkah

1 cup	sesame seeds	250 mL
3 tbsp	whole coriander seeds	45 mL
2 tbsp	whole cumin seeds	25 mL
1 cup	unsalted dry-roasted peanuts	250 mL
1 tsp	sea salt	5 mL

1. In a small, heavy skillet or saucepan over medium heat, toast sesame seeds, stirring constantly until pale brown, 1 to 2 minutes. Be careful not to burn the seeds. Set aside to cool.

2. In same skillet, combine coriander and cumin seeds. Toast over medium heat until seeds begin to pop and their fragrance is released, 1 to 2 minutes. Let cool.

3. In a food processor or using a mortar and pestle, grind or pound toasted spices until finely ground. Add sesame seeds and peanuts and pulse or pound until texture resembles coarse sand but not a paste. Tip into a small bowl and stir in salt to taste.

4. Store dukkah in a small jar with lid in the refrigerator or a cool, dark place for up to 2 months.

Healthy pumpkin seeds are the main ingredient in this easy-to-make snack.

Sweet Toasted Pumpkin Seeds

- *Preheat oven to 400°F (200°C)*
- *Rimmed baking pan, lightly oiled*

3 cups	raw pumpkin seeds	750 mL
3 tbsp	olive oil	45 mL
2 tbsp	organic cane sugar	25 mL
¼ tsp	ground cinnamon	1 mL
Pinch	ground nutmeg	Pinch

1. In a bowl, combine pumpkin seeds, oil, sugar, cinnamon and nutmeg. Spread evenly on prepared baking sheet and roast in preheated oven, stirring once or twice, for about 20 minutes, until crisp and puffy.

2. Store toasted pumpkin seeds in an airtight container in the refrigerator for up to 2 weeks.

Orange-Spiked Power Cereal

I love the orange-kissed flavor of this all-natural high-energy cereal. With no sugars except for those naturally occurring in the dried fruit and the nectar, this is a healthy alternative to commercially prepared cereals, which often use genetically modified sugars.

Variations

- Tailor this great-tasting snack to your own tastes by using any nuts, seeds and dried fruit.
- Use lemon zest in place of the orange zest.

- *Preheat oven to 300°F (150°C)*
- *2 rimmed baking sheets*

4 cups	large-flake rolled oats	1 L
1 cup	chopped unsulfured dried prunes or apples	250 mL
1 cup	coarsely chopped almonds	250 mL
1 cup	unsweetened shredded coconut, optional	250 mL
¾ cup	unsalted raw sunflower seeds	175 mL
½ cup	whole-grain teff	125 mL
½ cup	chopped unsulfured dried apricots	125 mL
½ cup	chopped raisins	125 mL
¼ cup	raw pumpkin seeds	50 mL
1 cup	agave nectar or brown rice syrup	250 mL
¼ cup	coconut oil	50 mL
½ cup	chopped dates	125 mL
2 tsp	ground cinnamon	10 mL
	Grated zest of 1 orange	

1. In a large bowl, combine oats, prunes, almonds, coconut, if using, sunflower seeds, teff, apricots, raisins and pumpkin seeds.

2. In a small saucepan, heat agave nectar and coconut oil over medium heat. Add dates, cinnamon and orange zest. Cook, stirring constantly, until dates are softened and mixture is thick, about 5 minutes. Pour over grains and mix well.

3. Divide mixture evenly between baking sheets and spread in a thin layer. Bake in preheated oven, stirring every 10 minutes, for 40 minutes or until grains and nuts are toasted and golden brown. Let cool on baking sheets, running a metal spatula under the grains to loosen them periodically as they cool.

4. Store cereal in an airtight container at room temperature for 2 to 3 weeks or in the refrigerator for up to 2 months.

Whole-Grain Power Bars

Taking their goodness from the homemade power cereal, these high-energy bars are a great snack for active people.

- *Preheat oven to 375°F (190°C)*
- *Rimmed baking sheet*
- *11- by 7-inch (2 L) baking pan*

1 cup	coarsely chopped walnuts	250 mL
½ cup	sesame seeds	125 mL
2 cups	Orange-Spiked Power Cereal (page 340) or granola	500 mL
1½ cups	unsweetened crisp brown rice cereal	375 mL
1 cup	dried cherries or cranberries	250 mL
¼ cup	flaxseeds	50 mL
2 tbsp	whole chia seeds	25 mL
1 tbsp	sea salt	15 mL
½ cup	brown rice syrup or agave nectar	125 mL
2 tbsp	coconut oil	25 mL
2 tsp	vanilla extract	10 mL

1. On baking sheet, combine walnuts and sesame seeds. Bake in preheated oven for 5 minutes or until lightly browned and toasted.

2. In a large bowl, combine Orange-Spiked Power Cereal, rice cereal, cherries, flaxseeds, chia seeds, salt and toasted walnuts and sesame seeds.

3. In a saucepan over medium-high heat, heat rice syrup until lightly simmering. Remove from heat and stir in coconut oil and vanilla. Stir until coconut oil is dissolved. Pour over grain mixture. Press into prepared baking pan and set aside for 15 minutes. Cut into 2-inch (5 cm) squares.

4. Store bars in an airtight container for up to 2 weeks or in the refrigerator for up to 1 month.

Corn Biscuits

This is an all-round great snack. You can double the recipe and freeze the extra biscuits.

Serving Suggestions

- Serve with strawberry jam for breakfast.
- Add Red Hot Hummus (page 184) or a nut butter at lunch or midday.
- Top with pesto or tapenade and thinly sliced vegetables and heat under the broiler for a light and quick dinner dish.

- *Preheat oven to 350°F (180°C)*
- *9-inch (2.5 L) square baking dish, lightly oiled*

1 cup	unbleached all-purpose flour	250 mL
1 cup	cornmeal	250 mL
1 ½ tsp	baking powder	7 mL
1 tsp	sea salt	5 mL
½ tsp	baking soda	2 mL
½ tsp	hot pepper flakes, or to taste	2 mL
½ cup	fresh or frozen corn kernels	125 mL
½ cup	rice milk or soy milk	125 mL
¼ cup	cider vinegar	50 mL
¼ cup	apple juice or water	50 mL
4 tbsp	vegetable oil	60 mL
3 tbsp	Fruit Purée (page 139) or applesauce	45 mL
½ cup	chopped Candied Nuts (page 157) or almonds	125 mL

1. In a bowl, whisk together flour, cornmeal, baking powder, salt, baking soda and hot pepper flakes. Stir in corn kernels.

2. In a separate bowl, whisk together rice milk, vinegar, apple juice, oil and Fruit Purée.

3. Make a well in dry ingredients and pour wet ingredients into it. Stir with a fork to blend well. Scrape into prepared dish and smooth top with the back of a spoon. Bake in preheated oven for 15 minutes. Spread nuts evenly over top and bake for 20 minutes longer or until a cake tester comes out clean when inserted in the center. Let cool slightly in dish. Cut into squares and serve warm or cool completely.

4. Store biscuits tightly wrapped in an airtight container for up to 4 days or in the refrigerator for up to 1 week. Store in the freezer for up to 1 month.

Sesame Nori Crackers

Sweet and salty with nutty overtones, this snack is great served on the side to add snap to soup, rice and noodle dishes.

- *Preheat oven to 350°F (180°C)*
- *Baking sheet, lined with parchment paper*

4	sheets nori	4
¼ cup	brown rice syrup	50 mL
¼ cup	grapeseed oil	50 mL
1 tbsp	Madras Curry Paste (page 255) or curry powder	15 mL
½ cup	toasted sesame seeds	125 mL
	Sea salt	

1. Tear each nori sheet into 3 long strips. Arrange in one layer on prepared baking sheet. In a bowl, whisk together rice syrup, oil and curry.

2. Using a pastry brush, paint the top of each strip liberally with syrup mixture. Sprinkle evenly with sesame seeds and salt. Bake in preheated oven for 10 minutes or until strips are dry and toasted on the top. Let cool.

3. Turn strips over and repeat Step 2. Transfer to a wire rack and let cool for at least 20 minutes.

4. Store crackers in an airtight container for up to 1 week.

Open-Face Black Bean Tostadas

The leftover Refried Rice and Beans makes it a snap to pull this satisfying snack together.

Variation

- In place of the Refried Rice and Beans use 1 cup (250 mL) vegan refried beans and ¼ cup (50 mL) cooked brown rice or chopped red onion.

2	10-inch (25 cm) corn tortillas	2
1 cup	Refried Rice and Beans (page 318) (see Variation, left)	250 mL
½ cup	shredded lettuce	125 mL
1	tomato, seeded and chopped	1
½	ripe avocado, sliced	½
¼ cup	black olives, optional	50 mL
¼ cup	Tofu Mayonnaise (page 178) or store-bought	50 mL

1. In a skillet over medium-high heat, toast tortillas for 30 seconds on each side. Place tortillas on serving plates. Spread ½ cup (125 mL) of the Refried Beans and Rice on each tortilla. Divide lettuce, tomato, avocado, olives, if using, and mayonnaise in half and pile each in that order over the tortillas.

Eggplant, Lettuce and Tomato Sandwiches

Easy to make, these ELT sandwiches are the answer to between-meal hunger cravings.

Tip

• Boston, Bibb or romaine lettuce or any fresh green will work in this sandwich.

4	crosswise slices (½ inch/1 cm) eggplant	4
	All-purpose flour	
2 tbsp	olive oil	25 mL
2	slices ripe tomato	2
2 tbsp	Almond Garlic Spread (page 179) or Tofu Mayonnaise (page 178) or store-bought	25 mL
2	large lettuce leaves (see Tip, left)	2

1. In a shallow dish, dust both sides of eggplant slices with flour. In a skillet, heat oil over medium-high heat. Add eggplant and cook about 2 minutes on each side or until tender, browned on both sides and soft inside but not flimsy and falling apart. Drain on paper towels.

2. Lay 2 eggplant slices on a work surface. Place a slice of tomato on each and spread 1 tbsp (15 mL) of the Almond Garlic Spread over each tomato slice. Place a lettuce leaf over each tomato slice and top with remaining eggplant slices.

Pear and Avocado Pitas

Warming the pitas makes them meltingly soft and nuttier in taste but to save time, this step may be omitted.

• *Preheat oven to 350°F (180°C)*

2	6-inch (15 cm) pita breads with pocket	2
2	ripe pears, chopped	2
1	ripe avocado, chopped	1
2 tbsp	freshly squeezed lemon juice	25 mL
4 tbsp	Red Hot Hummus (page 184), Vegetable Raita (page 187) or store-bought	60 mL
4 tbsp	chopped red onion	60 mL
1 cup	alfalfa sprouts	250 mL

1. Wrap pita breads in foil and warm in preheated oven for about 10 minutes.

2. In a bowl, combine pears, avocado and lemon juice. Set aside. Cut each pita in half and open up the pockets. Spread inside of each with 1 tbsp (15 mL) hummus. Divide pear-avocado mixture into 4 portions and spoon into pitas. Add 1 tbsp (15 mL) onion and ¼ cup (50 mL) alfalfa sprouts to each pita.

Desserts

Soy Ice Cream

• *Ice cream maker*

10 oz	firm silken tofu	340 g
1⅔ cups	soy milk	400 mL
⅓ cup	brown rice syrup or pure maple syrup	75 mL
2 tsp	vanilla extract	10 mL
½ tsp	sea salt, optional	2 mL

1. In a blender or food processor, combine tofu, soy milk, rice syrup, vanilla and salt, if using. Process on high until blended and smooth.

2. Transfer to ice cream maker and follow the manufacturer's instructions to process into a creamy frozen dessert. Store ice cream tightly covered in the freezer for up to 3 weeks.

Vanilla Poached Pears with Cinnamon Rice Cream

2 cups	white grape juice	500 mL
¼ cup	white wine	50 mL
2 tbsp	freshly squeezed lemon juice	25 mL
2	ripe pears, halved lengthwise	2
1	vanilla bean	1

Cinnamon Rice Cream

2 cups	Sweet Lemon Rice (page 349)	500 mL
½ cup	coconut cream	125 mL
½ tsp	ground cinnamon	2 mL

1. In a saucepan, combine grape juice, wine and lemon juice. Bring to a boil over medium-high heat. Add pears and vanilla bean. Cover, reduce heat to medium-low and simmer for 10 to 15 minutes or until pears are tender-crisp. Remove from heat and let stand in poaching liquid until ready to serve or overnight

2. *Cinnamon Rice Cream:* In a bowl, combine Sweet Lemon Rice, coconut cream and cinnamon. Spoon cream into serving bowls. Top with pears and drizzle with some of the poaching liquid.

Oatmeal Coconut Cookies

- *Preheat oven to 400°F (200°C)*
- *2 baking sheets*

If you use spelt flour, the cookies will be thin, lacy and crisp. If you use whole wheat flour, they will be a bit firmer, but still crisp around the edges. Don't crowd the cookies because they spread out and require lots of space on the baking sheet.

2 tbsp	ground flaxseeds	25 mL
½ cup	rice milk or soy milk, divided	125 mL
¾ cup	spelt flour or whole wheat flour (see Intro, left)	175 mL
½ tsp	baking soda	2 mL
½ tsp	baking powder	2 mL
¼ tsp	sea salt	1 mL
¼ tsp	ground nutmeg	1 mL
½ cup	coconut oil (see Tip, left)	125 mL
⅔ cup	lightly packed brown sugar	150 mL
½ tsp	vanilla extract	2 mL
1 cup	large-flake rolled oats	250 mL
½ cup	unsweetened shredded coconut	125 mL

Tip

- Coconut oil is a non-hydrogenated, naturally saturated oil from coconuts and does not contain trans fatty acids. It is a significant plant source of lauric acid, which has antiviral properties. Because coconut oil remains solid at room temperature, it replaces butter for cookies and cakes, but it is not as soft as room-temperature butter. For creaming, use a warm bowl and position it near the preheating oven. Do not put the bowl directly over heat because the coconut oil will quickly melt back into a liquid. If this happens, move to a cooler spot and let it firm up again before creaming. Refrigerate remaining coconut oil after opening.

1. In a bowl, combine flaxseeds and 3 tbsp (45 mL) of the rice milk. Let stand for 10 minutes or until gelatinous.

2. Meanwhile, in a bowl, combine flour, baking soda, baking powder, salt and nutmeg. Stir well with a wire whisk or fork.

3. In a large bowl, using a wooden spoon, cream together coconut oil and brown sugar. Beat in remaining rice milk, vanilla and flaxseed mixture. Stir dry ingredients into sugar mixture. Add rolled oats and coconut and mix until combined.

4. Using 2 spoons, drop about 2 tbsp (25 mL) of the dough onto baking sheets, about 2 inches (10 cm) apart. Bake in preheated oven for 8 minutes or until lightly browned around edges. Let cool on baking sheets for about 10 minutes before transferring to a wire rack to cool completely.

Any roasted stone fruit will be delicious with this dessert.

Tip

• This pudding is best when baked and served the same day. If making the pudding ahead, cover and refrigerate. Bring to room temperature and reheat before serving with roasted peaches or other stone fruit.

Baked Rice Pudding with Roasted Peaches

• *Preheat oven to 350°F (180°C)*
• *8-cup (2 L) baking dish*
• *Rimmed baking sheet, lightly oiled*

½ cup	rice milk or soy milk	125 mL
2 cups	cooked brown rice	500 mL
1	can (12 oz/341 mL) sliced peaches, drained and chopped	1
¼ cup	raisins	50 mL
1	banana	1
¼ cup	frozen pineapple or orange juice concentrate	50 mL
1 tsp	vanilla extract	5 mL
6	fresh peaches, halved	6
3 tbsp	organic cane sugar	45 mL

1. In a saucepan, heat rice milk over high heat to just under a gentle boil. Let cool slightly.

2. Meanwhile, in a bowl, combine rice, canned peaches and raisins. In a blender, combine banana, pineapple juice concentrate, vanilla and rice milk. Blend until smooth. Add to rice mixture. Scrape into baking dish and bake in preheated oven for 30 minutes. Remove from oven and increase heat to 400°F (200°C). Let rice pudding cool or serve warm or at room temperature.

3. Arrange peach halves, cut side down on prepared baking sheet. Roast in preheated oven for 10 to 15 minutes or until soft. Let cool on baking sheet. Remove skins and slice peaches into a bowl. Toss with sugar and serve with rice pudding.

Sweet Lemon Rice

Not too sweet and infused with lemon essence, this rather sticky rice confection is the perfect foil for fresh fruit, raw or poached.

I	can (14 oz/400 mL) coconut milk, divided	I
⅓ cup	organic cane sugar	75 mL
	Grated zest and juice of I lemon	
¼ tsp	sea salt	I mL
I cup	jasmine or long-grain white rice	250 mL
I tsp	ground cinnamon, optional	5 mL

1. In a heavy-bottomed saucepan, bring ½ cup (125 mL) of the coconut milk to a boil over high heat. Add sugar and stir until dissolved. Reduce heat and simmer for 15 minutes. Do not stir the sugar-milk mixture, but gently swirl the pan once or twice during cooking. The syrup should be reduced in volume and thickened.

2. Meanwhile, pour remaining coconut milk into a 2-cup (500 mL) measuring cup and add water until it reaches a scant 2 cups (500 mL). In a saucepan, combine coconut milk-water mixture with lemon zest and juice and salt. Bring to a boil over high heat. Stir in rice. Cover, reduce heat to low and cook for 20 minutes or until rice is tender and liquid is absorbed. Add coconut milk-syrup and stir well. Garnish with cinnamon, if using.

Serving Suggestions

- Serve ¼ cup (50 mL) of Sweet Lemon Rice with a spoonful of Strawberry Pecan Crisp (page 352) per serving.

- For every serving, pour ¼ cup (50 mL) rice milk over and stir in 1 tbsp (15 mL) raisins or chopped dried apricots or walnuts.

Black Blondies

The batter is fairly stiff yet the bars are soft and chewy when baked. Use a high-quality vegan dark baking chocolate — that's what gives this treat its soft, rich and dark interior.

- *Preheat oven to 350°F (180°C)*
- *8-inch (2 L) square baking pan, lightly oiled and lined with parchment paper*

⅓ cup	rice milk or soy milk	75 mL
3 tbsp	ground flaxseeds	45 mL
1 tbsp	freshly squeezed lemon juice	15 mL
½ cup	whole wheat flour	125 mL
½ cup	unbleached all-purpose flour	125 mL
1 tsp	baking powder	5 mL
1 tsp	baking soda	5 mL
5 tbsp	vegan margarine	75 mL
¾ cup	lightly packed brown sugar	175 mL
3 tbsp	applesauce	45 mL
1 tsp	vanilla extract	5 mL
½ cup	coarsely chopped semisweet vegan chocolate	125 mL
½ cup	coarsely chopped pecans, optional	125 mL

1. In a small bowl, whisk together rice milk and flaxseeds. Whisk in lemon juice and let stand for 10 minutes or until gelatinous.

2. In a bowl, combine whole wheat and all-purpose flours, baking powder and baking soda. Whisk to mix well and set aside.

3. In a large bowl, using a wooden spoon, cream together margarine and brown sugar. Add applesauce and vanilla and beat well. Add flaxseed mixture and beat well. Stir in half of the dry ingredients and beat well. Add remaining dry ingredients and stir to mix well. Stir in chocolate pieces and pecans, if using.

4. Scrape into prepared pan and spread evenly. Bake in preheated oven for 45 minutes or until a cake tester inserted in the center comes out clean. Let cool in pan and cut into 2-inch (5 cm) squares.

Strawberries with Balsamic Drizzle

Purchase the very best balsamic vinegar; it should say "Product of Modena" on the label. This thick, richly flavored nectar goes a long way and is much better than the less expensive caramel-colored imitation.

Variation

• Use cubed watermelon or melon in place of the strawberries.

| 4 cups | sliced strawberries | 1 L |
| 2 tbsp | balsamic vinegar (see Intro, left) | 25 mL |

1. Spoon strawberries into serving bowls and drizzle with vinegar.

Fruited Rice Spring Rolls

Fresh fruit combined with lemon-spiked rice is wrapped up in thin, softened rice paper for these surprise dessert packages.

Variation

• Substitute 1 1/2 cups (375 mL) leftover cooked rice and sweeten to taste with agave nectar or brown rice syrup in place of the Sweet Lemon Rice.

1 1/2 cups	Sweet Lemon Rice (page 349)	375 mL
1 tsp	agave nectar	5 mL
1 tsp	grapeseed oil	5 mL
10	strawberries, finely sliced, 12 slices reserved	10
4	kiwifruits, diced	4
1	mango, diced	1
12	8-inch (20 cm) rice-paper rounds	12
1 cup	Lemon Sauce (page 362) or Strawberry Sauce (page 362), optional	250 mL

1. In a bowl, combine Sweet Lemon Rice with agave nectar and oil. Fold in strawberries, kiwifruits and mango.

2. *Assemble spring rolls:* Fill a shallow dish with warm water. Dip one rice-paper round in water for about 30 seconds, until soft. Place on a flat surface and spoon about 2 tbsp (25 mL) of the fruited rice mixture on each wrapper and top with a strawberry slice. Fold up the bottom and fold down the top. Roll spring roll tightly and set on a tray with seam down. Repeat with remaining rice-paper rounds and fruited rice mixture, cover and refrigerate for up to 4 hours. Serve with Lemon Sauce, if desired.

Strawberry Pecan Crisp

Be sure to use fresh bread crumbs in this crisp because they help to soak up the juices from the cooked strawberries. Even with the flour and bread crumbs, this is a very "soupy" dessert, great for serving over Soy Ice Cream (page 346) or Sweet Lemon Rice (page 349).

Variation

• Substitute blueberries or blackberries for strawberries.

• *Preheat oven to 375°F (190°C)*
• *8-inch (2 L) square baking dish, lightly oiled*

6 cups	strawberries, halved (about 2 lbs/1 kg)	1.5 L
2 cups	fresh whole wheat bread crumbs	500 mL
¼ cup	organic cane sugar	50 mL
⅓ cup	unbleached all-purpose flour	75 mL
½ tsp	grated lemon zest	2 mL
2 tbsp	freshly squeezed lemon juice	25 mL
1 tbsp	balsamic vinegar	15 mL
1 tbsp	chopped fresh tarragon	15 mL

Pecan Crisp Topping

¼ cup	vegan margarine	50 mL
½ cup	organic cane sugar	125 mL
½ cup	large-flake rolled oats	125 mL
½ cup	chopped pecans	125 mL
¼ tsp	ground nutmeg	1 mL
¼ tsp	sea salt	1 mL
2 cups	Soy Ice Cream (page 346), optional	500 mL

1. In prepared dish, toss together strawberries, bread crumbs, sugar, flour, lemon zest and juice, vinegar and tarragon.

2. *Pecan Crisp Topping:* In a bowl, cream together margarine and sugar. Add oats, pecans, nutmeg and salt and mix until crumbly. Spread evenly over strawberries. Bake in preheated oven for 40 minutes or until berries are bubbly and topping is browned. Let cool and serve with Soy Ice Cream, if desired.

Dark Chocolate Pudding

The flaxseeds give a gelatinous texture to this rich pudding — no matter how finely ground they are, they still swell, and tiny bits add a chewy texture to the otherwise silky pudding. Dark chocolate provides antioxidant benefits, so it is the best type of chocolate to use.

Tip

• If using chocolate with a high percentage of cacao (70%) or more, use the full amount of sugar. If using a chocolate with a lower percentage, you will need to add less sugar.

2 cups	soy milk or rice milk, divided	500 mL
2 tbsp	ground flaxseeds	25 mL
2 to 4 tbsp	organic cane sugar (see Tip, left)	25 to 60 mL
6 oz	bittersweet (dark) chocolate, chopped (see Tip, left)	175 g
1 tsp	vanilla extract	5 mL
Pinch	sea salt	Pinch
10 oz	silken tofu, drained	300 g

1. In a bowl, combine 1 cup (250 mL) of the soy milk and flaxseeds. Let stand for 10 minutes or until gelatinous.

2. Meanwhile, in a saucepan, heat remaining soy milk over high heat until steaming. Stir in sugar and chocolate. Reduce heat to medium-low and slowly melt the chocolate, whisking constantly. When chocolate is completely melted, remove pan from heat and stir in vanilla and salt.

3. Whisk flaxseed mixture and stir into chocolate mixture. Cook over medium heat, stirring constantly, for 2 minutes or until mixture has thickened. Remove from heat and whisk in tofu.

4. Pour into dessert cups and cover with plastic wrap. Chill in the refrigerator for at least 1 hour or overnight.

In baked goods, use espresso powder or finely ground espresso beans because it makes this cake dark and flavorful. Do try to find espresso powder because you can also use it as a garnish for puddings and even rice dishes.

Tip

• Espresso powder is dehydrated brewed espresso coffee — like regular instant coffee but stronger. It is used in baked chocolate goods to enrich the chocolate and give a deep color and is also used as a garnish for puddings and drinks. If espresso powder is not available, substitute finely ground espresso beans in baked products.

The difference between the espresso powder and the ground beans is that the powder dissolves while the beans do not.

Chocolate Cake with Lemon Cream

- *Preheat oven to 350°F (180°C)*
- *9-inch (2.5 L) square baking pan, lined with parchment paper*

1¼ cups	all-purpose flour	300 mL
⅓ cup	unsweetened cocoa powder	75 mL
¼ cup	organic cane sugar	50 mL
1½ tsp	baking powder	7 mL
1 tsp	finely ground espresso beans or powder (see Tip, left)	5 mL
½ tsp	baking soda	2 mL
¼ tsp	salt	1 mL
½ cup	brown rice syrup or pure maple syrup	125 mL
½ cup	strong brewed coffee	125 mL
⅓ cup	olive oil	75 mL
¼ cup	Fruit Purée (page 139) or applesauce	50 mL
6 oz	firm tofu or ½ cup (125 mL) Soy Sour Cream (page 145)	175 g
1½ tsp	vanilla extract	7 mL
1 tsp	cider vinegar	5 mL
1 cup	Lemon Cream (page 362) or Strawberry Sauce (page 362)	250 mL

1. In a bowl, sift together flour, cocoa powder, sugar, baking powder, espresso powder, baking soda and salt.

2. In a blender, combine rice syrup, coffee, oil, Fruit Purée, tofu, vanilla and vinegar. Blend until smooth. Pour wet ingredients into flour mixture and whisk until smooth.

3. Pour batter into prepared pan and spread evenly. Bake for 20 minutes. Rotate pan and bake for another 20 minutes or until cake pulls away from sides of pan and a cake tester inserted in the center comes out clean. Let cool in pan. Serve with Lemon Cream.

A not-too-sweet dessert that is a positive addition to the day's healthy grain and soy servings.

Tip

• Cool or chill the rice before combining with the Lemon Cream.

Lemon Cream Rice Pudding

| 3 cups | Lemon Cream (page 362) | 750 mL |
| 2 cups | cooked brown rice | 500 mL |

1. In a bowl, combine Lemon Cream and rice. Serve at room temperature or chilled.

This is one of those desserts that can be pulled together at the last moment from foods at hand. Use any fresh fruit in combination with canned or frozen to make this meal finale.

Variation

• Substitute fresh mint or lemon balm for the tarragon.

Tropical Fruit with Orange Liqueur

I	mango, coarsely chopped	I
I	papaya, coarsely chopped	I
I	banana, diced	I
I	orange, sectioned and coarsely chopped	I
I	nectarine, coarsely chopped	I
I tbsp	chopped fresh tarragon or chervil	15 mL
¼ cup	orange liqueur	50 mL

1. In a bowl, combine mango, papaya, banana, orange, nectarine and tarragon. Toss with orange liqueur.

Poached Peaches with Lavender Custard

People will wonder what the "spice" is here as long as you don't use too much lavender. The fragrant flowery taste complements the bland flavor of the custard.

Tip

• Use only organic lavender, which has not been chemically treated.

4	peaches, halved	4
¾ cup	apple juice	175 mL
½ cup	white wine	125 mL

Lavender Custard

½ cup	soy milk or rice milk	125 mL
1	piece (3 inches/7.5 cm) vanilla bean	1
1	piece (2 inches/5 cm) licorice root, optional	1
1 tbsp	dried lavender buds (see Tip, left)	15 mL
12 oz	silken tofu	375 g

1. In a saucepan, combine peach halves, apple juice and wine. Bring to a boil over medium heat. Reduce heat and simmer for 10 minutes or until the tip of a knife meets with some resistance when inserted. Remove from heat and let peaches stand in the poaching liquid until ready to serve or overnight.

2. *Lavender Custard:* In a saucepan over medium-low heat, combine soy milk, vanilla bean, licorice, if using, and lavender. Cover, reduce heat and simmer until bubbles form around outside edge of pan. Let cool with cover on. Strain and discard vanilla, licorice and lavender. In a blender or food processor, process tofu until smooth. With the motor running, add cooled soy milk through opening in lid. Blend until smooth.

3. Using a slotted spoon, lift peaches into bowls and top with custard. Custard will keep tightly covered in the refrigerator for up to 2 days.

The garlic is barely perceptible in the orange-flavored sauce, but if it is detected, guests will think the caramelized garlic is chopped nuts.

Baked Bananas with Garlic Citrus Caramel Sauce

- *Preheat oven to 375°F (190°C)*
- *9-inch (2.5 L) baking dish, lightly oiled*

2	bananas	2
4 tbsp	brown sugar	60 mL
¼ cup	Garlic Citrus Caramel Sauce (below)	50 mL

1. Peel and slice bananas lengthwise and arrange, cut sides up, in prepared dish. Sprinkle each half with 1 tbsp (15 mL) of the brown sugar. Bake in preheated oven for 15 minutes or until bananas are soft.

2. Place bananas on dessert plates and drizzle with Garlic Citrus Caramel Sauce.

Lightly spiked with orange, this sauce is actually mild tasting, virtually odorless and surprisingly versatile. For desserts, drizzle it over soy ice cream or use it to add a finishing touch to pies and cakes. A small amount goes a long way, but for more of a good thing, double all of the ingredients except the garlic.

Garlic Citrus Caramel Sauce

6	cloves garlic, coarsely chopped	6
¼ cup	organic cane sugar	50 mL
2 tbsp	water	25 mL
1 tbsp	grated orange zest, optional	15 mL
½ cup	freshly squeezed orange juice	125 mL

1. In a small, heavy-bottomed saucepan, combine garlic, sugar and water. Stir over low heat until sugar is dissolved. Increase heat to medium-high and bring to a boil. Reduce heat and boil gently without stirring, for 7 minutes, or until sauce is a light amber color. Swirl pan occasionally to move garlic pieces around, but otherwise do not disturb the boiling sauce.

2. Remove pan from heat and gradually stir in orange juice. Return to medium heat, mash garlic bits with the back of a wooden spoon and boil for 8 to 10 minutes or until sauce is thick and syrupy and reduced to about ¼ cup (50 mL). Strain sauce or serve with the bits of caramelized garlic. Add grated orange zest, if using.

Spiced Apple Cake with Coconut Pecan Glaze

The spicy taste is rich and not too hot, but adjust the hot pepper to taste. Use spelt or other flours in place of the buckwheat flour if desired.

Tip

• If using sweetened coconut, use less sugar.

• *Preheat oven to 350°F (180°C)*
• *9-inch (2.5 L) square baking pan, oiled and lined with parchment paper*
• *Rimmed baking sheet*

¼ cup	large-flake rolled oats or Kamut flakes	50 mL
2	apples, grated	2
¼ cup	organic cane sugar	50 mL
1½ cups	unbleached all-purpose flour	375 mL
½ cup	buckwheat or whole wheat flour	125 mL
1 tsp	baking powder	5 mL
1 tsp	baking soda	5 mL
1 tsp	Garam Masala Spice Blend (page 254) or store-bought	5 mL
Pinch	ground nutmeg	Pinch
Pinch	hot pepper flakes	Pinch
¼ tsp	sea salt	1 mL
¼ cup	grapeseed oil	50 mL
¾ cup	pure maple syrup	175 mL
¼ cup	soy milk	50 mL
1 tbsp	freshly squeezed lemon juice	15 mL
1 cup	coarsely chopped dates	250 mL

Coconut Pecan Glaze

1¼ cups	pecan pieces	300 mL
1 cup	coconut milk or rice milk	250 mL
½ cup	unsweetened shredded coconut (see Tip, left)	125 mL
½ cup	organic cane sugar	125 mL
¼ cup	chopped dates	50 mL
1 tbsp	freshly squeezed lemon juice	15 mL
1 tsp	vanilla extract	5 mL

1. In a food processor or blender, chop oats to a fine powder. Transfer to a bowl. Add apples, sugar, all-purpose and buckwheat flours, baking powder, baking soda, garam masala, nutmeg, hot pepper flakes and salt. Stir well to combine.

2. In another bowl, whisk together oil, maple syrup, soy milk and lemon juice. Pour into dry ingredients and stir until mixed. Fold in dates. Pour batter into prepared pan and spread evenly. Bake in preheated oven for 35 to 40 minutes or until a tester inserted in the center comes out clean. Reduce oven temperature to 325°F (160°C). Let cake cool in pan for 10 minutes and turn out onto a cooling rack.

3. *Coconut Pecan Glaze:* Spread pecan pieces in one layer on baking sheet and toast in preheated oven for 8 to 10 minutes or until lightly browned. Let cool and pulse in a food processor or blender until coarsely chopped (or chop by hand).

4. In a saucepan, combine coconut milk, coconut, sugar and dates. Cook over medium heat, stirring constantly, for 12 minutes or until slightly thickened. Remove from heat and add lemon juice and vanilla. Fold in toasted pecans. Spread topping over warm cake and let cool before cutting into squares. Store cake in an airtight container in the refrigerator for up to 3 days.

Parsnip Carrot Cake

After creating this recipe I stumbled upon a blog at cakespy.com where five different vegetables were tested in a carrot cake recipe. The results were interesting, with radish and parsnip in the lead, sugar snap peas a close second and broccoli and Brussels sprouts definitely not favored. Parsnips are a natural in cakes and other baked goods since they have higher levels of natural sugars.

- *Preheat oven to 325°F (160°C)*
- *8-inch (2 L) baking pan, lightly oiled and lined with parchment paper*

2	medium parsnips, shredded	2
2	medium carrots, shredded	2
1 cup	water	250 mL
1 cup	organic cane sugar	250 mL
1/3 cup	raisins	75 mL
1 tsp	ground cinnamon	5 mL
1 tsp	finely grated fresh gingerroot	5 mL
1/2 tsp	sea salt	2 mL
1/4 tsp	ground cloves	1 mL
1/2 cup	shortening	125 mL
1/4 cup	pure maple syrup	50 mL
2 cups	all-purpose flour	500 mL
2 tsp	baking powder	10 mL
1 tsp	baking soda	5 mL
2 cups	applesauce, optional	500 mL

1. In a saucepan, combine parsnips, carrots, water, sugar, raisins, cinnamon, ginger, salt and cloves. Bring to a boil over medium-high heat. Reduce heat and cook, stirring occasionally, for 5 minutes or until vegetables are soft. Remove from heat and add shortening, stirring until melted. Let cool and add maple syrup.

2. Meanwhile, in a bowl, combine flour, baking powder and baking soda.

3. Scrape parsnip-carrot mixture into flour mixture. Stir just enough to moisten dry ingredients; do not overmix. Pour into prepared baking pan. Bake for 40 minutes or until edges of cake start to pull away from sides of pan and a toothpick inserted in the center comes out clean. Let cool in pan. Cut into 2-inch (5 cm) squares and serve with applesauce, if desired.

Christmas Sugarplums

Clement Clarke Moore wrote *The Night before Christmas,* with its famous line "While visions of sugarplums danced in their heads," in 1833. The dictionary defines a sugarplum as a kind of sweetmeat or a small round or oval piece of sugary candy. This recipe is my idea of the treat Moore's literary children were dreaming about.

- *75 candy paper or foil liners*

⅓ cup	freshly squeezed orange juice	75 mL
30	pitted dates, chopped	30
20	pitted prunes, chopped	20
10	dried figs, chopped	10
2 tbsp	freshly squeezed lemon juice	25 mL
¼ cup	dark rum or sherry	50 mL
¼ cup	pure maple syrup	50 mL
1 tsp	vanilla extract	5 mL
1 tsp	ground cinnamon	5 mL
¼ tsp	ground nutmeg	1 mL
¼ tsp	ground cloves	1 mL
1½ cups	raisins	375 mL
1 cup	pecans, chopped	250 mL
1 cup	chopped drained maraschino cherries	250 mL
1 cup	chopped candied citrus peel	250 mL
1 cup	chopped dried apricots	250 mL
2 tbsp	chopped candied ginger	25 mL
1 tsp	sea salt	5 mL
	Organic cane sugar for dusting	

1. In a saucepan over medium heat, bring orange juice to a boil. Add dates, prunes, figs and lemon juice. Reduce heat and simmer, stirring frequently, for 6 minutes or until fruit is very soft.

2. Remove from heat and stir in rum, maple syrup, vanilla, cinnamon, nutmeg and cloves.

3. Meanwhile, in a large bowl, combine raisins, pecans, cherries, citrus peel, apricots, ginger and salt. Scrape warm fruit mixture into raisin mixture and stir well to combine. Cover and chill in the refrigerator for 10 to 15 minutes or until slightly firm.

4. Scoop 1 tbsp (15 mL) of the mixture and form a ball. Roll in sugar. Drop into candy paper. Store between sheets of waxed paper in a tightly closed container in the refrigerator for up to 3 weeks. Serve at room temperature.

Lemon Sauce

½ cup	Fruit Purée (page 139)	125 mL
1 tsp	grated lemon zest	5 mL
⅓ cup	freshly squeezed lemon juice	75 mL
¼ cup	brown rice syrup or corn syrup	50 mL

1. In a blender, combine Fruit Purée, lemon zest, lemon juice and rice syrup. Blend until smooth. Store sauce in a sterilized jar with a lid in the refrigerator for up to 1 month.

Lemon Cream

1 cup	Lemon Sauce (above)	250 mL
2 cups	Soy Sour Cream (page 145)	500 mL

1. In a bowl, fold Lemon Sauce into Soy Sour Cream. Chill for 20 minutes.

Strawberry Sauce

1 cup	fresh or frozen (not thawed) strawberries, chopped	250 mL
½ cup	organic cane sugar	125 mL

1. In a bowl, mash strawberries using a fork or potato masher. Add sugar and stir until dissolved. Cover and let stand at room temperature until ready to use, for up to 1 hour or cover and refrigerate for up to 4 days.

Umeboshi Sauce

2 lbs	ripe black or red plums, quartered	1 kg
2 cups	organic cane sugar	500 mL
	Juice of half a lemon	
1 tbsp	dried lavender buds, optional	15 mL
1 tbsp	rice vinegar	15 mL
½ tsp	sea salt	2 mL
½ tsp	ground cinnamon	2 mL

Japanese ume fruit are similar to apricots, although they are often called plums. When dried and pickled, they make a salty condiment called umeboshi. Ume vinegar, or *umezu*, is the juice that collects as the ume are pressed. Here we are taking some artistic license with the name. Use this sweet sauce with poached fruit, as a garnish for sweet bars or puddings and to perk up steamed vegetables.

1. In a saucepan, combine plums, sugar, lemon juice, lavender, if using, vinegar, salt and cinnamon. Bring to a boil over medium-high heat. Reduce heat and simmer for 1½ hours or until thick.

2. Let cool and press through a fine sieve, discarding solids. Store sauce in a sterilized jar with a lid in the refrigerator for up to 1 month.

Apricot Coulis

10	fresh apricots, stoned and quartered	10
3	navel oranges, peeled and chopped	3
1	lemon, chopped	1
1½ cups	organic cane sugar	375 mL
1	piece (2 inches/5 cm) vanilla bean, split	1
2 tbsp	dried lavender buds, optional	25 mL
½ tsp	ground coriander	2 mL
½ tsp	ground cinnamon	2 mL

This is a good sauce to make for finishing off desserts or to use in other recipes as a sweetener.

1. In a saucepan, combine apricots, oranges, lemon, sugar, vanilla bean, lavender, if using, coriander and cinnamon. Bring to a boil over medium-high heat. Reduce heat and simmer, stirring occasionally, for 1½ hours or until thick.

2. Let cool and press through a fine sieve, discarding solids. Store coulis in a sterilized jar with a lid in the refrigerator for up to 1 month.

Glossary

Adaptogen: A substance that builds resistance to stress by balancing the functions of the glands and immune response, thus strengthening the immune system, nervous system and glandular system. Adaptogens promote overall vitality. *Examples: astragalus and ginseng.*

Alterative: A substance that gradually changes a condition by restoring health.

Analgesic: A substance that relieves pain by acting as a nervine, antiseptic or counterirritant. *Examples: German chamomile, meadowsweet and nutmeg.*

Anodyne: A substance that relieves pain. *Example: Clove.*

Anthocyanins: See Phenolic compounds, page 366.

Antibiotic: Meaning "against life," an antibiotic is a substance that kills infectious agents, including bacteria and fungi, without endangering health. *Examples: garlic, green tea, lavender, sage and thyme.*

Antihistamine: A substance that relieves the physical effects of histamines.

Anti-inflammatory: A substance that controls or reduces swelling, redness, pain and heat, which are normal bodily reactions to injury or infection. *Examples: German chamomile and St. John's wort.*

Antimicrobial: A substance that destroys or inhibits the growth of disease-causing bacteria or other microorganisms.

Antioxidant: A compound that protects cells by preventing polyunsaturated fatty acids (PUFAs) in cell membranes from oxidizing, or breaking down. Antioxidants do this by neutralizing free radicals (see Free radical, page 365). Vitamins C and E and beta-carotene are antioxidant nutrients, and foods high in them have antioxidant properties. *Examples: alfalfa, beet greens, dandelion leaf, garlic, parsley, thyme and watercress.*

Antipyretic: A substance that reduces fever. *Examples: German chamomile, sage and yarrow.*

Antiseptic: A substance used to prevent or reduce the growth of disease germs in order to prevent infection. *Examples: cabbage, calendula, clove, garlic, German chamomile, honey, nutmeg, onions, parsley, peppermint, rosemary, salt, thyme, turmeric and vinegar.*

Antispasmodic: A substance that relieves muscle spasms or cramps, including colic. *Examples: German chamomile, ginger, licorice and peppermint.*

Astringent: A drying and contracting substance that reduces secretions from the skin. *Examples: cinnamon, lemons, sage and thyme.*

Beta-carotene: The natural coloring agent (carotenoid) that gives fruits and vegetables (such as carrots) their deep orange color. It converts in the body to vitamin A. Eating foods high in beta-carotene helps prevent cancer, lowers the risk of heart disease, increases immunity, lowers the risk of cataracts and improves mental function. Beta-carotene is high in squash, carrots, yams, sweet potatoes, pumpkins and red peppers.

Betaine: A phytochemical that nourishes and strengthens the liver and gallbladder. It is found in high concentrations in beets.

Boron: A trace mineral that boosts the estrogen level in the blood, boron is also thought to help prevent calcium loss that leads to osteoporosis and to affect the brain's electrical activity. It is found in legumes, leafy greens and nuts.

Carbohydrates: An important group of plant foods that are composed of carbon, hydrogen and oxygen. A carbohydrate can be a single simple sugar or a combination of simple sugars. The chief sources of carbohydrates in a whole-food diet are grains, vegetables and fruits. Other sources include sugars, natural sweeteners and syrups.

Carcinogen: A cancer-causing substance.

Carminative: A substance that relaxes the stomach muscles and is taken to relieve gas and gripe. *Examples: clove, dill, fennel, garlic, ginger, parsley, peppermint, sage and thyme.*

Carotenoid: See Beta-carotene, above.

Cathartic: A substance that has a laxative effect. See also Purgative, page 367. *Examples: dandelion, licorice and parsley.*

Chlorophyll: Found only in plants, chlorophyll has a unique structure that allows it to enhance the body's ability to produce hemoglobin, which, in turn, enhances the delivery of oxygen to cells.

Cholagogue: Promotes the secretion of bile, assisting digestion and bowel elimination. *Examples: dandelion root, licorice and yellow dock.*

Choline: A phytochemical that researchers believe improves mental function, and is therefore helpful for people with Alzheimer's disease. Good sources of lecithin (which contains choline) are dandelion, fenugreek, ginkgo, sage and stinging nettle.

Cruciferous vegetables: The name given to the *Brassica* genus of vegetables, which includes broccoli, Brussels sprouts, cabbage, cauliflower, collard greens, kale, bok choy, rutabagas, turnips and mustard greens. The plants in this family were named *Cruciferae* because their flower petals grow in a cross shape.

Decoction: A solution made by boiling the woody parts of plants (roots, seeds and bark) in water for 10 to 20 minutes.

Demulcent: A soothing substance taken internally to protect damaged tissue. *Examples: barley, cucumbers, fenugreek, figs, honey and marshmallow.*

Depurative: Herbs taken to cleanse the blood. *Examples: burdock, dandelion root, garlic, onion, stinging nettles and yellow dock.*

Diaphoretic: A substance that induces sweating. *Examples: cayenne, cinnamon, German chamomile and ginger.*

Digestive: A substance that aids digestion. (See also Digestive System, page 20.)

Diuretic: A substance that increases the flow of urine. These are meant to be used in the short term only. *Examples: Cucumbers, burdock (root and leaf), dandelion (leaf and root), fennel seeds, lemons, linden, parsley and pumpkin seeds.*

Dysmenorrhea: Menstruation accompanied by cramping pains that may be incapacitating in their intensity.

Elixir: A tonic that invigorates or strengthens the body by stimulating or restoring health.

Ellagic acid: A natural plant phenol (see Phenolic compounds, page 366) thought to have powerful anticancer and antiaging properties. It is found in cherries, grapes, strawberries, and other red, orange or yellow fruits; nuts; seeds; garlic; and onions.

Emetic: A substance taken in large doses to induce vomiting to expel poisons. Small quantities of some emetics, such as salt, nutmeg and mustard, are used often in cooking with no ill effects.

Emmenagogue: A substance that promotes healthy menstruation. *Examples: calendula and German chamomile.*

Enzymes: The elements found in food that act as the catalysts for chemical reactions within the body, allowing efficient digestion and absorption of food and enabling the metabolic processes that support tissue growth, support high energy levels and promote good health. Enzymes are destroyed by heat, but using fruits and vegetables raw in smoothies leaves enzymes intact and readily absorbable.

Essential fatty acids (EFAs): Fat is an essential part of a healthy diet — about 20 fatty acids are used by the human body to maintain normal function. Fats are necessary to maintain healthy skin and hair, transport the fat-soluble vitamins (A, D, E and K) and signal the feeling of fullness after meals. The three fatty acids considered the most important, or essential, are omega-6 linoleic, omega-3 linolenic and gamma linolenic acids. Evidence suggests that increasing the proportion of these fatty acids in the diet may increase immunity and reduce the risks of heart disease, high blood pressure and arthritis. The best vegetable source of omega-3 EFAs in the diet is flaxseeds. Other sources of EFAs are hemp (seeds and nuts), nuts, seeds, olives, avocados and oily fish.

Expectorant: A substance that relieves mucus congestion caused by colds and flu. *Examples: elder, garlic, ginger, hyssop and thyme.*

Febrigue: Herbs that help reduce fever. *Examples: German chamomile, sage and yarrow.*

Fiber: An indigestible carbohydrate. Fiber protects against intestinal problems and bowel disorders. The best sources are raw fruits and vegetables, seeds and whole grains.

Types of fiber include *pectin*, which reduces the risk of heart disease (by lowering cholesterol) and helps eliminate toxins. It is found mainly in fruits, such as apples, berries and citrus fruits; vegetables; and dried legumes. *Cellulose* prevents varicose veins, constipation and colitis and plays a role in deflecting colon cancer. Because cellulose is found in the outermost layers of fruits and vegetables, it is important to buy only organic produce and leave the peels on. The *hemicellulose* in fruits, vegetables and grains aids in weight loss, prevents constipation, lowers the risk of colon cancer and helps remove cancer-forming toxins from the intestinal tract. *Lignin*, a fiber known to lower cholesterol, prevent gallstone formation and help people with diabetes, is found only in fruits, vegetables and Brazil nuts.

When raw fresh whole fruits or vegetables are used in smoothies, the pulp, or fiber, is still present in the drink and provides all the health benefits listed above.

Flavonoids: These phytochemicals (e.g., genistein and quercetin) are antioxidants that have been shown to inhibit cholesterol production. They are found in cruciferous vegetables (see Cruciferous vegetables, page 364), onions and garlic.

Food Combining: See page 26.

Free radical: A highly unstable compound that attacks cell membranes and causes cell breakdown, aging and a predisposition to some diseases. Free radicals come from the environment as a result of exposure to radiation, ultraviolet (UV) light, smoke, ozone and certain medications. Free radicals are also formed in the body by enzymes and during the conversion of food to energy. See also Antioxidant, page 367.

Gluten: A protein found in wheat that is responsible for keeping bread dough from collapsing during baking. It may cause allergic reactions in some people. Winter hard wheat (used for bread flour blends) contains more gluten than summer soft wheat (used for cake and pastry flours).

Hemicellulose: See Fiber, above.

Hepatic: Herbs that strengthen, tone and stimulate secretive functions of the liver. *Examples: dandelion, lemon balm, milk thistle, rosemary and turmeric.*

Hypotensive: A substance that lowers blood pressure. *Examples: garlic, hawthorn, linden flower and yarrow.*

Immunostimulant: A substance that assists the immune system.

Indole: A phytochemical found in cruciferous vegetables (see Cruciferous vegetables, page 364) that may help prevent cancer by detoxifying carcinogens.

Isoflavone: A phytoestrogen, or the plant version of the human hormone estrogen, that is found in nuts, soybeans and legumes. Isoflavones help prevent several types of cancer — including pancreatic, colon, breast and prostate cancers — by preserving vitamin C in the body and acting as antioxidants.

Lactose intolerance: Deficiency of the enzyme lactase, which breaks down lactose, the sugar in both cow's and human milk. If you don't have sufficient lactase, milk sugar will ferment in the large intestine, causing bloating, diarrhea, abdominal pain and gas.

Laxative: A substance that stimulates bowel movements. Laxatives are meant to be used in the short term only. *Examples: dandelion root, licorice root, prunes, rhubarb and yellow dock.*

Lignin: See Fiber, page 365.

Limonene: A type of Limonoid (see Terpene) thought to assist in detoxifying the liver and prevent cancer. *Examples: grapefruit, lemons, limes and tangerines.*

Limonoid: A subclass of terpenes (see Terpene, page 367) found in citrus fruit rinds.

Lutein: A carotenoid (see Beta-carotene, page 364) found in beet greens; collard greens; mustard greens; and other red, orange and yellow vegetables.

Lycopene: An antioxidant carotenoid (see Beta-carotene, page 364) that's relatively rare in food. High levels are found, however, in tomatoes, pink grapefruit and watermelon. Lycopene is thought to reduce the effects of aging by maintaining physical and mental function and to reduce the risk of some forms of cancer.

Lysine: An amino acid that controls protein absorption in the body. Lysine is higher in amaranth than any other complex carbohydrate.

Macrobiotic diet: Eating whole food that is seasonal and produced locally. Whole grains, vegetables, fruits (except tropical fruits), legumes, small amounts of fish or organic meat, sea herbs, nuts and seeds are appropriate foods for North Americans who eat macrobiotically.

Metabolism: The rate at which the body produces energy (or burns calories). It is measured by the amount of heat produced by the body, at rest or engaged in various activities, while maintaining its normal temperature.

Milk allergy: Many individuals, especially babies and young children, have allergic reactions to the protein in cow's milk, which causes wheezing, eczema, rashes, mucus buildup and asthma-like symptoms.

Mucilage: A thick, sticky, glue-like substance found in high concentrations in some herbs, which contains and helps spread the active ingredients of those herbs while soothing inflamed surfaces. *Examples: marshmallow and slippery elm.*

Mucopolysaccharides: Carbohydrates that aid in blood clotting and stimulate the body's immune system to increase resistance to infection. *Example: spelt.*

Nervine: A substance that eases anxiety and stress and nourishes the nerves by strengthening nerve fibers. *Examples: German chamomile, lemon balm, oats, skullcap, St. John's wort, thyme and valerian.*

Nonreactive cooking utensils: The acids in foods can react with certain materials and promote the oxidation of some nutrients, as well as discolor the materials themselves. Nonreactive materials suitable for brewing teas are glass, enameled cast iron or enameled stainless steel. While cast-iron pans are recommended for cooking (a meal cooked in unglazed cast iron can provide 20% of the recommended daily intake of iron), and stainless steel is a nonreactive cooking material, neither is recommended for brewing or steeping teas.

Omega-3 Fatty Acids: Polyunsaturated fatty acids found in oily fish and some vegetables, important for heart health. The body doesn't manufacture them. (See also Essential Fatty Acids, page 365.)

Organosulfides: Compounds that have been shown to reduce blood pressure, lower cholesterol levels and reduce blood clotting. *Examples: garlic and onions.*

Pectin: A type of fiber that helps to lower both cholesterol and colon cancer. Apples are high in pectin.

Phenolic compounds: Found in red wine, phenolic compounds, including catechins, anthocyanins, ellagic acid and tannins, can prevent the oxidation of "bad" low-density lipoprotein (LDL) cholesterol, thus reducing the risk of heart disease.

Phytochemicals: Chemicals that come from plants. *Phyto*, from the Greek, means "to bring forth" and is used as a prefix to mean "from a plant."

Proanthocyanidins: Phytonutrients that may contribute to the maintenance of urinary tract and heart health. *Examples: apples and cranberries.*

Protein: The building block of body tissues. Protein is necessary for healthy growth, cell repair, reproduction and protection against infection. Protein consists of 22 parts called amino acids. Eight of the 22 amino acids in protein are especially important because they can not be manufactured by the body. Those eight are called essential amino acids.

A food that contains all eight essential amino acids is said to be a complete protein. Protein from animal products — meat, fish, poultry and dairy products — is complete. The only accepted plant sources of complete protein are soybeans and soy products, but research is establishing new theories that the protein content of legumes may be complete enough to replace animal protein.

A food that contains some, but not all, eight essential amino acids is called an incomplete protein. Nuts, seeds, legumes, cereals and grains are plant products that provide incomplete proteins. If your meals include foods from two complementary incomplete protein sources, your body will combine the incomplete proteins in the right proportions to make a complete protein. For example, many cultures have a tradition of using legumes and whole grains together in dishes. Scientifically, this combination provides a good amino-acid (complete protein) balance in the diet, because legumes are low in methionine but high in lysine, and whole grains are high in methionine but low in lysine. When eaten together, the body combines them to make complete proteins. Nuts and seeds must be paired with dairy or soy proteins in order to provide complete proteins.

Purgative: A substance that promotes bowel movements and increased intestinal peristalsis. *Example: Yellow dock.*

Quercetin: See Flavonoid, page 365.

Resveratrol: A fungicide that occurs naturally in grapes and has been linked to the prevention of clogged arteries by lowering blood cholesterol levels. Resveratrol is found in red wine and, to a lesser extent, in purple grape juice.

Rhizome: An underground stem that is usually thick and fleshy. *Examples: ginger and turmeric.*

Rubefacient: A substance that, when applied to the skin, stimulates circulation in that area, bringing a good supply of blood to the skin and increasing heat in the tissue. *Examples: cayenne, garlic, ginger, mustard seeds; and oils of peppermint, rosemary and thyme.*

Sedative: A substance that has a powerful quieting effect on the nervous system that relieves tension and induces sleep. *Examples: German chamomile, lettuce, linden, lavender and valerian.*

Stimulant: A substance that focuses the mind and increases activity. *Examples: basil, cayenne, cinnamon, peppermint and rosemary.*

Styptic: Herbs causing capillaries to contract and thereby stop superficial hemorrhage bleeding. *Examples: calendula and cayenne.*

Tannin: A chemical constituent in herbs that causes astringency (see Astringent, page 364) and helps stanch internal bleeding. See also Phenolic compounds, page 366. *Examples: coffee, tea and witch hazel.*

Tea: Strictly speaking, "tea" refers to a solution made by pouring boiling water on the fermented leaves and stems of a plant which have been allowed to dry after fermentation (green or black tea). The term is often used when referring to a solution made by pouring boiling water on any plant's leaves, petals or stems. (See also Tea, page 122.)

Terpene: A class of phytochemicals found in a wide variety of fruits, vegetables and herbs that are potent antioxidants. Ginkgo biloba is a good source of some terpenes. Limonoids (see Limonoid, page 366), which are found in citrus fruit rinds, are a subclass of terpenes.

Therapeutic dose: Amount recommended by herbalist for healing certain ailments, usually higher and for longer periods of time than herbs used in cooking (which maintain health). Standardized amounts of specific herbs are used.

Tincture: A liquid herbal extract made by soaking an herb in alcohol and pure water to extract the plant's active components. Some herbalists maintain that tinctures are the most effective way to take herbs, because they contain a wide range of the plant's chemical constituents and are easily absorbed.

Tisane: The "official" term used for a solution made by steeping fresh or dried herbs in boiling water. The term is interchangeable with the word *tea* when herbs are used.

Tonic: An infusion of herbs that tones or strengthens the system. Often tonics act as alteratives (see Alterative, page 364). Taken either hot or cold, tonics purify the blood and are nutritive. Tonic herbs support the body's systems in maintaining health. *Examples: alfalfa, astragalus, dandelion (root and leaf) and ginseng.*

Vasodilator: A substance that relaxes blood vessels, increasing circulation to the arms, hands, legs, feet and brain. *Examples: peppermint and sage.*

Volatile oil: Essential component found in the aerial parts of an herb. Often extracted to make essential oils, volatile oils are antiseptic and very effective at stimulating the body parts to which they are applied.

Vulnerary: An herbal remedy that helps to heal external wounds and reduce inflammation. *Examples: aloe vera, calendula, comfrey, marshmallow root and slippery elm bark powder.*

Whole foods: The most nutrient-rich form of foods. They are as close to their natural state as possible. (See also Whole Foods, page 59.)

Wildcrafting: The practice of gathering herbs from the wild. Many plants today are endangered because of excessive wildcrafting. To avoid contributing to this problem, buy herbs that are organically cultivated.

Sources

Vegan Products

Dixie Diners' Club
P.O. Box 1969
Tomball, TX 77377
Tel (800) 233-3668
or (281) 516-3535
Fax (800) 688-2507
www.dixieusa.com
Distributors of "Health food that tastes like junk food."

Follow Your Heart
Dairy alternative food products including cheddar
cheese, sour cream, salad dressings, and chicken
free chicken.
www.followyourheart.com

Native Seeds/S*E*A*R*C*H
526 N. Fourth Avenue
Tucson, AZ 85705
Tel (866) 622-5561
Fax (502) 622-5591
www.nativeseeds.org
Source for native foods of southwest: beans, chile
powder, whole and smoked chiles, salsas and sauces,
agave nectar, herbs and teas.

Omega Nutrition Flax Seed Oil
www.omeganutrition.com
Fresh-pressed organic and Kosher flax oils including
Hi-Lignan®Flax Oil, Garlic-Chili Flax Oil and
Orange Flax Oil Blend.

Pangea
2381 Lewis Avenue
Rockville, MD 20851
Tel (800) 340-1200
Fax (301) 816-8955
www.veganstore.com
Source for a wide range of household products and
vegan food items including dairy alternatives.

Tofutti
www.tofutti.com
Dairy free products available in many
alternative/whole food stores in North America.
Products include cheese, sour cream, ice cream and
cream cheese.

Vegan, Herb and Organic Associations, Organizations, Agencies

American Vegan Society
P.O. Box 369
Malaga, NJ 08328
Tel (856) 694-2887
Fax (856) 694-2288
www.americanvegan.org
Educational member-based organization.

Canadian Organic Growers (COG)
Box 6408, Station J
Ottawa, ON
Canada, K2A 3Y6
Tel (613) 231 9047
www.cog.ca
Canada's national information network for organic
farmers, gardeners and consumers.

Herb Society of America (HSA)
9019 Chardon Road
Kirtland, OH 44094 USA
Tel (440) 256 0514
Fax (440) 256 0541
www.herbsociety.org
A well-organized group of herb enthusiasts with
6 Districts and many active local units.

International Herb Association (IHA)
910 Charles Street
Fredericksburg, VA 22401 USA
Tel (540) 368 0590
Fax (540) 370 0015
www.iherb.org
A professional organization of herb growers and
business owners.

Organic Trade Association (OTA)
P.O. Box 547
Greenfield, MA 01302-0547 USA
Tel (413) 774 7511
Fax (413) 774 6432
www.ota.com
Promotes awareness and understanding of organic
production, as well as providing a unified voice for
the industry.

Herb Farms and Herb Mail-Order Sources

Frontier Natural Brands
3021 78th Street
PO Box 299
Norway, IA 52318
Tel (319) 227-7996
Fax (319) 227-7966
www.frontiercoop.com
Supplier of bulk herbs.

Gilbertie's Herb Gardens
7 Sylvan Lane
Westport, CT 06880
Tel (800) 874-3727
www.gilbertiesherbs.com
The largest herb plant grower in the US.

Laurel Farm Herbs
Main Road, Kelsale
Saxmundham
Suffolk IP17 2RG, UK
Tel 01728 668 223
Fax 01728 668 468
www.theherbfarm.co.uk
Wide range of herb plants for shipping.

Mountain Rose Herbs
85472 Dilley Lane
Eugene, OR 97405 USA
Tel (800) 879 3337
Fax (510) 217 4012
www.mountainroseherbs.com
Bulk organic herbs, oils, butters, clays, teas
(mail order).

Richters Herbs
357 Highway 47
Goodwood, ON
Canada, L0C 1A0
Tel (905) 640 6677
Fax (905) 640 6641
www.richters.com
Herb specialists with over 800 varieties, selling herbs
since 1969. Mail order seeds, plants, books. Free
color catalogue, seminars and herbal events.

Related Consumer Websites

www.cog.ca
Canadian Organic Growers, a national membership-based organization representing farmers, gardeners and consumers in all provinces. Click on "Where to Buy Organics" for lists of Canadian organic growers and retailers.

www.davidsuzuki.org
A site dedicated to helping people choose solutions that will benefit the planet.

www.earthsave.org
Educates people about the powerful effects our food choices have on the environment, our health and all life on Earth and encourages a shift toward a healthy, plant-based diet.

www.peta.org/accidentallyVegan/default.asp
List of vegan food products: breakfast, beverages, snacks, condiments, baked goods, refrigerated & frozen, baking and staples.

Priya Kothari's blog
(http://365daysveg.wordpress.com) is one of the best vegetarian recipe sources online and her photographs are beautiful.

www.vrg.org/nutshell/faqingredients.htm
FAQs about food ingredients that help sort through the vegetarian and vegan issues surrounding ingredients and additives.

www.OrganicConsumers.org
Activist organization with information and action strategies for organic, genetically modified foods, irradiation, mad cow and other issues.

www.rodaleinstitute.org
In the mid 1900s, J. J. Rodale developed an emphasis on health and organic gardening through his publications and the Rodale family institute.

www.thinkvegetables.co.uk
A very good source of information about vegetables with a nutrient search and recipes for each vegetable.

www.whfoods.com
The "world's healthiest foods" site is provided by the George Mateljan Foundation, a non-profit organization that lists the nutrients and scientific information on whole foods. Recipes, tips and other non-biased information are available here.

Bibliography

American Vegan Society. *Here's Harmlessness.* Malaga, N.J.: American Vegan Society, 1993.

Ameye, L.G., et al. *Osteoarthritis and Nutrition. From neutraceuticals to functional foods: a systemic review of the scientific evidence.* Arthritis Research and Therapy 2006 July 19;8(4): R127.

Applegate, L. *101 Miracle Foods That Heal Your Heart.* Paramus, NJ: Prentice Hall Press, 2000.

Balch, P., Balch J. *Prescription for Dietary Wellness.* Greenfield, IN: PAB Books, 1993.

Baumel, S. *Dealing with Depression Naturally.* New Canaan, CN: Keats Publishing, Inc, 1995.

Berkson, D.L. *Healthy Digestion the Natural Way.* New York, NY; John Wiley & Sons, Inc., 2000.

Boik, J. *Cancer & Natural Medicine (A Textbook of Basic Science and Research).* Princeton MN: Oregon Medical Press, 1995.

Carper, Jean. *Food your Miracle Medicine.* New York NY: Harper Collins Publishers Inc, 1993.

Challem, J., et al. *The Complete Nutritional Program to Prevent and Reverse Insulin Resistance Syndrome X.* New York, NY: John Wiley & Sons Inc, 2000.

Crocker, Pat. *Oregano.* Neustadt ON: Riversong Studios, 2005.

_____ *The Vegetarian Cook's Bible.* Toronto ON: Robert Rose, 2007.

_____ *Tastes of the Kasbah.* Neustadt ON: Riversong Studios, 2005.

_____ *The Smoothies Bible.* Toronto ON: Robert Rose, 2003.

_____ *The Juicing Bible.* Toronto ON: Robert Rose, 2000.

Dalais F.S., et al. *Effects of a diet rich in phytoestrogens on prostate-specific antigen and sex hormones in men diagnosed with prostate cancer.* Urology. 2004 Sept; 64(3): 510-5.

Davis, Holly. *Nourish.* Toronto ON: Ten Speed Press, 1999.

DeBaggio, Thomas and Arthur O. Tucker, Ph.D. *The Big Book of Herbs.* Emmaus, PA: Rodale Press, 1997.

Dikasso D., et al. *Investigation on the antibacterial properties of garlic (Allium sativum) on pneumonia causing bacteria.* Ethiopian Medical Journal 2002 July; 40(3): 241-9.

Duke, James, Ph.D. *The Green Pharmacy.* Loveland, CO: Interweave Press, 2000.

Elkins, Rita. *Depression and Natural Medicine.* Pleasant Grove, UT: Woodland, Publishing Inc., 1995.

Estruch R., et al. *Effects of a Mediterranean-Style Diet on Cardiovascular Risk Factors.* Annals of Internal Medicine. 2006; 145: 1-11.

Fang, N., et al. *Inhibition of growth and induction of apoptosis in human cancer cell lines by an ethyl acetate fraction from shiitake mushrooms.* Journal of Alternative and Complementary Medicine 2006 Mar; 12(2):125-32.

Foster, Steven. *Herbal Renaissance: Growing, Using and Understanding Herbs in the Modern World.* Layton, Utah: Gibbs Smith, 1992.

Foster, Steven and Rebecca Johnson. *National Geographic Desk Reference to Nature's Medicine.* Washington, D.C.: National Geographic, 2006.

Fulghum, Bruce D. and M. Grossan. *The Sinus Cure.* New York, NY: Ballantine Books, 2001.

Gerras, Charles, Editor. *Rodale's Basic Natural Foods Cookbook.* Emmaus, PA: Rodale Press, 1978.

Goldberg, B. *Alternative Medicine Guide to Heart Disease, Stroke and High Blood Pressure.* Tiburon, CA: Future Medicine Publishing, 1998.

Halyorsen, B.L., et al. *Content of redox-active compounds (ie, antioxidants) in foods consumed in the United States.* American Journal of Clinical Nutrition 2006 Jul; 84(1): 95-135.

Hoffman, D. *Healthy Heart Strengthen your Cardiovascular System Naturally.* Pownal, VT: Storey Books, 2000.

Hoffmann, D. *Holistic Herbal.* Boston, MA: Element Books Limited, 1996.

Hudson et al. *Characterization of potentially chemoprotective phenols in extracts of brown rice that inhibit the growth of human breast and colon cancer cells.* Cancer Epidemiology Biomarkers and Prevention 2000 Nov; 9(11): 1163-70.

Hudson, T. *Women's Encyclopedia of Natural Medicine.* Los Angeles, CA: Keats Publishing, 1999.

Ivker, R.S., Nelson, T. *Asthma Survival.* New York, NY: Tarcher/Putman, 2001.

James, M.J., et al. *Dietary polyunsaturated fatty acids and inflammatory mediator production.* American Journal of Clinical Nutrition 2000 Jan; 71(1 Suppl): 343S-8S. Review.

Joseph, James A., Ph.D., Daniel A. Nadeau, M.D., and Anne Underwood. *The Color Code. A Revolutionary Eating Plan for Optimum Health.* New York, NY: Hyperion, 2002.

Judd, J.T., et al. *Dietary trans fatty acids: effect on plasma lipids and lipoproteins of healthy men and women.* American Journal of Clinical Nutrition, April 1994; 59:861-868.

Kaur, S.D. *The Complete Natural Medicine Guide to Breast Cancer.* Toronto, ON: Robert Rose Inc, 2003.

Kendall-Reed, P. and S. Reed. *Healing Arthritis.* Toronto, ON: CCNM Press, 2004.

Kumar, N.B., et al. *The specific role of isoflavones in reducing prostate cancer risk.* Prostate. 2004 May 1; 59(2): 141-7.

Kumar, P., et al. *Effect of quercetin supplementation on lung antioxidants after experimental influenza virus infection.* Experimental Lung Research 2005 June; 31(5): 449-59.

Lininger, S., Wright, J., Austin, S., Brown, D., Gaby, A. *The Natural Pharmacy*. Rocklin, CA: Prima Health Division of Publishing, 1998.

Logan, A. *Neurobehavioral Aspects of Omega-3 fatty acids: possible mechanisms and Therapeutic Value in Major Depression*. Alternative Medicine Review 2003;8(4): 410-425.

Lycopene. Alternative Medicine Review 2003; 8(3): 336-342.

Makabe, H., et al. *Anti-inflammatory sesquiterpenes from Curcuma zedoaria*. Journal of Asian Natural Products Research 2006 June; 20(7): 680-5.

Marcus, Erik. *Vegan: The New Ethics of Eating*. Ithaca, N.Y.: McBooks Press, 1997.

Mickleborough, T.D., et al. *Protective effect of fish oil supplementation on exercise-induced bronchoconstriction in asthma*. Chest. 2006 Jan; 129(1): 39-49.

Miller, A.L., et al. *Homocysteine Metabolism: Nutritional Modulation and Impact on Health and Disease*. Alternative Medicine Review 1997; 2(4): 234-254.

Mozaffarian, D., et al. *Fish Consumption and Stroke Risk in Elderly Individuals: The Cardiovascular Health Study*. Archives of Internal Medicine 2005; 165(2): 200-206.

Murray, M. *Diabetes and Hypoglycemia*. Rocklin, CA: Prima Health, 1994.

_____*Natural Alternatives to Prozac*. New York, NY: Quill, 1996.

_____*Pizzorno J. Encyclopedia of Natural Medicine 2nd Edition*. Rocklin, CA: Prima Health Division of Publishing, 1998.

Nez Heatherley, Ana. *Healing Plants, A Medicinal Guide to Native North American Plants and Herbs*. Toronto ON: Harper Collins Publishers Ltd., 1998.

O'Connor, D.J. *Understanding Osteoporosis and Clinical Strategies to Assess, Arrest and Restore Bone Loss*. Alternative Medicine Review 1997; 2(1): 36-47.

Ody, Penelope. *The Complete Medicinal Herbal*. Toronto, ON: Key Porter Books, 1993.

_____with A. Lyon and D. Vilinac. *The Chinese Herbal Cookbook. Healing Foods for Inner Balance*. Trumbull, CT: Weatherhill Inc., 2001.

Penny, M., Etherton, K. *Evidence that the antioxidant flavonoids in tea and cocoa are beneficial for cardiovascular health*. Current Opinion in Lipidology. Feb 2002; 13(1): 41-49.

Physicians Committee for Responsible Medicine, Melina V. *Healthy Eating for Life to Prevent and Treat Cancer*. New York, NY: John Wiley & Sons Inc., 2002.

Pitchford, Paul. *Healing with Whole Foods: Oriental Traditions and Modern Nutrition*. Berkeley CA: North Atlantic Books, 1993.

Prousky, J. *Anxiety Orthomolecular Diagnosis and Treatment*. Toronto, ON: CCNM Press, 2003.

Quercetin. Alternative Medicine Review 1998; 3(2): 140-143.

Robertson, Robin and Jon Robertson. *The Sacred Kitchen. Higher Consciousness Cooking for Health and Wholeness*. Novato, CA: New World Library, 1999.

Schroder, F.H., et al. *Randomized, double-blind, placebo-controlled crossover study in men with prostate cancer and rising PSA: effectiveness of a dietary supplement*. European Urology 2005 Dec; 48(6):922-30.

Sinclair, S. *Male Infertility: Nutritional and Environmental Considerations*. Alternative Medicine Review 2000; 5(1):28-38.

Stepaniak, Joanne. *The Vegan Sourcebook*. Los Angeles: Lowell House, 1998.

Sussman, Vic. *The Vegetarian Alternative*. Emmaus PA: Rodale Press, 1978.

Turner, Lisa. *Meals That Heal*. Rochester VT: Healing Arts Press, 1998.

Vanderhaeghe, L.R. and K. Karst. *Healthy Fats for Life Preventing and Treating Common Health Problems with Essential Fatty Acids*. Kingston, ON: Quarry Health Books, 2003.

_____Bouic, P.J.D. *The Immune System Cure*. Toronto, ON: Prentice Hall Canada, 1999.

_____*Healthy Immunity Scientifically Proven Natural Treatments for conditions A-Z*, Toronto. ON: Macmillan, 2001.

Whitaker, J. *The Memory Solution*. Garden City Park, NY: Avery Publishing Group, 1999.

Zampieron, E., E. Kamhi and B. Goldman. *Alternative Medicine Guide to Arthritis*. Tiburon, CA: AlternativeMedicine.com Books, 1999.

Library and Archives Canada Cataloguing in Publication

Crocker, Pat
    The vegan cook's bible / Pat Crocker.

Includes bibliographical references and index.
ISBN 978-0-7788-0217-4

1. Vegan cookery. 2. Veganism. 3. Health. I. Title.

TX837.C749 2009   641.5'636   C2008-907503-X

Index

Also available by the same author

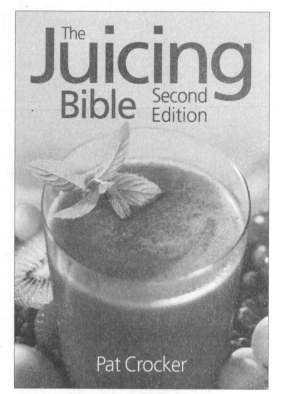

ISBN 978-0-7788-0181-8

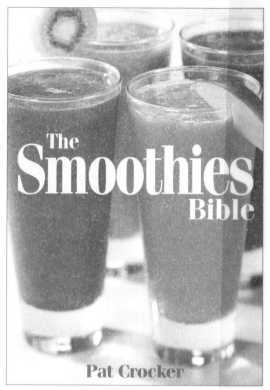

ISBN 978-0-7788-0063-7

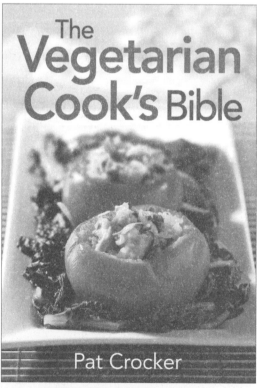

ISBN 978-0-7788-0153-5